Family and HIV/AIDS

Willo Pequegnat • Carl C. Bell

Editors

Family and HIV/AIDS

Cultural and Contextual Issues
in Prevention and Treatment

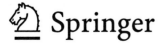 Springer

Editors
Willo Pequegnat
National Institute of Mental Health
Bethesda, MD, USA
wpequegn@mail.nih.gov

Carl C. Bell
Community Mental Health
Council, Inc.; The Institute for
Juvenile Research, Department of
Psychiatry, School of Medicine
University of Illinois Chicago, IL, USA
carlcbell@pol.net

ISBN 978-1-4614-0438-5   e-ISBN 978-1-4614-0439-2
DOI 10.1007/978-1-4614-0439-2
Springer New York Dordrecht Heidelberg London

Library of Congress Control Number: 2011937061

Printed on acid-free paper

Springer is part of Springer Science+Business Media (www.springer.com)

*This book is dedicated to the many resilient
families who are successfully preventing
HIV transmission in their members
and who are successfully ensuring that their
HIV seropositive members are living
a rewarding life.*

Foreword

In the *Surgeon's General Report on Youth Violence* in 2000, we put forth the science that showed that by improving parenting, we can reduce violence in communities. Certainly the importance of quality parenting cannot be overstated. Some would argue that parenting should be a required course for high school graduation since it is the most important job that most of us will ever have.

This book takes on the very vital and complex issue of the role of parenting in reducing risky behaviors that increase the spread of HIV/AIDS, and how this role may vary with race and culture.

Beyond the prevention of behaviors that increase the risk of HIV/AIDS, this book is about sexual health and healthy sexuality which is a formula for success in life and relationship. The recent 2009 Institute of Medicine's Report entitled *Preventing Mental, Emotional and Behavioral Disorders Among Young People: Progress and Possibilities* highlights the explosion in randomized controlled trials showing that prevention and health promotion are vital options for the USA to consider at this time in our history (National Research Council and Institute of Medicine 2009). Also, thanks to the National Institute of Mental Health Consortium on Families on HIV/AIDS, there is now sound evidence that family strengthening–prevention interventions can increase the likelihood that youth can be prevented from engaging in risky behaviors that lead to HIV and related infection.

This book clearly and succinctly addresses contextual issues that influence health outcomes and risky behaviors that we see in certain populations. It also addresses strategies for HIV prevention in special populations (African Americans, Latinos, youth in sub-Saharan Africa, homosexuals, bisexuals, lesbians, youth). We should face the fact that the causes of behavior are multidimensional and that without a model of health behavior change which involves multiple levels of cultural, social class, ethnicity, family dynamics, developmental stages, and others, our methods of reducing risk factors from becoming predictive of bad outcomes will certainly fail.

Clearly we need to consider "parents as teachers first" and help them to understand their obligations and opportunities to educate themselves and their children about risk to their offspring's well-being. In that reflection, we must consider the influence of mothers and fathers and how these parents can influence a child's life course toward risk and protective factors. Clearly there are several examples of even single parenting resulting in successful outcomes when those parenting behaviors are carried out appropriately. We also must consider how couples work together to avoid putting themselves and their partners at risk for developing HIV/AIDS.

But what about the children who wind up as orphans because their parents die from AIDS or other causes? I have visited such orphanages in Africa. In addition, how do we work with communities to gain their support in our public health work to prevent HIV infections from continuing to spread? These are some of the issues that are well addressed in this book.

Hence, in addition to issues of prevention, this text addresses the issue of how families can help with medication compliance once a family member find himself or herself infected with the HIV virus. Also questions of how gay, bisexual, and lesbian youths address these serious issues when confronted with them are addressed. Furthermore, how should mentally ill youth and their families approach the issue of HIV/AIDS?

Finally, how can we disseminate, adapt, and implement the evidence-based programs we already know that work quite well? This group of distinguished researchers addresses these and other challenging questions plaguing us as we deal with the HIV/AIDS epidemic that continues to impact those who continue to engage in risky sexual and other behaviors.

Atlanta, GA   David Satcher

Preface

After three decades of confronting the HIV epidemic, we finally have a National HIV/AIDS Strategy based on three primary goals to which President Obama is committed. They are: (1) reducing the number of people who become infected with HIV, (2) increasing access to care and optimizing health outcomes for people living with HIV, and (3) reducing HIV-related health disparities. This book brings together the results of a research effort supported by the National Institute of Mental Health (NIMH) and Centers for Disease Control and Prevention (CDC) and provides guidance to address all these goals.

The book *Working with Families in the Era of AIDS* (Pequegnat and Szapocznik 2000) presented the interventions being tested in NIMH-supported studies but no results were available. Now there are so much data that we have 15 chapters describing what is known about the context and culture of families addressing the challenge of HIV infection and presenting the findings from efficacious interventions. The authors of these chapters are experts in prevention research and provide guidance on interventions with a range of family configurations.

The recent 2009 Institute of Medicine's *Preventing Mental, Emotional, and Behavioral Disorders Among Young People: Progress and Possibilities* highlights the explosion of randomized controlled trials demonstrating that prevention and health promotion are viable options to improve the public health of US citizens (National Research Council and Institute of Medicine 2009).

Together these two documents provide the impetus for the recommendations in this book. The purpose of this book is to encourage researchers and service providers to become more involved in family-oriented approaches that can prevent the spread of HIV infection and its negative consequences and promote good health. We hope that these interventions will be used in effectiveness studies and that large community public health agencies and nongovernment organizations will find the evidence-based programs compelling enough to offer to their clients.

Community Collaboration

Because this group of researchers is committed to community-based research and to collaborating with members of the community, we feel that these interventions can be successfully adopted in public health agencies and clinics. Because of this collaborative approach, the interventions are community friendly and culturally appropriate. Without this community engagement in these research programs, the findings in this book would not have been possible.

Focus of Book

This book focuses on families confronting HIV infection and provides a review of findings about these families and efficacious prevention programs that can be adapted for different populations. These HIV prevention programs engage families and support their resolve to help their family members to prevent HIV transmission by encouraging healthier lifestyles with respect to drug use and sexual behavior among family members.

The book focuses heavily, but not exclusively, on African American women and their daughters because most of the studies have been conducted with these populations. We have made an effort to also focus on men and boys; Hispanic families and their children; and lesbian, gay, and bisexual youth and their families.

There are three chapters in the first section which presents a context for the rest of the book. Dr. Pequegnat provides a comprehensive overview of the family systems research that has been conducted over the last 15 years. Drs. Bell and McBride advocate for using the family as model of prevention of mental and physical health problems; they argue that the causes of behavior are multidetermined, and without a model of health behavior change that involves multiple levels of culture, society, social class, ethnicity, family dynamics, developmental stages, and personality and biologic dynamics, our programs to address HIV risk factors in families will fail. Dr. Brown and his colleagues admonish us not to forget the contextual issues (e.g., home, school, neighborhood, church, substance abuse treatment clinics, and mental health settings) that are determinant of behaviors in families.

The next section of the book has seven chapters and examines the role of family members in preventing and adapting to HIV. Parents are teachers and we need to help them understand their responsibility to educate themselves and their children about risks to their children's well-being. Drs. Krauss and Miller make the case that parents can be effective HIV/AIDS educators for their children. Drs. Dancy and DiIrio document the fact that mothers are influential in preventing HIV/STD risk behaviors, such as early sexual debut. Fathers have often been overlooked as important AIDS educators in their children's lives but Dr. Icard and his colleagues make the case for their important role. The couple is the bedrock of families and Drs. El-bassel and Remien describe important strategies to implement effective couple-based HIV prevention and treatment. Dr. Alison examines the major concerns about orphans and vulnerable children and their families in sub-Saharan Africa. Dr. McKay and her colleagues explore the way that families are embedded in communities that can be supportive in helping families in preventing and adapting to HIV. If investigators and service providers do not gain the support of communities, our public health work to prevent HIV infection from spreading will not be effective. As effective HIV medical treatment comes on line, adherence is a major concern and Dr. Simoni and colleagues describe how families can play a role with members who are struggling with a complex treatment regimen.

In the third section, there are three chapters that explore the ethnic, cultural, and gender issues associated with families. Dr. Murry and colleagues examine the ethnic and cultural issues in developing effective family-based prevention programs with African American and Hispanic youth. While we often hear about the estrangement between gay, lesbian, and bisexual youth from their families, Drs. Mustanski and Hunter provide evidence that parents are participants in their HIV prevention. A population that has a double risk is adolescents who are experiencing mental problems and Dr. Donenberg and her colleagues describe how family-based HIV prevention programs can reach them.

There are two chapters in the fourth section which are focused on the important topic of ensuring that efficacious family-based programs are implemented in front line HIV/AIDS care where they can benefit the greatest number of affected families. Dr. Rotheram and her colleagues provide a model of how to translate family-focused evidence-based practice into HIV/AIDS care. Drs. Rapkin and Mellins discuss some of the facilitators and barriers to implementing family-based efficacious programs into clinics and provide a successful model that indicates the multiple health and mental health benefits to families addressing HIV.

Bridging Research and Practice

We hope that the synthesis of research focused on different family configurations will be useful to service providers in public health agencies and NGOs that are on the front line of mounting combination behavioral and biomedical approaches. Moving beyond the individual and recognizing that a client is embedded in a system can ensure implementation of recommendations of health care providers.

Acknowledgments

We would like to acknowledge the major contribution from the NIMH Consortium on Families and HIV/AIDS. This group designed and sponsored 18 years of annual conferences where these results were presented and new initiatives were developed.

We would like to thank Dr. Jose Szapocznik who was a major driver in the beginning of this effort to conduct research that recognized that individuals at risk for and with HIV live in families and these cultural and contextual issues must be considered in all prevention efforts.

References

National Research Council and Institute of Medicine. Preventing mental, emotional, and behavioral disorders among young people: progress and possibilities. In: O'Connell ME, Boat T, Warner KE, editors. Committee on prevention of mental disorders and substance abuse among children, youth and young adults: research advances and promising interventions. Washington, DC: The National Academic Press. 2009. http://www.iom.edu/CMS/12552/45572/45572/64120.aspx.

Pequegnat W, Szapocznik J Working with families in the era of HIV/AIDS. Thousand Oaks, CA: Sage; 2000.

Bethesda, MD   Willo Pequegnat
Chicago, IL   Carl C. Bell

Contents

Part I
Overview of Family and HIV
and Mental Health

Chapter 1
Family and HIV/AIDS: First Line of Health Promotion and Disease Prevention

Willo Pequegnat and the NIMH Consortium on Families and HIV AIDS*

Abstract This chapter provides an overview of both the field of family-based research and of this book. The epidemiology of HIV affecting family members is briefly described to indicate the severity of the problem. We use the NIMH Consortium on HIV/AIDS definition of family which is "a network of mutual commitment" and we describe the different configurations of families. There is a description of what has been documented in the literature about family process, stigma, disclosure, social capital and social support, and psychological distress of families and HIV/AIDS. This chapter also addresses the multiple roles of parents and family members: (1) as AIDS educators; (2) as monitors, (3) as providers of warmth and support; and (4) as communicators about sex and relationships. There is a description of the role of families in adapting to HIV infection in family members and negotiating other family issues, such as homosexuality, high-risk sexual behavior, and alcohol and substance abuse. There is a discussion of issues about stigma and disclosure, family dynamics, stress and coping, handling complex medical regimes, and maintaining custody of children in families experiencing HIV infection. Other chapters in this book are referenced so that a more in-depth review of the issues can be explored.

* *Current members*: Susannah Allison, Ph.D., NIMH; Laurie Bauman, Ph.D., Albert Einstein College of Medicine; Carl C. Bell, M.D., Community Mental Health Council, Chicago; Cheryl A. Boyce, Ph.D., NIDA; James Bray, Ph.D., Baylor College of Medicine; Larry Icard, D.S.W., Temple University; Loretta Jemmott, Ph.D., University of Pennsylvania; Beatrice Krauss, Ph.D., Hunter College; Celia Lescano, Ph.D., Brown University; Mary McKay, Ph.D., Mount Sinai School of Medicine; Velma McBride Murry, Ph.D., University of Georgia; Hilda Pantin, Ph.D., University of Miami; Willo Pequegnat, Ph.D., NIMH; Bruce Rapkin, Ph.D., Albert Einstein College of Medicine, Gail E.Wyatt, Ph.D. *Emeritus members*: Ralph DiClemente, Ph.D., Emory University; Colleen DiIorio, Ph.D., Emory University; Roberta Paikoff, Ph.D., University of Illinois, Chicago; Mary Jane Rotheram-Borus, Ph.D., UCLA; José Szapocznik, Ph.D., University of Miami.

W. Pequegnat and C.C. Bell (eds.), *Family and HIV/AIDS: Cultural and Contextual Issues in Prevention and Treatment*, DOI 10.1007/978-1-4614-0439-2_1,
© Springer Science+Business Media, LLC 2012

1.1   Introduction

In recent years, researchers and health professionals have increasingly recognized the importance of the family in health promotion and disease prevention. The family is the first line in preventing HIV transmission among its members, providing education and reinforcing risk-reducing HIV-related behaviors in its members. The family is also the de facto caretaker for HIV-infected members. Effective treatments for HIV and related opportunistic infections have made HIV infection a chronic illness for individuals with access to them. Health care and mental health service providers are being challenged by the need for comprehensive family-based programs because multiple family members can be at risk and already infected (Crystal and Kersting 1998). HIV seropositive persons often have other family members who are HIV-infected and a constellation of family members who are affected. AIDS is changing the demographics of families in the United States and, in a more pronounced way, internationally.

1.2   Epidemiology of HIV Infection and AIDS

Because AIDS was first diagnosed in 1981 among homosexuals and drug users in the United States, family issues initially received little attention, because it was assumed that these groups were alienated from their families (Macklin 1988; Mayes and Cochran 1988). In the third decade of the AIDS epidemic, however, trends have emerged that have made the family prominent in both preventing the spread of HIV and in adapting to its consequences. First, as an epidemic ages, the age at which persons become infected is reduced, so 50% of all new HIV infections occur among young people aged 10–24 (WHO 2005). Second, women, especially monogamous, minority women, who are the capstones of their families, represent an increasing number of new HIV cases. African American gay men who are still in contact with their families are experiencing HIV prevalence rivaling sub-Saharan Africa. A positive trend is that perinatal transmission has essentially been eliminated in the U.S. due to widespread provision of good prenatal care and therapy to both mother and child and children who were perinatally infected are living into adulthood.

At the end of 2005, the Centers for Disease Control and Prevention (CDC) estimated that 437,982 people were living with AIDS in the United States: of these 44% were black, 35% white, 19% Hispanic, and 1% other race/ethnicity (Centers for Disease Control and Prevention (CDC) 2005). Seventy-seven percent of adults and adolescents living with AIDS are men. Men are more likely to have acquired HIV through homosexual contact (59%), women more likely through heterosexual contact (65%). During the 1990s, the epidemic shifted steadily toward African Americans and Hispanics, and especially women, and away from MSM, although this group still represents the largest single exposure group. In absolute numbers, blacks have outnumbered whites in new AIDS diagnoses and deaths since 1996, and in the number of people living with AIDS since 1998 (Centers for Disease Control and Prevention (CDC) 2005).

1.3 Definition of Family

Families experiencing high exposure to HIV come from a broad range of cultural groups and social settings and their structure is more complex than genetics (Pequegnat and Sczapocznik 2000; Mellins et al. 1996). Family networks include foster parents, extended family members, and non-blood members who function as relatives. A family can be a single seropositive mother who lives with her children, some of whom are seropositive and others seronegative; she may live with a boyfriend who may not be the father of any of the children. A family can be a grandmother taking care of her grandchildren because their parents have died of AIDS. A family can be a mixed serostatus couple – either two men or a man and a woman – who have close friends who assume multiple familial roles. A family can be a couple who are both seropositive, who are deciding whether to have a child or not. A family can be a stable social network of injection drug users in an urban area who inject together in shooting galleries and fulfill both instrumental and social support roles associated with extended family members. These myriad configurations required a thoughtful consideration of what is meant by "family," and led the NIMH Consortium on Families and HIV/AIDS to adopt the definition of family as a network of mutual commitment (Pequegnat and Bray 1997; Pequegnat and Sczapocznik 2000).

Despite the fact that family membership using the above definition can be fluid, it is essential to specify who is a member of the family when providing clinical services or conducting research. Members of the family can be identified through a genogram that includes both biological and nonbiological significant others (Mellins et al. 1996; Mitrani et al. 2000) (see genogram in Fig. 1.1). Additional relevant criteria for network of mutual commitment include: (1) blood relation or extended kinship (including fictive kin) or both; (2) perceived strength and duration of the relationship; (3) perceived support (including financial, emotional, and instrumental [e.g., transportation, child care, and other types of assistance]), and (4) perceived conflict. Although it is standard to include three generations in genograms, including four generations with minority families captures more of their extended family composition. In order to determine the best routes to intervene with the family, it is useful to develop an ecogram (Mitrani et al. 2000; Mellins et al. 1996) (see ecogram in Fig. 1.2).

1.4 Families as the Focus of Health Research

Families who are infected and affected by AIDS are often burdened with chronic poverty, homelessness, and drug abuse, as well as the social consequences of belonging to a cultural and ethnic minority or an ostracized group (Mellins and Ehrhart 1994). The complexities of these families create methodological difficulties for basic and applied research. Multiple constructs must be considered in designing research and providing services to these families. The salience of these constructs depends on whether the family is mobilized to prevent or adapt to HIV.

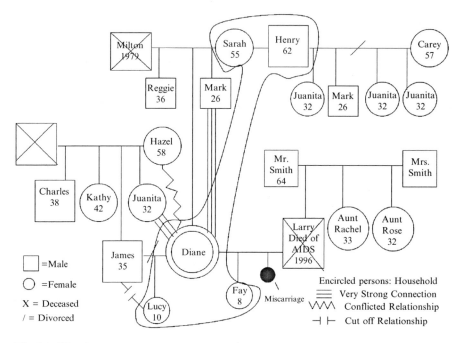

Fig. 1.1 Diane's genogram

1.4.1 Family Process

Family process, which refers to the dynamic interactions among family members, must be evaluated to understand the role of families in preventing and adapting to HIV/AIDS (Robbins et al. 1998). Certain family dynamics are consistently related to positive or negative adjustment and health of family members. Reciprocal communication, problem solving, warm affect, social support (within and outside the family), and caregiving are predictive of positive outcomes (Bray 1995; Hadley et al. 2009), while conflict and negative affect are associated with behavioral problems (Donenberg et al. 2001; Szapocznik and Kurtines 1993).

Parenting dynamics (supervision, monitoring, parental control) are most related to prevention of HIV risk behaviors in children and young adults. Three components of parent–child relationships were assessed by Mellins and colleagues (2007) in a study of risk and resilience in HIV-negative youth with and without mothers: (1) involvement (spending time and showing interest in the child and the child's activities); (2) communication (parent empathy and conversation across situations); and (3) autonomy (the extent to which the caregiver is willing to promote the child's independence). There were no differences in participation in "sexual possibility situations" (unsupervised times when the youth could engage in risky behavior) (see Paikoff 1995) between youth with and without seropositive mothers (Lewis et al. 2006). However, low scores on these parent–child relationship factors were significantly associated with the onset of sexual and drug risk behavior. Another

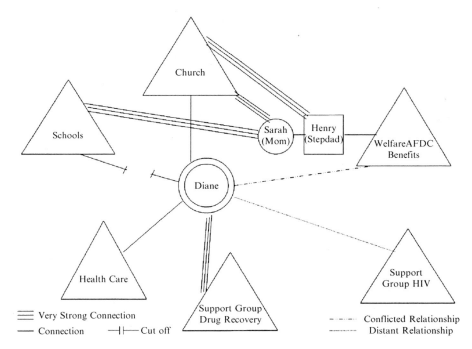

Fig. 1.2 Diane's ecogram

study, CHAMPSA, measured parenting dynamics by measuring caregiver monitoring, communication, comfort, and communication frequency, and found proximal outcomes indicating these parenting dynamics supported health promotion activities that were antithetical to being at risk for developing HIV. Compared to controls, the experimental families had greater caregiver monitoring (e.g., family rules, caregiver communication comfort, and caregiver communication frequency) (Bell et al. 2008) (see Chap. 2).

Stanton and colleagues examined the relationship of parental monitoring and communication to adolescent risk involvement, over time, in a sample of urban African American families (Li et al. 2000; Yang et al. 2007). Perceived parental monitoring had protective effects on adolescent risk involvement with peers over 2 years. The protective effect on girls' sexual abstinence increased significantly over time. The probability of girls engaging in sex increased among those who perceived problems with familial communication, while it remained stable for those perceiving less problem communication. These findings confirm the protective effect of perceived parental monitoring on adolescent risk involvement. They also extend previous findings by showing the importance of consistent parental monitoring and communication. Moreover, a supportive, communicative family environment, in which expectations regarding risk are clearly articulated, encourages adolescents to internalize their parents' values and norms, and in turn avoid risky behaviors (Brody et al. 2000). In this regard, studies targeting rural African American families have identified ways in which parents protect youth from involvement in HIV-related risk behavior (Brody et al. 2006; Murry et al. 2007). In particular, attachment to parents, parental monitoring, and family communication are strong protective factors against high-risk sexual behavior among African American youth (DiClemente et al. 2001; Miller et al. 1999; Perrino et al. 2000).

Rapkin and colleagues (2000) evaluated family communication style and problem solving on outcomes for families coping with AIDS. Their study corroborated findings from other studies showing that problem solving interventions can facilitate engagement of the family in social support groups and relationships with a case manager. This intervention also contributed to families maintaining their sense of well-being despite multiple problems.

1.4.2 Stigma

In the psychological literature, stigma is usually studied as a social process that negatively affects the individual (Herek 1998). In families with HIV or living in high HIV seroprevalence areas, stigma is a more complex issue. Stigma can be experienced by the entire family, especially when HIV was contracted through sex or drugs, stigma about HIV can be a source of conflict and shame for all family members. AIDS manifests at least four of the characteristics associated with a stigmatized disease: (1) cause is perceived to be the bearer's responsibility; (2) perceived to be fatal; (3) puts other people at risk; and (4) apparent to others and therefore upsetting (Herek 1999).

Stigma and shame are major factors driving the AIDS epidemic. Because of stigma, seropositive individuals fear to disclose, even to their families. Failure to disclose can have serious consequences: high-risk behavior with sexual partners, failure to seek and obtain social support from family and friends, and failure to seek life-saving medical care (Nyblade et al. 2004). Stigma may have a role in cutting off discourse about HIV – even conversations about prevention. Krauss and colleagues (2006) found little to no relationship within a household between parent's and children's knowledge about HIV and worries about HIV prior to the intervention. Youth had significantly more worries compared to their parents. The item most endorsed by youth was "someone I know has HIV and hasn't told me" (see Chap. 4). In the CHAMPSA study, the investigators found less stigma toward HIV-infected people in both caregivers and children in the group that received the intervention as compared to the control condition (Bell et al. 2008).

Stigma among seropositive women led to poorer parenting, isolation of children from adults and other children, and child behavior problems (Bauman et al. 2002). HIV-positive mothers reporting high levels of HIV-related stigma have been found to score significantly lower on measures of physical, psychological, and social functioning compared to mothers not experiencing high levels of stigma (Murphy et al. 2006a), and mothers' levels of depression were significantly higher when perceived stigma was high. Stigma can be associated with increased anxiety, depression, and somatization (Lee et al. 2002). It also contributed to mothers deciding not to disclose their HIV status in order to protect their children from stigma, but they were also motivated by concern that the children might inadvertently tell others

(Lester et al. 2002). Parents frequently identified the public perception of AIDS as a debilitating and frightening illness as a factor in their anticipation of disclosure having a negative effect on their children.

HIV-related stigma affects not only persons living with HIV but also their families, including children, and communities. Even children as young as six years of age have been found to be aware of "stigma by association" and are concerned about other people finding out about their mothers' serostatus for both self-protection reasons (i.e., worry that others would think badly of them), and because they want to protect their mothers (Murphy et al. 2002a). Adolescents aware of their mother's HIV-positive serostatus who perceive high levels of stigma have been found to be more likely to participate in delinquent behavior compared to adolescents reporting low HIV-related stigma (Murphy et al. 2006b). Krauss and colleagues conducted a study to determine whether an interactive training given to community parents would significantly increase their children's reported comfort in interacting with persons living with HIV (Krauss et al. 2006). For children of trained parents (regardless of whether the parent–child dyad was mother and daughter or son or father and daughter or son), significant increases in comfort were observed from baseline to 6-month follow-up, on 14 of 22 reported daily activities with persons living with HIV. This increased comfort predicted the number of recent experiences of interacting with a person living with HIV, even after controlling for closeness to the person living with HIV and number of persons with HIV that the child is aware of, living or deceased. This study demonstrated that training parents to be HIV health educators is significantly associated with changes in their children's behavior and shows promise for reducing HIV-related stigma and social isolation among families.

1.4.3 Disclosure

Conflict, domestic violence, increased risk-taking behaviors, failure to access social support, and poor custody planning can be results of secrets and lies. Disclosure of HIV status is inhibited by fear of stigma that may result in rejection by family and friends. Disclosure is a process, not an event, because there are multiple issues relating to what is being disclosed (early HIV diagnosis, latest CD4 count, HAART failure), to whom (male to male or female partner, mother to child) and whose status (parent's HIV, child's HIV). The conditions under which people make decisions related to these issues are a vital part of research on families living with HIV/AIDS. Often disclosure is implicit. A mother will drop hints to her children and friends about her poor health and assume that they understand what she is sharing.

Disclosure has important implications for family process because lack of disclosure can circumscribe family engagement (Mitrani et al. 2003). Seeking and securing social support for HIV-positive individuals and their families is inextricably related to disclosure. Families cannot participate in some prevention programs because certain topics can only be discussed with family members to whom the HIV diagnosis has been disclosed (Mitrani et al. 2003).

A longitudinal study by Murphy and colleagues (2002a, b) studied the long-term impact of mothers' disclosing their HIV status to their children (6–11 years old). Disclosing mothers reported higher levels of interpersonal problems and negative mood in their children than nondisclosing mothers. Disclosing mothers perceived their children to have lower self-esteem than their children reported. Children of nondisclosing mothers actually scored lower on self-esteem measures. It could be that mothers were reporting on their children's initial distress and difficulty but that this resolved over time. These findings indicate that therapeutic interventions for children following maternal disclosure – such as children's social support groups – might assist children during a potentially short-lived, stressful period. In a study by Lee and colleagues (2002), disclosure by mothers increased adolescent daughters' distress, perhaps initiating their anticipatory bereavement, even though disclosure was not correlated with level of maternal health. These findings might be explained by HIV's association with fear of stigma and loss of social support, and awareness of transmission risk within families.

Disclosing the child's HIV status to the child raises a different set of issues. Lester and colleagues (2002) found that parents feared to disclose to their child because they feared for the child's safety and well-being due to stigma in the community. Parents identified a range of factors that influenced their personal decision to tell their child, which included parental stage of illness, parental communication style, concern about the child's anticipated emotional distress, potential for stigma if the child inadvertently revealed the HIV within the family outside family, the child's developmental status, child's questions, and belief in the child's right to know (Lester et al. 2002). They carefully evaluated the impact of disease severity and disclosure on the psychological well-being of children. Most parents believed that children under the age of six could not understand the concept of death and dying. Most chose to disclose to their children between the ages of 6 and 10, identifying their children's rights, treatment adherence, and family communication as important factors in this decision. Most parents felt that children over the age of 11 needed to be aware of their medical diagnosis. In one study, Murphy and colleagues (2006a, b) found that the mean age of disclosure to children was 10 (range 5–14) among mothers who could recall the exact age when their child learned of their HIV status. In a sample of 90 families, by age 12–13, 84% of the children had been informed of their mothers' serostatus.

Mellins and colleagues (2002) administered quantitative and qualitative interviews about disclosure to 75 caregivers of seropositive 3- to 13-year-old children, as well as to all seropositive children in the study who knew their diagnosis. Many children had not been told about their HIV status because of parental concern about their mental health and other psychosocial issues, including ten children over the age of 10. On average, children to whom their parents had disclosed were older and tended to have lower CD4 count. Parents were more likely to disclose their children's HIV status as their children became symptomatic and immune compromised and their medication regimen became more complex, requiring greater cooperation from the child.

In addition to the issues posed by parent to child or adolescent disclosure, "Who Should I Tell?" is another critical question for HIV-infected adolescents (see Wiener and Lyon 2006). Newly diagnosed adolescents were more likely to disclose to their mothers than to their fathers. Adolescents who decided to tell friends or romantic partners were more likely to receive social support, have good social self-concept, and have fewer behavioral problems or post-traumatic stress symptoms. Proper prevention education is vital for both recent and long-time infected adolescents, to ensure safer sex practices. Families and health care providers need to guide and train sexually active adolescents, particularly those desiring a child, on how to disclose to their partners and families, which is an ethical challenge even for adults.

Moreover, Lee and his colleagues examined the associations between parental HIV disclosure and mental health outcomes among HIV-affected adolescents (Lee et al. 2007a), using the baseline data of HIV-affected adolescents from the intervention study by Rotheram-Borus and her colleagues (Rotheram-Borus et al. 2001). Parental HIV disclosure was significantly associated with adolescents' reported level of depression (Lee et al. 2007b). This finding underscores the need for careful planning on the part of parents prior to disclosing. In addition, it is crucial to ensure that adolescents have adequate social support to cope with parental HIV disclosure (see Chap. 14).

Appropriate disclosure outside the immediate family may confer some benefits to families in terms of their physical and mental health. Research in the larger social ecologies of families with HIV has not been conducted, which limits guidelines for advising families on when to disclose.

1.4.4 Social Capital and Social Support

"Social capital" refers to the connections between and within social networks, including interpersonal trust, norms of reciprocity, and membership in voluntary organizations in a community. Some researchers consider it to be an explanatory factor in the health achievements of societies. Social capital variables have been associated with cross-sectional variation in mortality rates of the U.S. (Kawachi et al. 1997). Evidence from other countries, including Sweden and Finland, has suggested links between community social capital, and lower prevalence of high-risk health behaviors, and mental health problems. Social capital has also been examined in relation to neighborhoods. The extent to which residents said that neighbors could be trusted and were willing to help their community was associated with higher collective efficacy (Sampson et al. 1997). This is important, because health-promoting effects of community social trust were significantly greater for individuals expressing higher trust of others. While the mechanism for linking social capital to health is still being identified, the epidemiology suggests that enhanced social support is an important determinant of longevity and quality of life (Kawachi and Berkman 2000; House et al. 1988).

Researchers have examined the effectiveness of social support from family and friends in extending life and providing comfort for HIV-infected individuals. Social support is viewed as either directly promoting health and health behaviors (William et al. 1981) or as buffering the adverse effect of stressors (Cohen and Wills 1985; House 1981).

Social support includes both functional and structural components (Metts et al. 1996). Functional support refers to perceived availability, actual receipt, reciprocity, and adequacy and satisfaction of that support. Structural support refers to sources of support (family of origin, family of procreation or choice, friends, health care providers, or other sources, such as support groups and churches). Other important factors include the size of the support network and links among network members (also known as density). Types of support include practical or instrumental (someone who would care for you when sick); emotional (someone in whom you can confide); affirmational (someone who lets you know he/she likes the things that you do or think); and informational (someone you can ask for advice). Different members of the social support network may provide different types of social support.

The benefits of social support may differ according to source. They can be tempered by the impact of one family member's stress on other members of the family (Feaster et al. 2000; Feaster and Szapocznik 2002). They found that social support from outside of the family to a new mother lowered the psychological distress of family members, whereas reports by the new mother of higher support from within the family increased other family members' feelings of coping adequacy. The new mother's report of her own hassles was negatively related to the family members' perceived adequacy of coping. The family members of HIV-positive new mothers, in particular, showed lower adequacy of coping when the new mother responded to the stress of the new birth with avoidance.

Social support benefits are not constant across the course of HIV infection. Changes may occur due to illness progression (changes in overall support and types of support, which can negatively impact family functioning and contribute to psychological distress experienced by persons living with AIDS and/or their caregivers (Pequegnat and Sczapocznik 2000). Understanding this reality, the CHAMPSA intervention targeted rebuilding the social fabric and found that, compared to those in the control groups, those in the experimental groups increased their primary social networks, which are an important consideration in combating the HIV epidemic (Bell et al. 2008) (see Chap. 2). In a study of the role of family in providing support and care of family members, Crystal and Kersting (1998) found that as HIV patients became sicker, more of their support and care transferred from the family to the public health system. Because social support provided by the family can have a beneficial impact on health and mental health of the seropositive family member, interventions that target improving the ability of the family to provide this support, even as the disease progresses, would improve the quality of life of persons living with HIV/AIDS.

Several studies have identified that social support is critical around the time of disclosure of the parent's or child's serostatus (Murphy et al. 2002a, b). If the family cannot adequately provide this, a social support group may be important for the children in handling their mothers' illness. Health care workers can provide support for mothers when they decide to disclose to their children (Lester et al. 2002). Children often lose social support when peers learn about their HIV infection and special planning may be needed before disclosing their HIV status. The research subjects in a study by Mellins and colleagues (2002) received mental health support from a family clinician, which provided a safety net during difficult periods and permitted them to develop a support system. Rotheram and colleagues reinforced the importance of social support when the adolescent's parent has died and the grieving child is being integrated into the family of the new caregiver (Rotheram-Borus et al. 2005a, b) (see Chap. 14).

Lee and his colleagues (2007a, b) examined the associations among social support and mental and behavioral outcomes among HIV-affected adolescents. Five distinct dimensions of social support were examined: size of social support, frequency of contact, perceived satisfaction with social support, positive social support, and negative role model influence (Rotheram-Borus et al. 1997). Adolescents who had more social support providers reported significantly lower levels of depression and fewer conduct problems; adolescents who had more negative influence from role models reported more behavior problems. Reductions in depression, multiple problem behaviors, and conduct problems were significantly associated with better social support.

1.4.5 Psychological Distress

Families who are at risk for and adapting to HIV are also at risk for serious mental health problems, and families with members who have mental health problems are at increased risk of HIV/AIDS. The effects of poor physical health may interact with other risk factors for poor mental health, such as stress, inadequate coping strategies, fear of disclosure, and limited social support. Elevated levels of depression among HIV-positive mothers have been associated with poor cohesion in the family and with poorer family sociability. Depression has also been associated with mothers' being less able to perform tasks that they typically would, and the children of more depressed mothers had increased household responsibilities (Murphy et al. 2002b). Some studies have shown that children of mothers with HIV/AIDS have elevated scores on a measure of children's behavior that is an indicator of the children being disruptive (Lee et al. 2007a). They found that the worse the mother's psychological distress, the more the children exhibited behavioral problems. However, only one aspect of mothers' health status – activity restrictions – was associated with negative impact on the mental health of their children. Rather than being a protective factor, in this study family cohesion was a risk factor for poor child mental health when other factors were controlled. Mothers with higher internalized stigma reported more behavioral problems in children who had been told about their HIV status. Bauman and colleagues (2007) found that every child in their study had one significant mental health problem at some point over their 4-year study.

Other studies have shown mixed results in children with and without seropositive mothers (Brackis-Cott et al. 2007; Lewis et al. 2006; Mellins et al. 2007). There were no significant differences in depressive symptomatology between children 10 and

14 years old with seropositive and those with seronegative mothers, but those children who knew their mother's diagnosis were more depressed (Brackis-Cott et al. 2007). Children with seropositive mothers may be at risk for a number of reasons other than their mother's HIV status – including growing up in high risk environments affected by poverty, substance abuse, family disruption, discrimination, and violence. As a result, it is not always clear what is associated with elevated levels of psychological distress, and future work needs to identify the role of HIV, as well as the role of other risk and protective factors. Moreover, fluctuations in the mothers' health may lead to differential findings. Stability in mothers' health over time has been linked with better child mental health indicators (Murphy et al. 2006b).

Families need interventions specific to psychosocial stressors of seropositive parents. In a study of seropositive parents, Rotheram-Borus and colleagues (2005a, b) found that being a custodial parent increased psychological stress and challenges to self-care, poorer medical adherence, and attendance at medical appointments. They were similar to non parents and noncustodial parents in mental health symptoms and treatment utilization for mental health and substance use problems (Goldstein et al. 2005). Noncustodial parents demonstrated the highest levels of recent substance use and substance abuse treatment.

Prior studies have demonstrated that when a parent becomes emotionally distressed, adolescent daughters (11–18 years old) are particularly vulnerable (Lee et al. 2002). Unexpectedly, Lee et al. (2002) found that despite high levels of distress (emotional distress, suicidal behavior, high-risk sexual and substance use) among seropositive mothers, their children did not exhibit more emotional distress, sexual risk, or substance use than would be expected in normative samples. This study suggests that developing family-based interventions that address mediators such as financial distress, illness disclosure, and parental bonding may help break the cycle of mental health problems in this population.

Another area of family function that can contribute to psychological distress is the rejection by family of young lesbian, gay, and bisexual who come out. In a study in San Francisco, Ryan and colleagues (2009) examined specific negative family reactions to sexual orientation and gender expression during adolescence as predictors of health problems in a sample of lesbian, gay, and bisexual young adults. Family rejecting reactions included 51 close-ended items such as, "Between ages 13 and 19, how often did your parents/caregivers blame you for any anti-gay mistreatment that you experienced." They found a link between these parental and caregiver behaviors and negative health problems among these youth, including depression, suicidal ideation and attempts, substance use, and sexual health risks (see Chap. 6).

1.5   Role of Family in Preventing the Spread of HIV

The increasing number of sexually active adolescents who do not consistently use condoms and the rising rate of HIV infection have re-invigorated public health efforts to provide them with information on protective sexual practices. Increased attention has been given to how families serve to promote or encourage adolescents to adopt responsible risk-reducing behavior (Biglan 1990; Brooks-Gunn and Paikoff 1993; Whitebeck et al. 1993; Bell et al. 2007; Pequegnat and Sczapocznik 2000; McKay and Paikoff 2007). Other researchers have focused on the impact that sociocultural factors and family systems have on perception of HIV/STD risk and risk reduction among poor, urban, ethnic minority families, particularly African Americans and Hispanics who are most at risk of acquiring HIV (Boyd-Franklin 1989; Donenberg et al. 2002, 2003, 2006; Nappi et al. 2009; Szapocznik and Kurtines 1993; Taylor and Wang 1997; Wilson and Donenberg 2004). Traditional models of HIV-risk and prevention have focused on cognitive mechanisms (e.g., Theory of Reasoned Action, Health Belief Model), but several studies suggest these may not be sufficient to explain HIV risk among youth (Donenberg et al. 2005; Mustanski et al. 2006). In fact, a broader social and personal model has been proposed to explain risk-taking among youth that includes the family and broader socio-ecological contexts (Bronfenbrenner 1986; Donenberg et al. 2007; Donenberg and Pao 2005).

Studies have consistently shown that powerful factors that protect rural African American youth from sexual risk behavior originate in the family environment, particularly in parents' caregiving practices (Brody et al. 2001, 2002; Murry and Brody 1999). Moreover, based upon patterns of family life established in African societies and modified in response to enslavement in America (Sudarkase 1988), reliance on family and extended kin networks has supported African Americans through multiple social transitions. African Americans' family-centered orientation protects adolescents from high-risk behaviors (Wills et al. 2003) (see Chap. 11).

1.5.1 Parents as AIDS Educators

Because families are the most proximal and fundamental social system influencing human development, they are the strategic point of entry for effective and lasting behavioral change that is the objective of family-based interventions (Bronfenbrenner 1986). Parents are adolescents' primary sex educators because they are best able to time their discussions to when their children are open to learn new information (Szapocznik and Coatsworth 1999). Most sex education programs, however, are directed toward adolescents individually and are provided through convenient venues, such as school and community agencies. Some students may understand and use information delivered this way, others may need repeated exposure to appreciate the relevance of prevention messages to their health practices. One option for matching readiness of youth with availability of information is to provide parents with information and skills, including training on developmentally appropriate ways of relating and communicating about sex to guide their adolescents in making responsible decisions regarding sexual behavior. Parents do a lot more than present information about sex, they communicate values, model appropriate behavior, encourage bonding to family and school, monitor the behavior of their children and their friends, and encourage children to form a long-term view of their behavior (Jordan and Donenberg 2006).

Because parental risky behaviors are closely associated with risky adolescent behaviors, parental risk appears to influence adolescent contraceptive use through its effect on parental self-efficacy (Wilder and Watt 2002). Hence, encouraging parents to behave well may be an effective model for adolescents' behavior. Alert parents can adapt their intervention to life conditions and risks their adolescents face.

Families influence adolescent sexual behavior in four primary ways, and these are often the focus of HIV prevention programs: (1) parental monitoring and control; (2) affective parenting behavior (warmth, support); (3) parental attitudes about sex; and (4) parent–adolescent communication (Donenberg and Pao 2005).

1.5.1.1 Parental Monitoring and Control

Parental monitoring and authoritative parental style are consistently associated with less risky sexual behavior, fewer sexual partners, less pregnancy, and increased condom use among youth (Li et al. 2000; Miller et al. 1999; Rai et al. 2003; Bell et al. 2008; Paikoff 1995). However, these affects may differ by child gender. In a study of youth seeking mental health services, Donenberg and colleagues (2002) found at low levels of parental permissiveness, rates of risky sex among boys and girls did not differ, but at high levels of permissiveness girls reported more sexual risk-taking than boys, and girls were more likely than boys to report having sex while using drugs and alcohol and having sex without a condom. Results suggest that parental monitoring and permissiveness are more strongly associated with sexual risk-taking in troubled girls than troubled boys, and they underscore a need for gender-sensitive, family-focused HIV-prevention programs. In another study, Donenberg and colleagues (2006) found that negative peer influence and high parental permissiveness were linked to greater risky sexual behavior but mainly among adolescents who reported using drug and alcohol use in the past 3 months.

1.5.1.2 Parental Warmth and Support

Family social environment has a profound impact on the healthy development of adolescents. Positive family factors protect against sexual risk behaviors (Leland and Barth 1993). Perceived parental warmth and support predict less adolescent risk-taking (Donenberg et al. 2003). Donenberg and colleagues (2003) found that together, parental hostile control, negative and positive peer influence, and youths' externalizing behavior problems correctly classified 87.4% of adolescents as initiating sexual activity under or over 14 years of age. Conversely, family conflict and early pubertal maturation are associated with earlier sexual debut (Paikoff 1995), and level of mother's coercive behavior and "love withdrawal" predict earlier age of first intercourse for women (Miller et al. 1997). Adolescents who say they have good relationships with their mothers, and who believe that their mother would approve of their using birth control are more likely to use birth control (Dittus and Jaccard 2000).

1.5.1.3   Parental Attitudes About Sex

Parents are the role models for their children's attitudes toward sex and sexual behavior, and influence their sexual debut, activity, and condom use. Frequent parent–child discussions about parent attitudes about sex and health topics are associated with more responsible sexual behaviors of the children (DiIorio et al. 2003; Dutra et al. 1999; Wills et al. 2003). In the absence of these discussions, adolescents overestimate the level of parental approval of their sexual behaviors, and mothers underestimate the amount of sexual activity of their adolescents (Jaccard et al. 1998). Youth report that parent–child discussions about sex are likely to delay sexual activity (Fox 1981; Darling and Hicks 1982; Stanton et al. 1993). Adolescents who believe that their mothers disapprove of premarital sex, whether or not the mother actually does disapprove, are less likely to initiate intercourse (Dittus and Jaccard 2000). With the exception of girls in single parent households, there was no effect of family structure on adolescent sexual initiation (David and Friel 2001). Mother–child relationship and mother's attitudes toward sexual behavior were more powerful. Perceived maternal disapproval of sexual intercourse, along with mother–child relationships characterized by high levels of warmth and closeness may be important factors related to delay of adolescents' first sexual intercourse (Sieving et al. 2000).

1.5.1.4   Parent–Adolescent Communication

Overall quality of parent–child communication is a critical determinant of risky sexual behaviors in adolescents (Leland and Barth 1993; Murry 1997; Yang et al. 2007). In general, parents and children do not speak sufficiently about sexuality (Hutchinson and Cooney 1998). Remarkably, children's perceptions of their relationships with their parents at ages 7-11 predict age of first sexual intercourse 11 years later (Miller et al. 1997). Mother–adolescent discussions regarding condom use prior to first sexual intercourse increase the chances that adolescents will use condoms during first and subsequent sexual intercourse (Christ et al. 1998; Christopherson 1994; Miller et al. 1998). Parental involvement in the adolescent's life initially mediates the negative effect of single-parent households on adolescent sexual risk-taking (Pearson et al. 2006).

Among youth seeking mental health services, parent–teen communication plays an important role in adolescent risky sexual behavior (Nappi et al. 2009; Wilson and Donenberg 2004). Nappi et al. (2009) used qualitative and quantitative data to examine the content and quality of parent–adolescent discussions and adolescent-reported condom use and number of sexual partners among 207 parent–teen dyads in psychiatric care. Dyads described the content of their communication and rated quality of family HIV/AIDS discussions. Results revealed that parents and teens discussed transmission, prevention, consequences, myths, and compassion. Parent-reported discussion of the consequences of risky sexual behavior was associated with greater sexual risk behavior, but only for girls. This finding corroborates a growing body of evidence indicative of the ineffectiveness of scare tactics to influence health behaviors (Taylor 2003). The girls in this study whose parents reported discussing the consequences of HIV/AIDS, both in the presence and absence of communication about protective behavioral skills, reported higher rates of sexual risk-taking. In terms of communication quality, sexual risk-taking was higher among teens who reported lower levels of parental comfort and openness during discussions about sex. This finding departs somewhat from Wilson and Donenberg (2004) who found high quality discussions contributed to greater reported risk-taking. However, differences may be more methodological than substantive, as Wilson and colleagues analyzed videotaped discussions and defined quality as the mutuality of the discussions. We defined quality as teens' perceived parental comfort and openness (e.g., "My mother/father tries to understand how I feel about topics like this."). Importantly, parents may send different messages about HIV/AIDS to sons versus daughters, and messages related to consequences may not effectively reduce risk among daughters. However, for boys *and* girls seeking psychiatric care, teaching parents *how* to discuss HIV/AIDS may promote safer sexual behavior.

1.5.2   Family-Based Primary Prevention Programs

Over the past 17 years, the National Institute of Mental Health has made a concerted effort to support a research program to develop family-based HIV prevention programs (Pequegnat and Sczapocznik 2000). The primary prevention programs have been based on systems theory and have borrowed heavily from Bronfenbrenner's (1986) social ecological theory. This work recognizes that adolescents' sexual behavior is part of their social development and that parents have a crucial role to play in guiding and shaping the social and sexual development of their children. Parents are the primary influence on children until adolescence, when youth begin to struggle for autonomy and peer norms have an increasing influence on their social behaviors. Parents, however, continue to have an enduring and direct impact on their children's risk-taking decisions (McKay et al. 2000).

In 1994, Paikoff and colleagues launched CHAMP I (Chicago HIV Prevention and Adolescence Mental Health Project) to address increased rates of adolescent HIV/AIDS exposure in minority neighborhoods (Paikoff 1995). A Collaborative Advisory Board was active in all aspects of this study, from reviewing the protocol to interpreting the data as it was analyzed (McCormick et al. 2000). Parents played a pivotal role in guiding adolescents' sexual behavior prior to their becoming sexually active, during a time when "sexual possibilities" are likely to increase (McKay et al. 2000). A "sexual possibility" is an opportunity to engage in risky behavior because they are not closely supervised. This family-based program had a dual education and skills-building approach: (1) parents-only groups developed skills that enhanced parent monitoring, discipline effectiveness, conflict resolution, support, and comfort in discussing sensitive topics; and (2) children-only groups developed skills to enhance social problem solving, such as an ability to identify risky situations and an ability to be assertive in handling sexual peer pressure (McBride et al. 2007a, b; McKay et al. 2004; Paikoff 1997). The overall objective was to promote comfort and communication about puberty, early sexual behavior, and HIV/AIDS (McBride et al. 2007a, b). CHAMP family programs were delivered by community members who co-facilitated multiple family groups with a university co-leader. When compared to the control group, families in CHAMP I showed increased family decision making, improvements in parental monitoring, family comfort in discussing sensitive topics, more neighborhood supports, and fewer disruptive difficulties with children (McKay et al. 2004, 2007a; McBride et al. 2007a, b). Parental anxiety and depression also decreased significantly from pre- to post-test (Paikoff 1997). The youth in the intervention families reported experiencing significantly less frequent and fewer sexual possibility situations than those in the comparison condition. Youth in the intervention group, however, reported significantly higher levels of family conflict than the comparison group, which could be due to the fact that they were having more discussions about important topics (McBride et al. 2007a, b).

Based on findings from the original study, CHAMP II (Southside of Chicago) was developed, consisting of a 12-week fourth- and fifth-grade family intervention, in partnership with urban parents (McKay et al. 2007a, b). Five hundred families with 324 children were randomly assigned to receive the CHAMP Family Program with 73% of the families completing the entire program. The high rate of participation was attributed to the intensive outreach strategies designed and implemented by the community collaborators. Sixty percent of the youth in the intervention families reported using condoms "every time" and 72% reported using condoms at last intercourse (Tolou-Shams et al. 2007). The youth also reported less aggressive and disruptive behaviors (Bannon and McKay 2007).

To further explore how to transfer this family-based prevention program, CHAMP III (Bronx, New York and Westside of Chicago) was designed to hand off the CHAMP program to community service agencies in Chicago and New York (Baptiste et al. 2007a). This work highlights the dissemination process of an evidence-based, efficacious intervention in the real world (McKay and Paikoff 2007).

CHAMP IV – also known as CHAMPSA or the AmaQhawe Family Project – is a culturally appropriate adaptation for families and communities in Durban, South Africa (Bhana et al. 2004). It is based on the Theory of Triadic Influence (TTI) and seeks to intervene in three sources of behavioral influence: (1) an intrapersonal stream, (2) a social normative stream, and (3) a cultural/attitudinal stream (Petraitis et al. 1995; Bell et al. 2007; Baptiste et al. 2007c). This study recruited 450 South African pre-adolescents (9–12 years old) and their adult caregivers from 20 equivalent schools (10 experimental and 10 control). The control group received an existing school-based HIV information curriculum.

Youth and families who participated in CHAMPSA were likely to be better informed about HIV/AIDS transmission, have less HIV stigmatizing attitudes, have greater parental monitoring of children's activities and adherence to the family rules, and have increased parental comfort communicating about difficult topics. There was also less neighborhood disorganization and greater neighborhood social control and cohesion. CHAMPSA has significant potential to enhance protective influences in communities (Bell et al. 2008). CHAMPSA is a potential model for adapting HIV intervention programs to meet local needs internationally (Baptiste et al. 2007c).

CHAMP was also adapted for the Caribbean, which has the second highest rate of HIV per capita in the world (Baptiste et al. 2005, 2007b). CHAMP V (Trinidad and Tobago) was a pilot study conducted with 32 parents/caregivers and youth (average age 12.5 years), attending two public schools, situated in high HIV/AIDS sero-prevalent counties. Comparing the mean change from pretest to posttest, youth in the CHAMP group reported increased frequency of discussions about HIV/AIDS, decreased frequency of discussions about gangs, and increased parental expectations that they be at a certain place at a particular time. As with other CHAMP programs, there was strong community participation in the design and administration of the pilot study (Baptiste et al. 2007b; Voisin et al. 2005).

While most family-based prevention programs have been developed for mothers, Krauss and colleagues (2000) designed PATH which is a prevention programs for both mothers and fathers, acknowledging fathers' important role in the sexual health of their 10- to 13-year-old preadolescents. This trial recruited 238 parent and 238 child participants in dyads (father–son; father–daughter; mother–daughter; mother–son). They were randomized to receive either a parent training program plus materials or materials only. Parents participated in four 3 hour group training sessions, given once a week, covering knowledge and safety skills regarding sex, drugs, and HIV; child development; parent–child communication. The initial parent training was followed by a parent child session in which each parent and child met alone with a facilitator. Parents chose activities to perform with their child and children had an opportunity to ask questions. The parent group met again after three months to discuss real-life situations that had occurred.

This study demonstrated that an intervention delivered by either a mother or father can reduce HIV-risk-associated sexual behaviors of adolescents (Krauss et al. 2002; Freidin et al. 2005). These interventions are aimed at fostering family involvement in the sexual health of adolescents, including delay of sexual intercourse, acquiring information about HIV/AIDS, interacting comfortably with community members and family who may have HIV, and ensuring HIV risk-reduction skills.

At the request of parents and youth, two 1.5 hour sessions on risk-reduction communication during the transition to adolescence were added to the "basic training." These sessions emphasize household safety, affirming findings that youth worry as much about their parents' risks as parents worry about youth's (Krauss et al. 2002). Aside from increased comfort in interacting with persons with HIV, findings indicate that children of trained parents have increased practical HIV knowledge, decreased unrealistic worry, and higher intention to use condoms at first and subsequent intercourse (Krauss et al. 1997). This intervention also demonstrated a protective effect in increased delay of first intercourse for male and female youth who have their first sexual experience at age 15 or younger (Krauss et al. 2007). In this study they found at baseline that HIV information was not shared within households. Six months post-intervention, children of parents offered training evidenced significantly more HIV knowledge and less unrealistic worries about HIV worry than children of parents not offered training – moderated through parent knowledge only for children of trained parents (Krauss et al. 2002). As the youth matured to age 15, approximately 25.3% of control and intervention youth became sexually active. The delay in sexual initiation, however, was longer for children of parents offered training (a protective effect of 25–30 months) and more uniform across genders (Krauss et al. 2007).

DiIorio and colleagues (2000) developed a prevention program for mothers and adolescents and a later one for fathers and sons. The primary objective of the mother–adolescent program, called *Keepin' it R.E.A.L.!* (Responsible, Empowered, Aware, Living) was to enhance the role of mothers in postponing sexual debut of their 11 through 14-year-old adolescents (DiIorio et al. 2000. Embedded within *Keepin' it R.E.A.L.!* are two programs – one based on social cognitive theory (SCT) and the other on problem behavior theory (PBT). The SCT program was built on the recognition that behavior is dependent on a dynamic interaction of personal, environmental, and behavioral factors (Bandura 1997). The facilitation of desirable behaviors, such as delaying the initiation of sexual intercourse, requires supporting the development of behavior-specific cognitive, behavioral, and efficacy skills. Thus, the SCT program included sessions on sexual health, HIV transmission and protection, communication skills, and peer pressure. The second program was built on PBT principles, which propose that problem behaviors in adolescents arise from common underlying psychological attributes or a predisposition (Jessor et al. 1997). The incorporation of PBT principles was reflected in the program by addressing a wide variety of adolescent behaviors including smoking, violence, sexual intercourse, and school performance. Both the SCT and the PBT programs were designed to be interactive with games, videos, role plays and skits to demonstrate and practice skills learned in the sessions. There were take-home activities in which each participant sets a personal goal to be accomplished by the following session. The efficacy of the two programs in reducing sexual involvement of adolescents was assessed in a study that compared the programs to each other and to a control group (DiIorio et al. 2007). The results of this study showed that although there were no differences in delay of sexual intercourse among the three groups, those who participated in the PBT program reported an increase in condom use, and those in the SCT and the control group demonstrated higher levels of knowledge about HIV. Mothers reported more comfort talking about sex with their adolescents and greater confidence in doing so over time. Mothers in the SCT program reported talking about more sex topics, and mothers in the SCT and PBT programs indicated a greater intent to discuss and more comfort discussing sexual topics than those in the control group. Mothers in the SCT program also demonstrated higher levels of HIV knowledge than mothers in the PBT and control groups.

The program for fathers, called *R.E.A.L. (Responsible, Empowered, Aware, Living)* was designed to enhance the father's role in postponing the sexual debut of their 11 through 14-year-old adolescent sons (DiIorio et al 2007). Fathers attended the program once a week for 7 weeks, bringing their sons for the final session. Similar to sessions for mothers in *Keepin' it R.E.A.L.!*, the sessions for fathers were interactive and included goal setting and take-home activities. The efficacy of the program was assessed in a study comparing the SCT program to a nutrition and exercise program for fathers. Adolescents whose fathers participated in the SCT program reported significantly higher rates of sexual abstinence, condom use, and intent to delay initiation of sexual intercourse. Fathers in the program reported significantly more discussions about sexuality and greater intention to discuss sexuality in the future with their sons. They also reported more confidence discussing sexual issues with their sons and more positive outcomes associated with those discussions.

Jemmott and colleagues (2000) designed a family-based prevention program to enable mothers to teach their sons about sex and to decrease their risky behavior. This program helps mothers examine their values related to sexuality and provide them with factual information to share with their sons. Activities are intended to increase mothers' understanding about developmental challenges and social stressors that their sons are experiencing and to improve their parental communication skills. Unfortunately, no results are yet available from this study.

Another intervention in which the parents assume the role of AIDS educators is *Familias Unidas*. An ecodevelopmental, Hispanic-specific, ecologically focused, parent-centered preventive intervention, *Familias Unidas* promotes protection for adolescents against HIV and substance use. This program promotes four major family processes operating at different systemic levels: (1) increasing family functioning (e.g., positive parenting), (2) promoting parent–adolescent communication, (3) fostering proactive connections between the family and other important systems such as peers and school, and (4) gathering external support for parents (Pantin et al. 2004). The group format of the intervention was designed to provide social support for Hispanic immigrant parents by introducing them to other parents in similar situations.

The *Familias Unidas* intervention has been evaluated in two separate randomized controlled trials. In the first randomized controlled trial, Pantin et al. (2003) found that this 9-month intervention was efficacious (in a sample of 167 Hispanic youth), relative to a no-intervention control group, in increasing parental involvement, parent–adolescent communication, and parental support for the adolescent; and in reducing adolescent behavior problems. Not surprisingly, active participation in the group was shown to predict engagement and retention in the intervention (Prado et al. 2006a), and in turn engagement and retention have been shown to facilitate improved outcomes for adolescents (decrease in behavior problems) and families participating in the intervention (Prado et al. 2006a, b). The intervention did not significantly impact adolescent school bonding/academic achievement (see Chap. 11).

In the second randomized controlled trial, evaluated the efficacy of *Familias Unidas + PATH* relative to (a) *English for Speakers of Other Languages (ESOL) + PATH* and (b) *ESOL + HEART*, a family-centered adolescent cardiovascular health intervention. In the *ESOL + PATH* and *ESOL + HEART* conditions, *ESOL* served as an attention control (i.e., equivalent dosage and contact hours) for *Familias Unidas*. In the *ESOL+HEART* condition, HEART served as an attention control for *PATH*. The outcomes examined in that study included substance use and unsafe sexual behavior, as well as family functioning (parental involvement, parent–adolescent communication, positive parenting, and family support).

The results showed that *Familias Unidas + PATH* were efficacious in reducing current illicit drug use relative to *ESOL+HEART*. The results also showed that *Familias Unidas + PATH* were efficacious, relative to both *ESOL+PATH* and *ESOL+HEART* in reducing current cigarette use. Moreover, *Familias Unidas + PATH* were efficacious, relative to *ESOL+PATH* in reducing unprotected sexual behavior at last sexual encounter. What is remarkable about these findings is that for both cigarette smoking and unsafe sex, the condition with only the module targeting the outcome in question was less efficacious than the intervention including *Familias Unidas*, the family strengthening intervention.

These findings suggest that targeting problem behaviors outside the context of a family intervention was not efficacious with our target sample. Post-hoc analyses also showed that adolescents in the *Familias Unidas* condition reported significantly lower rates of sexual transmitted diseases than adolescents in the two control conditions. Finally, the effects of *Familias Unidas + PATH* on smoking and illicit drug use were partially mediated by improvements in family functioning. Specifically, improvements in positive parenting (reward contingencies offered by parents) and in parent–adolescent communication explained some of the effects of intervention condition on cigarette and illicit drug use.

A third and fourth trial of the *Familias Unidas* intervention are ongoing. In the first of these, Pantin and colleagues are evaluating the efficacy of *Familias Unidas* (relative to community referrals) in reducing HIV-risk behaviors and substance use in a sample Hispanic youth with behavior problems. In the second of these two studies, Prado is evaluating the efficacy of a 6-week version of the *Familias Unidas* intervention, relative to prevention as usual services. This streamlined version of the intervention targets those family processes that have been found to mediate the effects of the *Familias Unidas* intervention on the two prior randomized trials.

Based on over a decade of longitudinal research with rural African American families and youth, Murry and associates designed a family-based preventive intervention to deter HIV-related risk behavior among rural African American youth. The Strong African American Families (SAAF) program is the only universal randomized prevention trial designed specifically for rural families and youth. Analyses of data gathered from 667 rural African American families with an 11-year-old youth supported SAAF's efficacy in deterring youths' vulnerability to HIV-related risk behavior 2 years post-intervention (Brody et al. 2006). The 7-week intervention includes separate programming for youth and their parents, as well as activities in which parents and youth engage together. Key curriculum content for the seven sessions is presented on videotapes, which Murry and Brody produced, depicting family interactions that illustrate targeted intervention concepts. SAAF was implemented in community settings during youths' transition to middle school, an important developmental juncture for preventive intervention (Jemmott et al. 1999; Kirby 2001). Results revealed that SAAF was efficacious in reducing rural African American youths' vulnerability to HIV-related risk behavior through the intervention's effect on parenting practices and its effect on youth intrapersonal protective factors. Specifically, families who participated in SAAF experienced increases in regulated-communicative parenting (Brody et al. 2004; Murry et al. 2005) and in youth intrapersonal protective processes, namely heightened racial identity, elevated self-esteem, increased acceptance of body image and physical attractiveness (Murry et al. 2005, 2007). SAAF-induced effects on parenting behavior deterred not only precursors to risk behavior such as risk-related attitudes, future orientation, self-regulatory capacity, and resistance efficacy (Gerrard et al. 2006), but also immediate HIV-related risk behavior (Brody et al. 2006), including early onset of substance use and sexual intercourse (Murry et al. 2007) and alcohol use trajectories (Brody et al. 2005). These findings support the SAAF curriculum's potential public health impact (see Chap. 11).

Project STYLE is a multi-site (Providence, Chicago, Atlanta) randomized controlled trial evaluating the comparative efficacy of three interventions: (1) family-based HIV prevention intervention, (2) adolescent-only HIV prevention intervention, and (3) general health promotion intervention; in increasing safer sexual behavior among 13- to 18-year-old adolescents with psychiatric disorders. All three interventions were delivered during a 1-day workshop in groups of 6–8 and led by two facilitators. In the family-based intervention, parents and teens were assigned at-home exercises that targeted communication and risk reduction whereas in the adolescent-only and health promotion interventions only the adolescents were given take-home exercises targeting adolescent risk reduction and health promotion, respectively. Participants in all three arms attended individualized 2-week follow-up appointments during which monitoring plans (family), risk plans (family and adolescent-only), and health promotion plans (health promotion) were reviewed and problem solving was used to remedy specific areas of difficulty. All participants attended a 3-month booster session with their same group members and facilitators to review material previously covered during the 1-day workshop. Assessments occurred at baseline, 3, 6, 12, 24, 30, and 36 months (see Chap. 13).

Initial findings revealed important associations. Contrary to reports of youth in outpatient care (Donenberg et al. 2001), sexual risk behavior was associated with a wide range of psychiatric disorders including internalizing problems (Brown et al. 2010).

In summary, these studies demonstrate that parents can be taught to be effective AIDS educators: they can effectively impart information as well as teach their children skills to protect themselves in risky situations. The studies also provide corroborative evidence that the quality of parent–child relations and communication is an important predictor of sexual risk behaviors. Across the studies, adolescents who reported low levels of parental support or more emotional distance from their families were more likely to engage in sexual behaviors at a younger age. Conversely, adolescents' belief that they have a close relationship with their parents was protective against early sexual intercourse.

1.6   Role of Family in Adapting to HIV

Although AIDS has become a chronic disease for many individuals in the U.S. who have access to HAART, adherence to treatment is challenging and can be complicated by persistent symptoms and side effects. Co-morbid conditions, such as substance abuse, mental illness, or other severe chronic conditions can further complicate the medical regimen and activities of daily living. Family-based prevention programs for families living with HIV/AIDS must address a complex array of problems, such as treatment adherence and family-based problem solving associated with HIV and, frequently, poverty.

1.6.1   History of Family Issues

A history of longstanding problems can damage the social environment of the family at a time when they need to be united. Families who are experiencing the highest rates of HIV infection may also have to deal with issues among members, with the patient's partner, or with the partner's children. Often families have not resolved issues associated with the seropositive person's exposure to HIV, including homosexuality, bisexuality, substance abuse use, and infidelity, prior to finding themselves in a caretaking role.

1.6.2   Communication

Family members may be reticent to discuss problems with the persons living with AIDS, for fear of worrying them and making them sicker. By the same token, persons living with AIDS may be reluctant to become a burden to their family members (Hays et al. 1990). Without communication, nothing is resolved, ensuring that the same issues arise again and again.

1.6.3   Stigma and Disclosure

Paramount among shared family issues was stigma and disclosure. Both the seropositive family member and other family members may experience stress from fear of repercussions if friends and neighbors find out the reason for the illness. They may initially lie and explain that it is cancer, a more socially acceptable illness. Problems in coping are compounded by the stigma of AIDS. Persons living with AIDS and their families may experience rejection from friends, loss of jobs, and harassment. Concerns about disclosure may inhibit parents with AIDS from seeking support; disclosing to their children, other family members, and friends; and making permanency plans for children who will be orphaned at their death (Smith and Rapkin 1995, 1996).

1.6.4 Family Dynamics

HIV changes family functioning in multiple areas (Krishna et al. 2005). Major adjustments in the lifestyle may be necessary if the ill family member lives at home. Siblings and spouses may have concerns, such as having their needs ignored as the family attends to the sick member. There may be anger in low-income families because everyone is expected to contribute to the household but the seropositive person is unable to work because of fatigue and unpredictable health. Families report changes in the roles and responsibilities when the families' primary support person becomes ill. Family members begin to play multiple roles, taking on increased responsibility as the illness progresses, resulting in increased role strain. There may be developmental or role changing issues: a previously independent adult may have to be reintegrated into the family for care, an adolescent with chronically ill parents, who is struggling for emancipation may need to provide care, and a mother who is recovering from drug addiction may need to redefine her role as mother and daughter. As illness progresses, some family members withdraw due to physical or emotional exhaustion or over identification with the patient (Carl 1986; Dunkel-Shetter and Wortman 1982; Flaskerud and Rush 1989; Namir et al. 1989).

There are also concerns about infecting other members of the family which inhibits family dynamics. In-person interviews were conducted with 344 parents from a nationally representative probability sample of adults receiving health care for HIV in the contiguous U.S. (Schuster et al. 2005). Questions were asked about parents' fear of transmitting HIV to their children, fear of catching an illness or opportunistic infection from their children, and avoidance of four types of interactions (kissing on the lips, kissing on the cheeks, hugging, and sharing utensils) because of these fears. Forty-two percent of parents feared catching an infection from their children, and 36.1% of parents feared transmitting HIV to their children. Twenty-eight percent of parents avoided at least one type of interaction with their children "a lot" because they feared transmitting HIV or catching an opportunistic infection. When parents who avoided physical interactions "a little" are included, the overall avoidance rate rises to 39.5%. Hispanic parents were more likely than African American parents and parents who were white or of other races or ethnicities to avoid interactions. Although many parents feared transmitting HIV to their children or catching an infection from their children, few were avoiding the most routine forms of physical affection. They were much more likely to avoid interactions suggestive of fear of contagion through saliva.

In a longitudinal study of the effects of having children take on responsibilities due to maternal HIV, it was found that those children who had taken on more responsibility for instrumental caretaking roles directly because of their mother's illness when they were young showed better autonomy development as early- and middle-age adolescents. Therefore, "parentification" of young children with a mother with HIV may not negatively affect later autonomy development.

It is interesting to note that patterns of family reliance differ according to population or site. In a study of public health services utilization in the New York City greater metropolitan area, Crystal and Kersting (1998) found that asymptomatic persons tended to rely on social support from their families, but as the disease progressed, the ill family members developed more complications and relied more on public health services. In contrast, a study in San Francisco revealed that seropositive gay men tend to rely first on their families of choice and extended support network, but as the disease progressed, they tended to rely more on their families of origin (Hays et al. 1990). These differences may be explained by proximity to family. In New York, a larger heterosexual population may have become exhausted or burdened with having to care for more than one seropositive family member. In San Francisco, on the other hand, the HIV-infected population was primarily homosexual men whose parents did not live in the area. As the disease progressed, the family of choice or the extended family may have become exhausted, and romantic partners may have become ill and died. The seropositive person would then seek the support of their families of origin, who often lived out of town and had not been previously been stressed with day-to-day care.

1.6.5   Maintaining Custody of Children

Data was collected from interviews of 538 parents with 1,017 children (0–17 years old) from a nationally representative sample of HIV-infected adults receiving health care in the U.S. (Schuster et al. 2005). Forty-seven percent of the children were in the custody of their HIV-infected parent at both survey waves, 4% were in the parent's custody at the first but not second survey wave, 42% were not in custody at either survey wave, and the parent of 7% gained custody between survey waves. Parents cited drug use (62%) and financial hardship (27%) as reasons for losing custody. Children of HIV-infected fathers, older parents, parents living without other adults, parents with low CD4 counts, drug-using parents, and parents with one hospital stay were less likely to be in their parent's custody at either survey wave.

1.6.6   Stress and Coping

AIDS places an enormous strain on family systems. Families must manage an unpredictable illness while handling other chronic and acute stressors, often with little or no specialized training, guidance, or support. Family stress levels depend on how well they problem solve and cope with these issues together. Several studies conducted prior to the advent of the newest HIV medications have provided an initial taxonomy of the stressful problems experienced by families affected by symptomatic

Table 1.1 Taxonomy of problems experienced by families living with HIV/AIDS

Course of HIV/AIDS and medical regimen
  Concerns about recurring acute illness episodes
  Difficulty in adhering to a complex medical regimen
  Difficulty in maintaining a predictable routine
  Complicated task of relating to multiple health and mental health providers
  Lack of good medical care and counseling
Family dynamics and emotions
  Isolation from other family members and friends, contributing to the deterioration of partner
    and family relationships
  Emotions associated with illness (e.g., depression, confusion, loneliness, fear, and suicidal
    ideation)
  Guilt about having infected others
Problems of living
  Anxiety about financial problems
  Lack of available and affordable housing and related services because of their known health
    status
  Possible need to address problems of substance abuse and changes in lifestyle
  Lack of respite from providing care and inadequate or unavailable alternative child care
  Need to plan for bereavement and future of the survivors
  Handling the stigma of a disease with moral overtones

AIDS cases (Pequegnat and Bray 1997). These stressors are still relevant when the seropositive family member is unable to tolerate treatment, unresponsive to such treatment, or has other conditions that make medication adherence difficult (e.g., substance abuse, mental illness), and consequently continues to manifest severe physical symptomatology (see Table 1.1).

Given the scope and uncertainty of the challenges they face, families affected by AIDS need flexible coping skills that can be applied to a variety of circumstances, including geographical distance; competing demands for family members' time, energy, or other resources (Stoller and Pugliesi 1989); lack of knowledge about how to be helpful (Good et al. 1990; Starrett et al. 1990); and history of negative interactions (Shinn et al. 1984; Fiore et al. 1983). Coping with AIDS is made more difficult when more than one family member in a household, or even in the close extended family, is HIV-infected, including children. Many families have already experienced significant losses due to AIDS and have not had an opportunity to adequately grieve significant losses due to AIDS that they have already experienced (Rotheram-Borus et al. 1997).

1.6.7   Complex Medical Regimen

Families affected by AIDS face multiple health care and psychosocial problems throughout the illness trajectory. Problems include complex medical management and care giving issues, disruption of family roles and routines, and concerns about the family's future as illness progresses. The course of illness and the efficacy of treatment may be unpredictable, making it impossible for families to know precisely what problems they will need to cope with and when.

Family members may feel helpless and overwhelmed by the needs of their ill family member for time, energy, or money; and they may feel lacking in good caregiving skills (Szapocznik et al. 2004). Family and caretakers can be instrumental in helping the patient maintain good medical treatment adherence (Lyon et al. 2003; Simoni et al. 2006).

Of course, problems related to AIDS co-occur with other issues facing the family. Given high levels of poverty, substance abuse, unemployment, and poor health care, at any given time, AIDS-related problems may not be the most pressing problems for families (Smith et al. 2001). In addition to the stressors experienced by all families, AIDS-affected families have challenges that require family solutions, such as caretaking for the ill family members, replacing the lost income, and reassigning roles filled by the seropositive person prior to the illness.

1.7   Family-Based Secondary Prevention Programs

Over the past 17 years, there has been a concerted effort by the National Institute of Mental Health (NIMH) to support a research program to develop family-based HIV prevention interventions (Pequegnat and Sczapocznik 2000). Secondary prevention programs have focused on developing interventions to help them cope with multiple problems, including stigma, medication adherence, changing parental roles, and custody planning.

There are compelling clinical and public health reasons for designing secondary prevention programs aimed at building supportive social networks, increasing coping skills, and reducing stress, risky sexual behaviors, and STDs. First, they could reduce unprotected sex and needle sharing. Second, they could improve quality of life among persons living with HIV by reducing stressors, enhancing coping skills, and requiring less need for expensive health care. Third, they could reduce risk of HIV transmission to seronegative sexual partners. Finally, they could reduce the risk of HIV transmission by women to their unborn children.

The original family-based intervention entitled Project TALC (Teens and Adults Learning to Communicate) designed for seropositive mothers and their children has extremely successful. The goal was to help parents make decisions regarding disclosure and custody, as well as to increase a family's ability to maintain positive daily routines while the parent is ill. The mothers are taught to problem solve stressful situations, maintain their parental role, and make custody arrangements for their children. The adolescents are taught to cope with emotional distress, maintain a healthy, drug-free lifestyle, and explore roles within the family. By 2 years after recruitment, the intervention adolescents and parents reported significantly fewer problem behaviors and less emotional distress than those in the standard care condition. Coping skills were significantly higher among youth, and parents had significantly more positive social support in the intervention condition, compared to standard care condition (Rotheram-Borus et al. 2001). Over four years following the delivery of the intervention, fewer adolescents became teenage parents and fewer parents were drug dependent in the intervention compared to the control condition (Rotheram-Borus et al. 2004). At six years, youth in the intervention condition reported significantly less substance use three and six years later. In addition, positive parental bonds reported at baseline reduced emotional distress at three years and increased positive future expectations at six years Rotheram-Borus et al. 2006).

Based on the success of this initial intervention for families living with HIV, Rotheram-Borus and colleagues began a series of adaptations of this intervention for different contexts. These adaptations rest on the premise that there are predictable challenges faced by all families affected by HIV (e.g., disclosure, social support, medication adherence, stigma, transmission behaviors), which are affected by the particularities of local culture and social context (Rotheram-Borus et al. 2005a, b). The first of these adaptations was in Los Angeles, CA. This adaptation accounted for therapeutic advances in the prevention and treatment of HIV illness as well as shifts in the population of infected mothers, which resulted in moving the intervention from New York to Los Angeles. Three hundred and thirty-nine HIV-positive women who were the mother or primary female caregiver of a child between the ages of 6 and 20 years and 257 adolescents between the ages of 12 and 20 years were recruited. At 6-month follow-up, more mothers demonstrated reductions in hard drug use in intervention compared to control. For adolescents, there was also a reduction in hard drug use and negative family-based life events among the intervention group, relative to control (Rice 2007).

Thailand has been the first international context for the adaptation of this intervention. Thailand has been extremely successful in mounting individual-based interventions to combat HIV/AIDS. Yet, the effect of HIV radiates throughout the family. Rotheram-Borus and Li initiated a study in Northern and Northeastern Thailand to adapt the cognitive-behavioral intervention developed by Rotheram-Borus and her colleagues. The adaptation of the intervention contents, tools, and activities was achieved through a series of workgroups involving a U.S. research team, the local Thai research team, and health care providers from Thai provincial, district levels. Adaptation of intervention tools and activities required careful reframing to fit the Thai culture. In particular, as a country deeply rooted in Buddhism, meditation emerged as a highly relevant and applicable relaxation activity in Thailand. Therefore, meditation was employed throughout the pilot sessions as a relaxation activity. In addition, meditation was applied as a stress management tool in several of the intervention sessions. Similarly, singing and dancing were incorporated as ice breaking activities; these were highly relevant and appropriate in Thai culture, thus promoting group cohesiveness and supportive environment. The team is currently mounting the main trial and providing the family-based intervention in northern and northeastern Thailand, focusing on family well-being, in a nonstigmatizing setting (Lee and Singparu 2007).

Different international contexts create unique challenges to the adaptation of the original family-based program. Work has been done in China to assess the needs of families affected by HIV. The studies illustrate that family is an intricate part of the disclosure process in China, and demonstrates the importance of including families in HIV/AIDS interventions. This is especially important and relevant in the context of China's new "four frees and one care" policy (Li et al. 2007). Moreover, because of the family challenges caused by HIV/AIDS, some children needed to find paid jobs outside the home in order to contribute to the family's income. Lack of money also impacted the family's capacity to provide children with ample, healthy, nutritious food. The stigma and discrimination these families and children faced only added to their difficulties. Together, these challenges affected children's normal developmental process and school performance, and some children were not able to attend school at all (Ji et al. 2007; Lin et al. 2008).

In the most recent international work on family-based secondary prevention, Rotheram-Borus and her collaborators have developed adaptations of the original family-based intervention for two different communities in South Africa. Unique challenges impact the development and delivery of effective interventions for families impacted by HIV in high-incidence developing world countries. For example, a vestige of South Africa's apartheid past is the fragmentation of ante- and postnatal care and TB and HIV testing and care into uncoordinated clinics. Working in KwaZulu-Natal and the Western Cape Provinces, Rotheram-Borus is investigating whether a clinic or neighborhood-based intervention is the optimal settings for the delivery of a family-based secondary prevention program. She is also exploring the impact of using positive social deviants (Mentor Mothers) as interventionists (Rotheram-Borus 2007; Trizzino 2007).

Rapkin and colleagues (2000) developed an intervention to teach AIDS-affected families problem solving skills. The Family Health Project (Rapkin et al. 2000) breaks down problem solving into its component elements and encourages families to follow these steps: (1) create a comfortable climate for problem solving, (2) identify the problem, (3) brainstorm, (4) weigh the consequences of various alternatives, (5) think through together the implementation of possible solutions, (6) set goals, and (7) evaluate solution outcomes. Both patients and family members in the experimental group reported that they were more likely to reinforce one another's problem solving efforts (Rapkin et al. 2007). They were also more likely to express uncertainty about problems. Although this result was unexpected, it may reflect the fact that the patients in the intervention group and their family members reported more unresolved problems. Despite this, they reported greater ability to care for themselves. Families receiving the intervention attended support groups more often than controls and were more likely to have a case manager. Consequently, these families were also more able to maintain their sense of well-being relative to the control group.

Taking another tack, Szpaocznik and colleagues designed an intervention, Structural Ecological Therapy (SET), to improve the quality of the social relations and supports of African American seropositive women (see Mitrani et al. 2000). The intervention focused on changing the quality of relationships, building family trust, increasing mutual support, and reducing blaming and personal attacks (family negativity). This social ecological perspective helped to rebuild a supportive network around the woman and her family that included the family's relation to kin and other neighborhood supports, faith communities, and HIV support groups. The first test of this approach was successful in reducing psychological distress and family hassles and, that reduction of family hassles was partially mediated by the reduction in distress (Szapocznik et al. 2004).

SET has been adapted to a variety of populations and target behaviors. It is being modified for use in helping seropositive men returning from prison reintegrate into their families (ecosystems). The goals are to mobilize participants' families and other ecosystem members, such as service providers, to support and motivate reduced HIV risk behavior and increased medical adherence. Participants and their ecosystem members meet with intervention staff in sessions designed to restructure their interactions and communication patterns, to better support participants' positive behavior change. Preliminary results indicate that men in SET are adapting much better to family life, reducing HIV risk behaviors, and increasing adherence to medication regimens after their release from prison.

Another adaptation of SET is being conducted that focuses on women being reintegrated into their families after drug treatment. Drug abuse and subsequent treatment frequently include prolonged separation from the family, who may feel betrayed due to prior episodes of sobriety that ended in relapse. This adaptation focuses on relapse prevention, HIV medication adherence, and reduction in HIV sexual risk behavior. Like the original adaptation of SET, it works to help seropositive women reestablish a parenting role with their young children, whose guardianship they may have lost because of their addiction, neglect, and time away in substance abuse treatment.

While SET reintegrates women and men into their existing social support systems, another program that helps seropositive women build new social support networks to enhance and prolong their lives. The WiLLOW Program: Women Involved in Life Learning from Other Women was designed to reduce HIV/STD risk behaviors and enhance psychosocial factors, such as expanding social networks of women living with HIV (Wingood and DiClemente 2000). These women who live in semirural areas feel isolated because of stigma and low rates of disclosure. The four-session, group-administered intervention emphasized gender pride, maintaining current and identifying new network members, HIV transmission knowledge, communication and condom use skills, and healthy relationships. Over the 12-month follow-up, women in the WiLLOW intervention relative to the comparison reported fewer episodes of unprotected vaginal intercourse and had a lower incidence of bacterial infections (Chlamydia and gonorrhea). Additionally, participants in the intervention reported greater HIV knowledge and condom use self-efficacy, more social network members, fewer beliefs that condoms interfere with sex, fewer partner-related barriers to condom use, and demonstrated greater skills in using condoms. This is one of the first trials to demonstrate reductions in risky sexual behaviors and incident bacterial STDS and to enhance HIV preventive psychosocial and structural factors. Centers for Disease Control and Prevention (CDC) has evaluated and classified WiLLOW as an "evidence-based intervention" and is disseminating it nationally as part of its Continuum of HIV Prevention Interventions for African American Women.

Adolescents whose parents are living with AIDS face daily challenges and stressors related to the stage of their parents' illness and adjustment following their parents' death. An intensive, cognitive-behavioral intervention was developed by Rotheram-Borus and colleagues (1997) that address coping at each phase of adjustment. The intervention targeted long-term social, behavioral, and mental health outcomes of the adolescent for both the mothers and their adolescents. Parents living with AIDS and their adolescent children participated in both joint and adolescent-only sessions in order to enhance their affective and behavioral skills for coping with the parents' illness. The intervention was delivered in three modules of 8–16 sessions each. In Module 1, parents were helped to recognize their emotional response to their own diagnosis, make decisions about illness status disclosure, and establish positive daily routines in their household. Module 2 focused on parenting, custody, and estate planning. Adolescents joined their parents for the last eight sessions, addressing their reactions to parental illness and daily routines. After the parent died, adolescents and their new custodial parents addressed issues of bereavement and adjustment in Module 3.

In order to address the disruptive social and economic circumstances of children whose mothers died from HIV, *Project Care* was designed to test the efficacy of a short-term preventive intervention (Bauman et al. 2000). The aims of the study were to reduce risk factors and increase protective factors in children to prevent psychological dysfunction after their mothers' AIDS-related death. The intervention enhanced disclosure and communication among seropositive mothers, the designated guardians, and the children. It enhanced stability and security of the child's future by developing an appropriate custody plan prior to parental death. It enhanced work with guardian and child after the death of mother to facilitate the transition to the new family. It also enhanced access to resources and social support. Thirty-five percent of mothers disclosed their HIV status to their children, ages 8–12 years old (Bauman et al. 2002). If they disclosed to one child, they usually disclosed to all the children.

In *Project Care* more than 50% of the mothers with HIV were depressed, which was significantly related to mothers' reports of having non-HIV-related medical conditions, spending time in bed in the past 2 weeks, having more activity restrictions, and having a lot of difficulty caring for their children due to ill health. Higher scores were also associated with lower education, more negative life events, and greater receipt of inadequate social support. Thus, higher distress was associated with inability to perform usual activities and mobilize social support. However, other HIV-related health factors, traditional background characteristics, and psychosocial measures (e.g., HIV stigma, parenting stress, family environment) failed to indicate who was most vulnerable (Silver et al. 2003). While maternal illness per se was not associated with childhood distress, maternal depression, inadequate maternal support, or poor mother–child relationships. However, the mothers' illness was associated with symptoms of poor mental health in the children. Children behavior problems were significantly related to the mother's psychological distress and marginally related to her having illness-related activity restrictions. They were not related to other measures of maternal physical health, stigma, or disclosure of their HIV status to the children. Two children's dispositional factors: productivity and independence; and two family factors: adaptability and a good parent–child relationship, were related to better functioning of the children. Paradoxically, family cohesion was a risk factor for poorer adjustment (Bauman et al. 2002).

Over the 2-year period, every child (100%) scored in the clinical range (12% once 25% twice, 26% three times, 27% four times, and 9% all five times). Most were identified by both maternal and child report (only on maternal report, 5%; only on child report, 8%). Chronicity of symptoms was not related to child age or gender, maternal health, parent–child relationship, maternal depression, or participation in *Project Care*. Two-thirds of the children received mental health services during the 2 years, but less than 25% received care at any one time. Half of the children with chronic symptoms never received counseling (Bauman et al. 2007).

An important area of family research that has not received enough attention is advance care planning for seropositive adolescents and their families. Lyon and colleagues conducted a focus group with parents who had lost an adolescent to HIV/AIDS, to collect ideas about a program that would make it easier for families to discuss these sensitive issues (Lyon et al. 2007). Parents reported that it would have been valuable to have a program to help them talk with their children about what kind of treatment they wanted and what end-of-life decisions (e.g., extent of care, after-death plans for children) should be made. Focus groups with HIV-positive adolescents also indicated that they would be interested in participation in such a program. Lyon and colleagues have completed the development of an NIMH-supported Family Centered Advance Care Planning Program (Lyon et al. 2007). Intermediate results indicate that families are finding the study satisfying and worthwhile. Furthermore, no problem solving session was needed to work through disagreements. Parents in the treatment program were more satisfied than their adolescents compared with parents and adolescents in the control group. Those receiving the intervention reported feeling "courageous" and feeling "like a load lifted off my mind." There were no adverse outcomes. Unexpected positive findings included families' requests for copies of the Five Wishes, an advance directive. Families spontaneously reported that now that they understood how the process worked, they wanted to complete one. Adolescence is a critical period for setting the stage for the development of a sexual code of ethics and for consolidation of a moral code of living. This is an under-researched area, an opportunity for families and providers to facilitate the growth of HIV-positive adolescents entrusted to their care.

In summary, there is a need to view the families of patients as partners in the treatment process. Until recently, families of patients were not viewed by the medical community as resources in the treatment of the patient. The family is deeply affected – physically and psychologically – by the trauma of serious illness, especially one as devastating as AIDS. The family – whether of origin or of choice – can provide powerful support, guidance, and solace when its considerable resources are marshaled. Although there are common concerns, coping strategies for different stresses may be required, depending on which members of the family are HIV-infected. Interventions can restructure familial interactions and communication patterns, enhance family problem solving skills, enhance a supportive social network, improve quality of life, and ensure HIV risk reduction.

1.8   Conclusions

In tackling problems related to preventing HIV infection and adapting to HIV/AIDS within families, it is important to understand HIV-related behaviors in the social context in which they were learned and reinforced. Noncontextual, fragmented approaches may complicate the problem and create a sense of hopelessness on the part of individuals, families, peers, and health care workers; rather than promote more effective use of family resources (Pequegnat and Sczapocznik 2000). Several family characteristics have shown consistent relationships with measures of health or illness regardless of the disorder. For example, high family conflict, too permeable or too rigid intra- and extra-familial boundaries, low levels of family organization, and poor spousal or partner support are associated with poor outcomes. When families are functioning in an adaptive way, parents are typically the family leaders, and when they are incapacitated by drug abuse, mental illness, or ill health, family social support may evaporate, which places its members at risk for a host of problems. Social isolation may result from the stigma associated with HIV infection, desire to remain anonymous, and not knowing how or with whom to disclose and talk about their concerns and the pressures they experience due to their HIV infection. Rejection may occur if neighbors and friends blame the seropositive person for their infection due to a high-risk lifestyle even though that may not be the case.

Family research provides a general framework for investigating the processes through which psychological, social, and cultural factors influence the health and well-being of all family members. Many of the conditions that contribute to the spread of HIV infection: poverty, drug abuse, and an inadequate health care system for the poor, need to be addressed with renewed initiatives in family research. Historically, research identifying aspects of the family system has been based on the report of one family member. Theories and conceptual frameworks that are culturally appropriate and integrate reports from multiple members of the family system are essential if we are to move family-based prevention work forward.

In the last 17 years, investigators have increasingly enlisted families in research to better understand family process and decision-making in order to prevent and adapt to AIDS. There is a better understanding of the nature of communication within families, the roles of family members in shaping opinion and behavior in the family, and the kinds of incentives under the control of parents and older siblings. Also, the psychological and social factors that characterize families and their response to illness have been identified. Based on the findings reported in this chapter, it is imperative that community-based program offer these evidence-based prevention programs for families. New organizations and health care systems must be created to respond to the special needs of AIDS patients and their families.

Acknowledgement A special word of thanks is due to Rayford Kytle at NIMH who did zeverything from literature searches to editing the original text.

References

Bandura A. A social cognitive approach to the exercise of control over AIDS infection. In: DiClemente R, editor. Adolescents and AIDS: a generation in jeopardy. Beverly Hills: Sage; 1997. p. 89–116.

Bannon WM, McKay MM. Addressing urban African American youth externalizing and social problem behavioral difficulties in a family oriented prevention project. In: McKay MM, Paikoff RL, editors. Community collaborative partnerships: the foundation for HIV prevention research efforts. Binghamton, NY: Haworth Press; 2007. p. 221–40.

Baptiste DR, Paikoff RL, McKay MM, Madison-Boyd S, Coleman D, Bell C. Collaborating with an urban community to develop an HIV and AIDS prevention program for Black youth and families. Behav Modif. 2005;29(2):370–416.

Baptiste D, Blachman D, Cappella E, Dew D, Dixon K, Bell CC, et al. Transferring a university-led HIV/AIDS prevention initiative to a community agency. Soc Work Ment Health. 2007a; 5(3/4):269–93.

Baptiste D, Voisin DR, Smithgall C, Martinez DDC, Henderson G. Preventing HIV/AIDS among Trinidad and Tobago teens using a family-based program: preliminary outcomes. In: McKay MM, Paikoff RL, editors. Community collaborative partnerships: the foundation for HIV prevention research efforts. Binghamton, NY: Haworth Press; 2007b. p. 333–54.

Baptiste D, Bhana A, Peterson I, Voisin D, McKay M, Bell C, et al. A community participatory framework for international youth-focused HIV/AIDS prevention in South Africa and Trinidad. J Pediatr Psychol. 2007c;31(9):905–16.

Bauman LJ, Draimin B, Levine C, Hudis J. Who will care for me? Planning the future care and custody of children orphaned by HIV/AIDS. In: Pequegnat W, Szapocznik J, editors. Working with families in the era of AIDS. Thousand Oaks, CA: Sage; 2000. p. 155–88.

Bauman LJ, Camacho S, Silver EH, Hudis J, Draimin B. Behavioral problems in school-aged of mothers with HIV/AIDS. Clin Child Psychol Psychiatry. 2002;7(1):39–54.

Bauman LJ, Silver EJ, Draimin BH, Hudis J. Children of mothers with HIV/AIDS: unmet needs for mental health services. Pediatrics. 2007;120:5.

Bell CC, Bhana A, Petersen I, McKay MM, Gibbons R, Bannon W, et al. Building protective factors to offset sexually risky behaviors among black South African youth: a randomized control trial. J Nat Med Assoc. 2008;100(8):936–44.

Bell CC, Bhana A, McKay MM, Petersen I. A commentary on the triadic theory of influence as a guide for adapting HIV prevention programs for new contexts and populations: the CHAMP-South Africa story. In: McKay MM, Paikoff RL, editors. Community collaborative partnerships: the foundation for HIV prevention research efforts. Binghamton, NY: Haworth Press; 2007. p. 243–61.

Bhana A, Petersen I, Mason A, Mahintsho Z, Bell C, McKay M. Children and youth at risk: adaptation and pilot study of the CHAMP (Amaqhawe) programme in South Africa. Afr J AIDS Res. 2004;3(1):33–41.

Biglan A. Social and behavior factors associated with high-risk sexual behavior among adolescents. J Behav Med. 1990;13:245–61.

Boyd-Franklin N. Black families in therapy: a multisystems approach. New York: Guildford Press; 1989.

Brackis-Cott E, Mellins CA, Speigel D, Dolezal C. The mental health risk of mothers and children: the role of HIV infection. J Early Adolesc. 2007;27:67–89.

Bray JH. Family assessment: current issues in evaluating families. Fam Relat. 1995;44:469–77.

Brody GH, Ge X, Katz J, Arias I. A longitudinal analysis of internalization of paternal alcohol-use norms and adolescent alcohol use. Appl Dev Sci. 2000;4:71–9.

Brody GH, Ge X, Conger R, Gibbons FX, Murry VM, Gerrard M, et al. The influence of neighborhood disadvantage, collective socialization, and parenting on African American children's affiliation with deviant peers. Child Dev. 2001;72:1231–46.

Brody GH, Murry VM, Gerrard M, Gibbons FX, Molgaard V, McNair L, et al. The Strong African American Families Program: translating research into prevention programming. Child Dev. 2004;75:900–17.

Brody GH, Murry VM, Kim S, Brown AC. Longitudinal pathways to competence and psychological adjustment among African American children living in rural single-parent households. Child Dev. 2002;73:1505–16.

Brody GH, Murry VM, McNair L, Chen Y-F, Gibbons FX, Gerrard M, et al. Linking changes in parenting to youth self-control: the Strong African American families program. J Res Adolesc. 2005;15:47–69.

Brody GH, Murry VM, Kogan SM, Gerrard M, Gibbons FX, Molgaard V, et al. The Strong African American Families program:A cluster-randomized prevention trial of long-term effects and a meditational model. Journal of Consulting and Clinical Psychology, 2006;74:356–66.

Bronfenbrenner U. Ecology of the family as a context for human development research. Dev Psychol. 1986;22:723–42.

Brooks-Gunn J, Paikoff RL. Sex is a Gamble, Kissing is a Game: Adolescent Sexuality and Health Promotion. In Millstein S., Petersen, A., and Nightingale, E., eds. Promoting the Health of Adolescents: New Directions for the Twenty-first Century. Oxford University Press, New York, NY; 1993.

Brown LK, Hadley W, Steward A, Lescano C, Whiteley L, Donenberg G, DiClemente R. Psychiatric disorders and sexual risk among adolescents in mental health treatment. Journal of Consulting and clinical Psychology, 2010;78(4):590–97.

Carl D. Acquired immune deficiency syndrome: A preliminary examination of the effects on gay couples and coupling. Journal of Martial and Family Therapy, 1986;12(3):241–47.

Centers for Disease Control and Prevention (CDC). HIV/AIDS surveillance report, vol. 17. Atlanta, GA: CDC; 2005.

Christ JJ, Raszka WV, Dillon CA. Prioritizing education about condom use among sexually active female adolescents. Adolescence. 1998;33(132):735–44.

Christopherson CR. Pubertal development, parent-teen communication, and sexual values as predictors of adolescent sexual intentions and sexually related behaviors. Dissertation Abstr Int A: Humanities Soc Sci. 1994;54(12A):45–99.

Cohen S, Wills TA. Stress, social support, and the buffering hypothesis. Psychol Bull. 1985; 98:310–57.

Crystal S, Kersting RC. Stress, social support, and distress in a statewide population of persons with AIDS in New Jersey. Soc Work Health Care. 1998;28(1):41–60.

Darling CA, Hicks MW. Parental influence on adolescent sexuality: implications for parents as educators. J Youth Adolesc. 1982;11:231–45.

David EC, Friel LV. Adolescent sexuality: disentangling the effects of family structure and family context. J Marriage Fam. 2001;63:669–81.

DiClemente RJ, Salazr LF, Crosby RA. A review of STD/HIV preventive interventions for adolescents: sustaining effects using an ecological approach. J Pediatr Psychol. 2001;32: 888–906.

DiIorio C, Resnicow K, Denzmore P, Rogers-Tillman G, Wang DT, Dudley WN, et al. Keepin' It R.E.A.L.! A mother-adolescent HIV prevention program. In: Pequegnat W, Szapocznik J, editors. Working with families in the era of AIDS. Thousand Oaks, CA: Sage; 2000. p. 113–32.

DiIorio C, Pluha E, Belcher L. Parent–child communication about sexuality: a review of the literature from 1980 to 2001. J HIV/AIDS Prev Educ Adolesc Child. 2003;5:7–31.

DiIorio C, McCarty F, Resnicow K, Lehr S, Denzmore P. REAL Men: a group-randomized trial of an HIV prevention intervention for adolescent boys. Am J Pub Health, 2007;97(6): 1084–9.

Dittus PJ, Jaccard J. Adolescents perceptions of maternal disapproval of sex: relationship to sexual outcomes. Am J Public Health. 2000;90(9):1426–30.

Donenberg GR, Pao M. Youths and HIV/AIDS: psychiatry's role in a changing epidemic. J Am Acad Child Adolesc Psychiatry. 2005;44(8):728–47.

Donenberg GR, Emerson E, Bryant FB, Wilson H, Weber-Shifrin E. Understanding AIDS-risk behavior among adolescents in psychiatric care: Links to psychopathology and peer relationships. Journal of the American Academy of Child and Adolescent Psychiatry. 2001;40(6):642–53.

Donenberg GR, Wilson HW, Emerson E, Bryant FB. Holding the line with a watchful eye: the impact of perceived parental permissiveness and parental monitoring on risky sexual behavior among adolescents in psychiatric care. AIDS Educ Prev. 2002;14(2):138–57.

Donenberg G, Bryant F, Emerson E, Wilson H, Pasch K. Tracing the roots of early sexual debut among adolescents in psychiatric care. J Am Acad Child Adolesc Psychiatry. 2003;42: 594–608.

Donenberg GR, Schwartz RM, Emerson E, Wilson HW, Bryant FB, Coleman G. Applying a cognitive-behavioral model of HIV risk to youths in psychiatric care. AIDS Educ Prev. 2005;17(3):200–16.

Donenberg GR, Emerson E, Bryant FB, King S. Does substance use moderate the effects of parents and peers on risky sexual behaviour? AIDS Care. 2006;18(3):194–200.

Donenberg GR, Paikoff R, Pequegnat W. Introduction to the special section on families, youth, and HIV/ Family-based intervention studies. J Pediatr Psychol. 2007;31(9):869–73.

Dunkel-Shetter CA, Wortman CB. The interpersonal dynamics of cancer: problems in social relationships and their impact on the patient. In: Friedman HS, DiMateo MR, editors. Interpersonal issues in health care. New York: Academic; 1982. p. 69–100.

Dutra R, Miller K, Forehand R. The process and content of sexual communication with adolescents in two-parent families: associations with sexual risk-taking behavior. AIDS Behav. 1999; 3:59–66.

Feaster DJ, Szapocznik J. Interdependence of the stress processes among African American family members: influence of HIV serostatus and a new infant. Psychol Health. 2002;17(3): 339–63.

Feaster D, Robbins M, Szapocznik J. Using individual level data in family assessment: hierarchical linear modeling with African American HIV+ mothers and their families. Miami, FL: University of Miami, Center for Family Studies; 2000.

Fiore J, Becker J, Coppel PB. Social network interactions: a buffer or stress? Am J Community Psychol. 1983;11:423–39.

Flaskerud JH, Rush CE. AIDS and traditional health beliefs and practices of black women. Nurs Res. 1989;39(2):96–107.

Fox JL. The family's role in adolescent sexual behavior. In: Ooms T, editor. Teenage pregnancy in a family context. Philadelphia, PA: Temple University Press; 1981. p. 73–130.

Freidin L, Hodorek S, Krauss B, O'Day J, Godfrey C. What they walked away with: what children say they learned from HIV-related conversations with their parents. Poster presented at the National institute of mental health annual international research conference on the role of the families in preventing and adapting to HIV/AIDS, Brooklyn, NY; July 2005.

Gerrard M, Gibbons FX, Brody GH, Murry VM, Cleveland MJ, Wills TA. A theory-based dual focus alcohol intervention for pre-adolescents: the Strong African American Families Program. Psychol Addict Behav. 2006;20:185–95.

Goldstein RB, Johnson MO, Rotheram-Borus MJ, Kirshenbau SB, Pinto RM, Kittel L, et al. Psychological distress, substance use, and adjustment among parents living with HIV. J Am Board Fam Pract. 2005;18(5):362–73.

Good MD, Good BJ, Schaffer C, Lind SE. American oncology and the disclosure on hope. Cult Med Psychiatry. 1990;12:59–79.

Hadley W, Brown LK, Lescano CM, Kell H, Spalding K, DiClemente RJ, et al. Parent-adolescent sexual communication: discussing condoms matters. AIDS and Behavior, 2009;13(5): 997–1104.

Hays RB, Catania JA, McKusick L, Coates TJ. Help seeking for AIDS-related concerns: a comparison of gay men of various HIV diagnoses. Am J Community Psychol. 1990;18: 743–55.

Herek G. Stigma and sexual orientation: understanding prejudice against lesbians, gay men, and bisexuals: psychological perspectives on lesbian and gay issues. In: Herek GM, editor. Bad science in the service of stigma: a critique of the Cameron group's survey studies. Thousand Oaks, CA: Sage; 1998. p. 223–55.

Herek G. AIDS and stigma. Am Behav Sci. 1999;42(7):1106–16.

House JS. Work, stress, and social support. Reading, MA: Addison-Wesley; 1981.

House JS, Landis KR, Umberson D. Social relationships and health. Science. 1988;241:540.

Hutchinson MK, Cooney TM. Patterns of parent-teen sexual risk communication: implications for intervention. Fam Relat. 1998;47:185–94.

Jaccard J, Dittus PJ, Gordon VV. Parent-adolescent congruency in reports of adolescent sexual behavior and in communication about sexual behavior. Child Dev. 1998;69(1):247–61.

Jemmott JBI, Jemmott LS, Fong GT, McCaffree K. Reducing HIV risk-associated sexual behavior among Africa American adolescents: testing the generality of intervention effects. Am J Community Psychol. 1999;27:161–75.

Jemmott LS, Outlaw F, Jemmott III JB, Brown EJ, Howard M, Hopkins BH. Strengthening the bond: the mother-son health promotion project. In: Pequegnat W, Szapocznik J, editors. Working with families in the era of HIV/AIDS. Thousand Oaks, CA: Sage; 2000. p. 133–51.

Jessor R, Van Den Bos J, Vanderryn J, Costa FM, Turbin MS. Protective factors in adolescent problem behavior: moderator effects and developmental change. In: Marlatt GA, VandenBos GR, editors. Addictive behaviors: readings on etiology, prevention, and treatment. Washington, DC: American Psychological Association; 1997. p. 239–64.

Ji GP, Li L, Lin CQ, Sun S. The impact of HIV/AIDS on families and children: a study in China. AIDS. 2007;21(8):S157–61.

Jordan K, Donenberg GR. Family context and HIV risk among youth in psychiatric care: what pediatricians can do. Curr Opin Pediatr. 2006;18(5):545–50.

Kawachi I, Berkman LF. Social cohesion, social capital, and health. In: Berkman LF, Kawachi I, editors. Social epidemiology. New York: Oxford University Press; 2000. p. 174–90.

Kawachi I, Kennedy BP, Prothrow-Stith D. Social capital, income inequality and mortality. Am J Public Health. 1997;87:1491–8.

Kirby D. Emerging answers: research findings on programs to reduce teen pregnancy (Summary). Washington D.C: National Campaign to Prevent Teen Pregnancy; 2001.

Krauss B, Tiffany J, Goldsamt L. Research notes: parent and pre-adolescent training for HIV prevention in a high seroprevalence neighbourhood. AIDS/STD Health Promot Exchange. 1997;1:10–2.

Krauss BJ, Godfrey C, Yee D, Goldsamt L, Tiffany J, Almeyda L, et al. Saving our children from a silent epidemic: the PATH program for parents and preadolescents. In: Pequegnat W, Szapocznik J, editors. Working with family in the era of AIDS. Thousand Oaks, CA: Sage; 2000. p. 89–112.

Krauss B, Godfrey C, O'Day J, Pride J, Donaire M. Now I can learn about HIV – effects of a parent training on children's practical HIV knowledge and HIV worries: a randomized trial in an HIV-affected neighborhood [Abstract]. XIV-th World AIDS conference, Barcelona, Spain. Abstract no. WePeD6344; 2002.

Krauss B, Godfrey C, O'Day J, Freidin E, Kaplan R. Learning to live with an epidemic: reducing stigma and increasing safe and sensitive socializing with persons with HIV. In: Lyon ME,

D'Angelo LJ, editors. Teenagers, HIV, and AIDS: insights from youth living with the virus. Westport, CT: Praeger; 2006. p. 83–103.

Krauss B, McGinniss S, O'Day J, Hodorek S, Bournea M, Kaplan R. Delaying tactics: parent HIV education as a protective factor for early sexual debut. Poster presented at NIMH international conference on the role of families in preventing and adapting to HIV/AIDS. San Francisco, CA; July 2007.

Krishna VAS, Bhatt RS, Chandra PS, Juvva S. Unheard voices: experiences of families living with HIV/AIDS in India. Contemp Fam Ther. 2005;27(4):483–505.

Lang DL, Crosby RA, DiClemente RJ, Salazar LF, Brown LK, Donenberg GR, et al. Neighborhood environment and prevalence of sexually transmitted infections among adolescents diagnosed with psychological disorders. American Journal of Community Psychology, 2010;46: 303–311.

Lee S-J, Singparu S. Adaptation of family-based HIV intervention in Thailand Presented at NIMH annual international research conference on the role of families in preventing and adapting to HIV/AIDS. San Francisco, CA: NIMH; 2007.

Lee MB, Lester P, Rotheram-Borus MJ. The relationship between adjustment of mothers with HIV and their adolescent daughters. Clin Child Psychol Psychiatry. 2002;7(1):171–84.

Lee S-J, Detels R, Rotheram-Borus M, Duan N. The effect of social support on mental and behavioral outcomes among HIV-affected adolescents. Am J Public Health. 2007a;97(10): 1820–6.

Lee S-J, Detels R, Rotheram-Borus M, Duan N, Lord L. Depression and social support among HIV-affected adolescents. AIDS Patient Care STDs. 2007b;21(6):409–17.

Leland NL, Barth RP. Characteristics of adolescents who have attempted to avoid HIV and who have communicated with their parents about sex. J Adolesc Res. 1993;8:58–76.

Lester P, Chesney M, Cooke M, Weiss R, Whalley P. When the time comes to talk about HIV: factors associated with diagnostic disclosure and emotional distress in HIV-infected children. J Acquir Immune Defic Syndr. 2002;31(3):309–17.

Lewis L, Mellins CA, Brackis-Cott E, Dolezal C. Developmental, ethnic and social influences on participation in sexual possibility situations for heterosexual early adolescent youth with HIV positive mothers. J Early Adolesc. 2006;(26):160–84.

Li X, Feigelman S, Stanton B. Perceived parental monitoring and health risk behaviors among urban low-income African-American children and adolescents. J Adolesc Health. 2000;27: 43–8.

Li L, Sun S, Wu ZY, Wu S, Lin CQ, Yan ZH. Disclosure is a family matter, field notes from China. J Fam Psychol. 2007;21(2):307–14.

Lin CQ, Li L, Ji GP. Children' body mass index and nutrition intake in HIV/AIDS affected families in China. Vulnerable Child Youth Stud. 2008;3(1):16–23.

Lyon ME, Trexler C, Akpan-Townsend C, Pao M, Selden K, Fletcher J, et al. A family group approach to increasing adherence to therapy in HIV-infected youths: results of a pilot project. AIDS Patient Care STDs. 2003;17:299–308.

Lyon ME, Briggs L, Garvie PA, McCarter R, Marsh J, Lee S, et al. Adaptation/development of a family-centered advance care planning intervention through community based participatory research. Paper presented at NIMH annual international research conference on the role of families in preventing and adapting to HIV/AIDS. San Francisco, CA; July 2007.

Macklin ED. AIDS: implications for families. Fam Relat. 1988;37(2):141–9.

Mayes VM, Cochran SD. Black gay and bisexual men coping with more than just a disease. Focus. 1988;4(1):1–3.

McBride CK, Baptiste D, Paikoff RL, Madison-Boyd S, Coleman D, Bell CC. Family-based HIV preventive intervention: child level results from the CHAMP family program. In: McKay MM, Paikoff RL, editors. Community collaborative partnerships: the foundation for HIV prevention research efforts. Binghamton, NY: Haworth Press; 2007a. p. 203–20.

McBride C, Baptiste D, Paikoff R, Madison S, Coleman D, Bell C, et al. Family-based HIV preventive intervention: child level results from the CHAMP family program. Soc Work Ment Health. 2007b;5(1–2):203–20.

McCormick A, McKay MM, Wilson M, McKinney L, Paikoff R, Bell C, et al. Involving families in an urban HIV prevention intervention: how community collaboration addresses barriers to participation. AIDS Educ Prev. 2000;12(4):299–307.

McKay M, Paikoff R, editors. Community collaborative partnerships: the foundation for HIV prevention research efforts in the United States and internationally. West Hazleton, PA: Haworth Press; 2007.

McKay MM, Baptiste D, Coleman D, Madison S, Paikoff R, Scott R. Preventing HIV risk exposure in urban communities: the CHAMP family program. In: Pequegnat W, Szapocznik J, editors. Working with families in the era of HIV/AIDS. Thousand Oaks, CA: Sage; 2000. p. 67–87.

McKay MM, Chasse KT, Paikoff R, McKinney LD, Baptiste D, Coleman D, et al. Family-level impact of the CHAMP Family Program: a community collaborative effort to support urban families and reduce youth HIV risk exposure. Fam Process. 2004;43(1):79–93.

McKay MM, Block M, Mellins C, Traube DE, Brackis-Cott E, Minott D, et al. Adapting a family-based HIV prevention program for HIV-infected preadolescents and their families. Soc Work Ment Health. 2007a;5(3/4):355–78.

McKay MM, Hibbert R, Lawrence R, Miranda A, Paikoff R, Bell CC, et al. Creating mechanisms for meaningful collaboration between members of urban communities and university-based HIV prevention researchers. In: McKay MM, Paikoff RL, editors. Community collaborative partnerships: the foundation for HIV prevention research efforts. Binghamton, NY: Haworth Press; 2007b. p. 147–68.

Mellins CA, Ehrhart AA. Families affected by pediatric acquired immunodeficiency syndrome: sources of stress. J Dev Behav Pediatr. 1994;15 suppl 3:S54–60.

Mellins CA, Ehrhardt AA, Newman L, Conard M. Selective kin: defining the caregivers and families of children with HIV disease. In: Jemmott LS, O'Leary A, editors. Women and AIDS: coping and care. New York: Plenum; 1996. p. 12–149.

Mellins CA, Brackis-Cott E, Dolezal C, Richards A. Patterns of HIV status disclosure to perinatally HIV-infected children and subsequent mental health. Clin Child Psychol Psychiatry. 2002;7:101–14.

Mellins CA, Dolezal C, Brackis-Cott E, Nicholson O, Warne P, Meyer-Bahlburg HFL. Predicting the onset of sexual and drug risk behavior in youth affected by maternal HIV disease: the role of contextual, self-regulation, and social interaction factors. J Youth Adolesc. 2007;36:265–78.

Metts S, Manns H, Kruzic L. Social support structures and predictors of depression in persons who are seropositive. J Health Psychol. 1996;1(3):367–82.

Miller BC, Norton MC, Curtis T, Hill EJ, Schwaneveldt P, Young MH. The timing of sexual intercourse among adolescents: family, peer, and other antecedents. Youth Soc. 1997;29(1): 54–83.

Miller KS, Levin ML, Whitaker DJ, Xu X. Patterns of condom use among adolescents: the impact of maternal-adolescent communication. Am J Public Health. 1998;88(10):1542–4.

Miller KS, Forehand R, Kotchick BA. Adolescent sexual behavior in two ethnic minority samples: the role of family variables. J Marriage Fam. 1999;61:85–98.

Mitrani VB, Szapocznik J, Batista CR. Structural ecosystems therapy with HIV+ African American women. In: Pequegnat W, Szapocznik J, editors. Working with families in the era of AIDS. Thousand Oaks, CA: Sage; 2000. p. 243–80.

Mitrani VB, Prado G, Feaster DJ, Robinson-Batista C, Szapocznik J. Relational factors and family treatment engagement among low-income, HIV-positive African American mothers. Fam Process. 2003;42(1):31–45.

Murphy DA, Roberts KJ, Hoffman D. Stigma and ostracism associated with HIV/AIDS: children carrying the secret of their mothers' HIV+ serostatus. J Child Fam Stud. 2002a;11: 191–202.

Murphy DA, Marelich WD, Dello Stritto ME, Swendeman D, Witkin A. Mothers living with HIV/AIDS: mental, physical, and family functioning. AIDS Care. 2002b;14(5):633–44.

Murphy DA, Austin EL, Greenwell L. Correlates of HIV-related stigma among HIV-positive mothers and their uninfected adolescent children. Women Health. 2006a;44(3):19–42.

Murphy DA, Greenwell L, Mouttapa M, Brecht ML, Schuster MA. Physical health of mothers with HIV/AIDS and the mental health of their children. J Dev Behav Pediatr. 2006b;27(5): 386–95.

Murphy DA, Greenwell L, Resell J, Brecht ML, Schuster MA. Early and middle adolescents' autonomy development: impact of maternal HIV/AIDS. Clin Child Psychol Psychiatry. 2008;13:253–77.

Murry VM. Black American adolescent females sexual activity patterns: abstainers mothers, and those-in-between. Afr Am Res Perspect. 1997;3:25–31.

Murry VM, Brody GH. Self-regulation and self-worth of Black children reared in economically stressed, rural, single parent families: the contribution of risk and protective factors. J Marriage Fam. 1999;67:627–42.

Murry VM, Brody GH, McNair L, Luo Z, Gibbons FX, Gerrard M, et al. Parental involvement promotes rural African American youths' self-pride and sexual self-concepts. J Marriage Fam. 2005;67:627–42.

Murry VM, Berkel C, Brody GH, Gibbons FX, Gerrard M. The Strong African American Families program: longitudinal pathways to sexual risk reduction. J Adolesc Health. 2007;41:317–418.

Mustanski B, Donenberg G, Emerson E. I can use a condom, i just don't: the importance of motivation to prevent HIV in adolescent seeking psychiatric care. AIDS Behav. 2006;10(6):753–62.

Namir S, Wolcott DL, Fawzy FI. Social support and HIV spectrum disease: clinical research perspectives. Psychiatr Med. 1989;7:97–105.

Nappi CM, McBride CK, Donnenberg GR. HIV/AIDS communication among adolescents in psychiatric care and their parents. J Fam Psychol. 2007;21(4):637–44.

Nappi CM, Thakral C, Kapungu C, Donenberg GR, DiClemente RJ, Brown L, et al. Parental monitoring as a moderator of the effect of family sexual communication on sexual risk behavior among adolescents in psychiatric care. AIDS Behav. 2009;13(5):1012–20.

Nyblade LC, Pande R, Banteyerga H, Bond V, Kilonzo G, Mbwambo J, et al. Family and community-level stigma impedes HIV prevention and care, and lowers the quality of life for people living with HIV and AIDS. Paper presented at international conference on AIDS, Bangkok, Thailand. Abstract no. ThPeD7783; July 2004.

Paikoff RL. Early heterosexual debut: situations of sexual possibilities during the transition to adolescence. Am J Orthopsychiatry. 1995;65(3):389–401.

Paikoff RL. Applying developmental psychology to an AIDS prevention model for urban African-American youth. J Negro Educ. 1997;65:44–59.

Pantin H, Coatsworth JD, Feaster DJ, Newman FL, Briones E, Prado G, et al. Familias Unidas: the efficacy of an intervention to promote parental investment in Hispanic immigrant families. Prev Sci. 2003;4:189–201.

Pantin H, Schwartz SJ, Sullivan S, Prado G, Szapocznik J. Ecodevelopmental HIV prevention programs for Hispanic adolescents. Am J Orthopsychiatry. 2004;74(4):545–58.

Pearson J, Muller C, Frisco M. Parental involvement, family structure and adolescent sexual decision making. Sociol Perspect. 2006;49:67–90.

Pequegnat W, Bray J. Families and HIV/AIDS: introduction to the special sections. J Fam Psychol. 1997;1(1):3–10.

Pequegnat W, Sczapocznik J, editors. Working with families in the era of AIDS. Thousand Oaks, CA: Sage; 2000.

Perrino T, Gonzalez-Soldevila A, Pantin H, Szapocznik J. The role of families in adolescent HIV prevention: a review. Clin Child Fam Psychol Rev. 2000;3(2):81–96.

Petraitis J, Flay BR, Miller TQ. Reviewing theories of adolescent substance use: organizing pieces in the puzzle. Psychol Bull. 1995;1(17):67–86.

Prado G, Schwartz SH, Pattatucci-Aragon A, Clatts M, Pantin H, Fernandez MI, et al. The prevention of HIV transmission in Hispanic adolescents. Drug Alcohol Depend. 2006a;84 Suppl 1:S43–53.

Prado G, Pantin H, Schwartz SJ, Lupei NS, Szapocznik J. Predictors of engagement and retention into a parent-centered, ecodevelopmental HIV preventive intervention for Hispanic adolescents and their families. J Pediatr Psychol. 2006b;31(9):874–90.

Rai AA, Stanton B, Wu Y, Li X, Galbraith J, Cottrell L, et al. The relative influence of perceived parental monitoring and perceived peer involvement on adolescent. J Adolesc Health. 2003;33(2):108–18.

Rapkin B, Munoz M, Murphy P. The family problem solving interventions for HIV/AIDS: a progress report submitted to NIMH. Unpublished report; 2007.

Rapkin BD, Bennett JA, Murphy P, Munoz M. The family health project: strengthening problem solving in families affected by AIDS to mobilize systems of support and care. In: Pequegnat W, Szapocznik J, editors. Working with families in the era of HIV AIDS. Thousand Oaks, CA: Sage; 2000. p. 213–42.

Rice E. Adaptation of an effective family-based HIV prevention and coping intervention in Los Angeles. Paper presented at NIMH annual international research conference on the role of families in preventing and adapting to HIV/AIDS. San Francisco, CA; July 2007.

Robbins MS, Szapocznik J, Alexandra JF, Miller J. Family systems therapy with children and adolescents. In: Hersen M, Bellack AS (series editors), Ollendick TH (editor). Comprehensive clinical psychology, vol. 5. Children and adolescents: clinical formulation and treatment. Oxford, UK: Elsevier Science; 1998. p. 149–480.

Rotheram-Borus MJ. International adaptation of evidence based prevention programs. Presented at NIMH annual international research conference on the role of families in preventing and adapting to HIV/AIDS. San Francisco, CA; July 2007.

Rotheram-Borus MJ, Murphy D, Draimin B, Miller S. An intervention for adolescents whose parents are living with AIDS. Clin Child Psychol Psychiatry. 1997;2(2):201–19.

Rotheram-Borus MJ, Lee MB, Gwadz M, Draimin B. An intervention for parents with AIDS and their adolescent children. Am J Public Health. 2001;91:1294–302.

Rotheram-Borus MJ, Lee MB, Leonard N, Lin YY, Franzke L, Lightfoot MA. Four-year behavioral outcomes of an intervention for parents living with HIV and their adolescent children. AIDS. 2004;17(8):1217–25.

Rotheram-Borus MJ, Flannery D, Rice E, Lester P. Families living with HIV. AIDS Care. 2005a;17:978–87.

Rotheram-Borus MJ, Weiss R, Alber S, Lester P. Adolescent adjustment before and after HIV-related parental death. J Consult Clin Psychol. 2005b;73(2):221–8.

Rotheram-Borus MJ, Stein JA, Lester P. Adolescent adjustment over six years in HIV-affected families. J Adolesc Health. 2006;39(2):174–82.

Ryan C, Huebner D, Diaz RM, Sanchez J. Family rejection as a predictor of negative health outcomes in White and Latino lesbian, gay, and bisexual young adults. Pediatrics. 2009;123(1): 346–52.

Sampson RJ, Raudenbush SW, Earls F. Neighborhoods and violent crime: a multilevel study of collective efficacy. Science. 1997;277:918–24.

Schuster MA, Beckett MK, Cornoa R, Zhou A. Hugs and kisses: HIV-infected parents' fears about contagion and the effects on parent-child interaction in a nationally representative sample. Arch Pediatr Adolesc Med. 2005;159:73–179.

Shinn M, Lehmann S, Wong NW. Social interaction and social support. Journal of Social Issues, 1984;40(4):55–76.

Sieving RE, McNeely CS, Blum RW. Maternal expectations, mother-child connectedness and adolescent sexual debut. Arch Pediatr Adolesc Med. 2000;154:809–16.

Silver EJ, Bauman LJ, Camacho S, Hudis J. Factors associated with psychological distress in urban mothers with late-stage HIV/AIDS. AIDS Behav. 2003;7(4):421–31.

Simoni JM, Frick PA, Huang B. A longitudinal evaluation of a social support model of medication adherence among HIV-positive men and women on antiretroviral therapy. Health Psychol. 2006;25:74–81.

Smith MY, Rapkin BD. Unmet needs for help among person with AIDS. AIDS Care. 1995;7(3):353–63.

Smith MY, Rapkin BD. Social support and barriers to family involvement in caregiving for persons with AIDS: implications for patient education. Patient Educ Couns. 1996;27: 85–94.

Smith L, Feaster DJ, Prado G, Kamin M, Blaney N, Szapocznik J. The psychosocial functioning of HIV+ and HIV− African American mothers. AIDS Behav. 2001;5:219–31.

Stanton B, Romer D, Ricardo I, Black M, Feigelman S, Galbraith J. Early initiation of sex and its lack of association with risk behaviors among adolescent African-Americans. Pediatrics. 1993;92(1):62–74.

Starrett RA, Bresler C, Decker JT, Water GT, Rogers D. The role of environmental awareness and social support networks in Hispanic elderly persons' use of formal social services. J Community Psychol. 1990;18:218–27.

Stoller EP, Pugliesi KL. Other roles of caregivers: competing responsibilities or supportive resources. J Gerontol. 1989;44:S231–8.

Sudarkase N. African and Afro-American family structure. In: Colle JB, editor. Anthropology from the nineties. New York: Collier MacMillan; 1988.

Szapocznik J, Coatsworth JD. An ecodevelopmental framework for organizing the influences on drug abuse: an ecodevelopmental model for risk and prevention. In: Glantz M, Hartel CR, editors. Drug abuse: origins and interventions. Washington, DC: American Psychological Association; 1999. p. 331–66.

Szapocznik J, Kurtines WM. Family psychology and cultural diversity: opportunities for theory, research and application. Am Psychol. 1993;48(1):400–7.

Szapocznik J, Feaster DJ, Mitrani VB, Guillermo Prado G, Smith L, Robinson-Batista C, et al. Structural ecosystems therapy for HIV-seropositive African American women: effects on psychological distress, family hassles, and family support. J Consult Clin Psychol. 2004;72(2): 288–303.

Taylor MM. The increasing importance of sexually transmitted diseases in HIV-infected persons. J Child Psychol Psychiatry. 2003;45(2):387–95.

Taylor RW, Wang MC, editors. Social and emotional adjustment of family relations in ethnic minority families. Mahwah, NJ: Erlbaum; 1997.

Tolou-Shams M, Paikoff R, McKirnan DJ, Holmbeck GN. Mental health and HIV risk among African American adolescents: the role of parenting. In: McKay MM, Paikoff RL, editors. Community collaborative partnerships: the foundation for HIV prevention research efforts. Binghamton, NY: Haworth Press; 2007. p. 27–58.

Trizzino J. Adaptation of an effective family-based HIV prevention and coping intervention for South African families. Presented at NIMH annual international research conference on the role of families in preventing and adapting to HIV/AIDS. San Francisco, CA; July 2007.

Voisin R, Baptiste D, Martinez D, Henderson G. Exporting a US-HIV/AIDS prevention program to a Caribbean-island nation: lessons from the field. Int Soc Work. 2005;49:75–86.

Whitebeck LB, Conger RD, Kao M. The influence of parental support, depressed affect, and peers on the sexual behavior of adolescent girls. J Fam Issues. 1993;14:261–78.

WHO. Make every mother and child count. Available via: http://www.who.int/world-health-day/previous/2005/en/ (2005). Cited 12 Mar 2011.

Wiener L, Lyon M. HIV disclosure: who knows? who needs to know? clinical and ethical considerations. In: Lyon ME, D'Angelo LJ, editors. Teenagers, HIV, and AIDS: insights from youth living with the virus. Westport, CT: Praeger; 2006. p. 83–103.

Wilder EI, Watt TT. Risky parental behavior and adolescent sexual activity at first coitus. Milbank Q. 2002;80(3):481–524.

Wills TA, Gibbons FX, Gerrard M, Murry VM, Brody GH. Family communication and religiosity related to substance use and sexual behavior in early adolescence: a test for pathways through self-control and prototype perceptions. Psychol Addict Behav. 2003;17:312–23.

Wilson HW, Donenberg G. Quality of parent communication about sex and its relationship to risky sexual behavior among youth in psychiatric care: a pilot study. J Child Psychol Psychiatry. 2004;45(2):387–95.

Williams AW, Ware JE, Donald CA. A model of mental health, life events, and social supports applicable to general population. Journal of health and Social Behavior, 1981;22:324–336.

Wingood GM, DiClemente RJ. The WiLLOW program: mobilizing social networks of women living with HIV to enhance coping and reduce sexual risk behaviors. In: Pequegnat W,

Szapocznik J, editors. Working with families in the era of AIDS. Thousand Oaks, CA: Sage; 2000. p. 281–98.

Yang H, Stanton B, Li X, Cottrel L, Galbraith J, Kaljee L. Dynamic association between parental monitoring and communication and adolescent risk involvement among African-American adolescents. J Natl Med Assoc. 2007;99(5):517–24.

Chapter 2
Family as the Model for Prevention of Mental and Physical Health Problems

Carl C. Bell and Dominica F. McBride

Abstract In this chapter, the authors discuss the family as a model for a prevention delivery system for a wide range of mental and physical health problems. Accordingly, the chapter highlights multiple examples of family-based prevention interventions that seek to prevent various mental and emotional disorders and behavioral problems of youth. Because family processes have a profound impact on bolstering and maintaining healthy behavior in adolescence, the chapter mainly focuses on family-based prevention interventions for adolescents that have been shown to decrease their risky sexual behaviors. Evidence exists that shows family-based interventions can prevent problems that occur during the prenatal and postnatal periods (e.g., maternal depression) and high-risk pregnancies among teenagers. These interventions thereby prevent other problems, such as genetic anomalies; poor maternal nutrition; maternal smoking, alcohol and drug use; exposure to neurotoxins; maternal depression or stress; low birth weight; and peri-natal insults (Institute of Medicine [IOM], 2009). In addition, there is research indicating that family-based prevention intervention strategies can prevent problems of child maltreatment, aggression, and other problem behaviors (e.g., substance abuse, antisocial behavior) (IOM 2009). Further, the potential of the family as a means to cultivate resiliency in children is underscored. Finally, efforts to move family-based prevention interventions into day-to-day life and how we can create a healthy future for our children are discussed.

2.1 Introduction

In this chapter, the authors will discuss the family as a model for a prevention delivery system for a wide range of mental and physical health problems. The chapter will highlight multiple examples of family-based prevention interventions that seek to prevent various mental and emotional disorders and behavioral problems of youth.

W. Pequegnat and C.C. Bell (eds.), *Family and HIV/AIDS: Cultural and Contextual Issues in Prevention and Treatment*, DOI 10.1007/978-1-4614-0439-2_2, © Springer Science+Business Media, LLC 2012

Adolescence is a phase in human development that has a significant influence on subsequent adult behavior. Because family processes have a profound impact on bolstering and maintaining health behavior in adolescence, the chapter will mainly focus on family-based prevention interventions for adolescents that have been shown to decrease their risky sexual behaviors. Available evidences support that family-based interventions can prevent problems that occur during the prenatal and postnatal period (e.g., maternal depression) and prevent high-risk pregnancies among teenagers. These interventions thereby prevent other problems, such as genetic anomalies; poor maternal nutrition; maternal smoking, alcohol and drug use; exposure to neurotoxins; maternal depression or stress; low birth weight; and perinatal insults (National Research Council and Institute of Medicine 2009). In addition, there is research indicating that family-based prevention intervention strategies can prevent problems of child maltreatment, aggression, and other problem behaviors (e.g., substance abuse and antisocial behavior) (National Research Council and Institute of Medicine 2009). Further, the potential of the family as a means to cultivate resiliency in children will be underscored. Finally, efforts to move family-based prevention interventions into day-to-day life and measures to create a healthy future for our children are discussed.

2.2 Introduction to the Family as a Vehicle for Prevention of Mental and Physical Health Problems

Because of the relatively slow development of the human brain, beginning at conception and ending in early adulthood, we are vulnerable during this period of our lives. From bottom up and from inside out, brain development starts with the vegetative, appetitive parts and ends with the cognitive, judgmental components of the central nervous system. Humans need families to ensure optimal survival and to provide cognitive, social, emotional, and behavioral competencies. Families are essential for developing survival skills, such as the capacity for connectedness, learning, socialization; for providing protection, monitoring, and self-esteem, and for sources of "mastery experiences for infants, children, adolescents, and young adults." Families have the potential to inculcate healthy behaviors and stave off illness-generating behaviors; therefore families are ideal systems to prevent mental, emotional, and physical health problems (Pequegnat and Stover 2000). The National Institute of Mental Health (NIMH) Consortium on Families and HIV/AIDS defines family as a network of mutual commitment (Pequegnat and Bray 1997; Pequegnat and Szapocznik 2000). Although many individuals are resilient and do well despite their family's limited capacity to provide mutual commitment, the family has a great deal of influence on the success of an individual's outcomes.

The "stress-diathesis model" is clear that behavior is multi-determined. Three major threads that determine behavior are genetics, environment, and their interaction.

Thus, if a child is born with genetics that protect the child from maladaptive reactivity to trauma, then a traumatogenic family will not overtly harm that genetically fortunate child. If, however, a child is born with genetics that make the child vulnerable to being overly and harmfully reactive to trauma, then the capacity of the family to protect the child from being exposed to trauma is critical to the child's development. Furthermore, should a child be exposed to trauma, how the family responds to a child that is genetically vulnerable to the impact of trauma is critically important. Finally, since we may not be able to identify who is who genetically, we need to nurture all children by protecting them from trauma or helping them cope with trauma should they get exposed.

For more than 15 years, the NIMH's Consortium on Families and HIV/AIDS has been developing family-based prevention strategies to prevent HIV infections in adolescents and young adults. In addition, family-based prevention strategies have also been applied to prevent high-risk pregnancy among teenagers; problems during the prenatal period and infancy (e.g., alcohol and drug use or maternal depression or stress); peri-partum depression; child maltreatment; and aggression and other problem behaviors, including substance abuse, antisocial behavior, and violence (National Research Council and Institute of Medicine 2009). This chapter largely draws on the work of members of the NIMH Consortium on Families and HIV/AIDS and the work described in the NRC and IOM's report on *Prevention of Mental Disorders, Substance Abuse, and Problem Behaviors in Children, Adolescents, and Young Adults* (2009). This report addresses the family's role in prevention of mental and emotional disorders, substance abuse, and problem behaviors in children, adolescents, and young adults.

2.3 Scope of the Problem

The capacity of the US to identify mental, emotional, and behavioral disorders in youth that could respond to family-based prevention interventions is sorely limited (National Research Council and Institute of Medicine 2009). As emphasized in Dr. Satcher's *Report of the Surgeon's Conference on Children's Mental Health: A National Action Agenda* (US Public Health Service 2000), we have information that half of all mentally ill adults recalled that their mental disorders began by their mid-teens, and three-quarters by the mid-20s (Kessler et al. 2005). Further, some studies show that the prevalence of behavioral and emotional difficulties among preschool children is similar to the rates observed for older children. McDermott and Weiss (1995) found 33% of children in nonselective, community samples evidence sub-clinical psychological symptoms, which have a detrimental impact on quality of life and compromise functioning in domains such as school, family life, or social relations outside the home. Mash (2003) found that 8–10% of preschool children had conditions that meet the DSM-IV criteria for diagnosable mental disorders. Fourteen to 22% had conditions that caused impairment but did not qualify for a formal DSM-IV diagnosis. The 2003 National Survey of Children's Health found the most commonly diagnosed problems among children 6–17 years of age were learning disabilities (11.5%), attention-deficit/hyperactivity disorder (ADHA; 8.8%), and behavioral problems (6.3%) (Blanchard et al. 2006). These results are close to other surveys for specific diagnoses, such as ADHD (7%) and learning disabilities (8–10%) (Dey and Bloom 2004), behavioral and conduct problems (5–7%) (Guevara et al. 2003), anxiety or depressive disorder (2–4%) (Costello et al. 2003), and alcohol or drug abuse (19–22%) (Office of Applied Studies 2003). As one would expect, Blanchard et al. (2006) found that, among preschoolers, speech problems (5.8%) and developmental delay (3.2%) were most common, and children with developmental problems had lower self-esteem, more depression and anxiety, and more problems with learning. In addition, these children missed more school and were less involved in sports and other community activities which are potential protective factors facilitated by the family that could mediate and moderate their increased risk. Blanchard et al. (2006) also found that, despite the rates of mental disorders, substance abuse, and problem behaviors of children and adolescents matching other surveys, rates of parental concerns about emotional, developmental, or behavioral problems were much higher. For example, 41% of parents surveyed had concerns about learning difficulties and 36% about depression or anxiety.

More recently, from a six-state study, using the ABLE (Attention, Behavior, Language, and Emotions) screening tool, we know parents identified 18.4% and pre-kindergarten teachers identified 10.5% of children with severe behavioral, emotional, and language problems (Barbarin 2007). By kindergarten, the proportion of children identified by their teachers with serious problems more than doubled to 23%, and inattention/over-activity and behavior problems were the greatest identified. However, fewer than 14% of public, pre-kindergarten, children identified with serious problems had received mental health services by the end of kindergarten (Barbarin 2007).

In 1982, we began developing significant evidence that relatively large proportions of children are exposed to domestic and community violence [i.e., experience trauma (Bell 1987; Bell and Jenkins 1991)]. Subsequent to this early work, numerous scientists confirmed the observations that at least 20% of youth experienced the trauma of witnessing violence in childhood, and, in some communities, the risk for exposure to violence is even higher (Jenkins and Bell 1997). In the late 1990s, the landmark Adverse Childhood Experiences (ACE) Study was conducted (Felitti et al. 1998) that highlighted the potential negative impact of adverse childhood experiences on youth's mental and physical health outcomes in adulthood (Division of Adult 2008).

The ACE study of 17,000 mostly European-American, middle-class, working adults revealed that more than half the respondents had experienced at least one category of adverse childhood exposure (psychological abuse, physical abuse, sexual abuse, violence against mother, living with household members who were substance abusers, living with household members who were mentally ill or suicidal, and living with ex-offender household members) (Division of Adult 2008). Furthermore, 6.2% of the sample reported experiencing four or more adverse childhood exposures increasing their risk for mental and physical health problems. Compared to those who had no exposure to adverse childhood experiences, persons who experienced four or more had: a 7.4-fold increased risk for alcoholism; a 10.3-fold increased risk for drug abuse; a 4.6-fold increased risk for depression; a 12.0-fold increased risk in suicide attempts; a 2.2-fold increased risk in smoking; a 2.2-fold increased risk poor self-rated health; a 3.2-fold increased risk in having 50 or more sexual partners; a 2.5-fold increased risk in sexually transmitted disease; a 2.2-fold increased risk in ischemic heart disease; a 1.9-fold increased risk cancer; a 3.9-fold increased risk in chronic lung disease (bronchitis and emphysema); a 1.6-fold increased risk in skeletal fractures; and a 2.4-fold increased risk in liver disease.

This work illustrates that childhood trauma places youth at risk for engaging in health behaviors that result in later adult mental and emotional disorders and behavior problems. It should be apparent that children exposed to adverse childhood experiences are several times more at risk for behaviors that would result in contracting HIV infections. It should also be apparent that, in addition to being at risk for increased mental and emotional disorders (i.e., depression and suicide attempts), children exposed to trauma are more at risk for developing chronic physical illness in adulthood. Thus, in an effort to ensure the public's health research scientists, health professionals, policy makers, and others should be figuring out how to protect children from trauma in childhood and/or how to prevent the negative impact of trauma in childhood.

Despite the enormity of the problem, we should not lose hope, and we can do this by taking a lesson contained in the IOM report on suicide prevention (Goldsmith et al. 2002). Drawing on the Adverse Childhood Experiences Study (1998), this milestone report appropriately noted that childhood trauma has emerged as a strong risk factor for suicidal behavior in adolescents and adults. The IOM Report on Reducing Suicide noted the official rate of child victimization in 1999 was approximately 12 per 1,000 (rates are even higher in surveys of children and parents) (Goldsmith et al. 2002, p 3 and 160). In 2003, young children (birth to 3 years of age) had the highest rate of victimization at 16.4 per 1,000 children in the national population (US Surgeon General 2005). Independent of psychopathology and other known risk factors, child sexual abuse has been reported in 9–20% of suicide attempts in adults. Despite the weak quality of data on suicide attempts, the goal for 2010 is to reduce adolescent suicide attempts by 1% each year (US Department of Health and Human Services [DHHS] 2000). One national school-based study of youth found high 1-year prevalence rates for suicide attempts (7.7%), ideation (20.5), and making a plan (15.7) (Kann et al. 1998). Joe et al. (2006) noted that the lifetime prevalence of suicide attempts among Caribbean black men was around 7.5%. According to a recent Centers for Disease Control and Prevention (CDC) report, the prevalence of attempted suicide for white and black high school students (7.3 and 7.6%, respectively) was roughly equal (Eaton et al. 2006). The lesson for hope here is simple. In examining the poor health outcome of suicide, we learn that 20,000/100,000 suffer a mental disorder; using high estimates, rates of suicide attempts are 8,000/100,000;

and the overall suicide rates are approximately 11–12/100,000 in the course of a year (US DHHS 1999). Clearly, there must be protective factors shielding the 7,988 suicide attempters and 19,988 mentally ill individuals from completing suicide; this reality illustrates the maxim, "Risk factors are not predictive factors due to protective factors."

2.4 Research Innovations to Address the Problem

"Families are the most central and enduring influence in children's lives … the health and well-being of children are inextricably linked to their parent's physical, emotional and social health, social circumstances, and childrearing practices" (Schor 2003). Because of the existence of the NIMH Consortium on Families and HIV/AIDS, we have a much better understanding of the reality that families have a significant influence on their children's sexual risk taking (Paikoff et al. 2007; Pequegnat and Szapocznik 2000). Research has determined that the quantity and quality of family communication with adolescents is a significant influence on risky sexual behaviors. Specifically, comfortable and frequent family communication tends to delay sexual debut (Bell et al. 2007, 2008; Biglan et al. 1990; Donenberg et al. 2003; McKay and Paikoff 2007; Pequegnat and Szapocznik 2000; Resnick et al. 1997; Wilson and Donenberg 2004). Depending on what parental expectations are and how adolescents perceive them, parental expectations also influence adolescent behavior. Adolescents listen when parents communicate their approval of responsible sexual behavior. When such communications are absent, adolescents misjudge their parents' in ways that suggest sexual risk taking is acceptable (Jaccard et al. 1998). Conversely, family conflict and negative affect are associated with behavioral problems (Szapocznik and Kurtines 1993), such as early sexual debut (Paikoff 1995), generally risky sexual behavior (Biglan et al. 1990), violence and conduct problems (Borduin et al. 1985; Brody et al. 2008; Henggeler et al. 1992; Farrington 1989; Gorman-Smith et al. 1996; Tolan and Lorion 1988), and drug use (Brody et al. 2004; Wills et al. 2003, 2007).

Research has also shown that parental monitoring and an authoritative parenting style are associated with adolescents who engage in less risky sexual behavior, have fewer sexual partners and less pregnancy, and increased condom use (Baumrind 1966; Bell et al. 2007, 2008; Biglan et al. 1990; Donenberg et al. 2002; Flay et al. 2004; Rai et al. 2003; Yang et al. 2007; Paikoff 1995). These family-based prevention interventions focus on improving parent–child communication and supportive parental behaviors, and increasing parental monitoring and limit-setting. Unfortunately, because of the variety of study designs, there are no meta-analyses of these programs. Fortunately, there is sufficient evidence that family-based HIV prevention interventions are efficacious and effective (Brody et al. 2002; DiIorio et al. 2007; Jemmott et al. 2005; Krauss et al. 1997; McKay and Paikoff 2007; Murry et al. 2005; Wills et al. 2003, 2007; see also Chap. 1).

At-risk behaviors do not occur in isolation. Thus, youth who engage in risky sexual behaviors are also likely to be engaging in risky behaviors involving substances, violence, suicide, and truancy and dropping out of school. Some studies have been assessing outcomes in multiple domains to describe this constellations of risk behaviors better (Brody et al. 2001, 2003, 2004, 2005, 2006a, b, 2008; Bannon and McKay 2007; Prado et al. 2007).

In summary, the evidence is very clear that family-based prevention interventions are ideal and effective for changing health behaviors in adolescents. Further, since there are such common threads (improving parent–child communication and supportive parental behaviors, and increasing parental monitoring and limit-setting) connecting various family-based interventions, it should be possible to adapt and implement such prevention interventions so they become ubiquitous, especially in high-risk populations.

2.5 Family-Based HIV Prevention Interventions

An example of a successful, cross-contextual (i.e., having success in different contexts) family-based HIV prevention intervention is the Chicago HIV Prevention and Adolescent Mental Health Project (CHAMP). CHAMP interventions are family-based prevention interventions designed to prevent HIV infections in young adolescents (youth in fourth and fifth grade) by engaging caregivers and their youth in 10–12 manualized, multiple-family group sessions. The sessions are designed to provide education and skill-building practice to increase knowledge about HIV, risky sexual behaviors and contexts, and essential caregiver skills (e.g., parental connectedness with youth, parenting styles, parental monitoring, and caregiver support from the community and peers) designed to protect youth from engaging in high-risk behaviors. The sessions also actively seek to strengthen caregiver comfort and frequency in talking about difficult topics, caregiver and youth connectedness, and caregiver skills in monitoring and disciplining their youth. The program also helps youth practice social and emotional skills of resisting sexual and drug use, peer pressure, and problem solving about how to avoid risky sexual situations (Bell et al. 2008; Baptiste et al. 2006; McBride et al. 2007; McKay et al. 2004; McKay and Paikoff 2007). Because a CHAMP research staff member and a member of the indigenous community deliver CHAMP family-based interventions in multiple-family groups held in the community and co-led, all of the CHAMP family-based interventions are adapted to the population and setting (McKay et al. 2007a). In addition, serious community partnership is a centerpiece of all CHAMP family-based interventions (McKay et al. 2007b).

In the original CHAMP that began in Chicago in 1993 (Madison et al. 2000; McCormick et al. 2000), 324 families were randomly assigned to the experimental condition and 315 families were assigned to the control condition (McBride et al. 2007). Nearly three-fourths of the families in the experimental condition completed the entire program. Compared to the control families, these families showed increased family decision making, improved caregiver monitoring, greater comfort in discussing sensitive topics, more neighborhood supports, and fewer disruptive difficulties with children, such as externalizing (aggressive and rule-breaking behavior) behaviors and social problems (McBride et al. 2007; Bannon and McKay 2007; McKay et al. 2004, 2007a). However, the youth in the experimental condition also reported significantly more family conflict than the control group presumably because they were having more serious conversations with their caregivers (McBride et al. 2007). More importantly, the youth in the experimental condition reported that they chose to be in fewer situations in which risky sexual behavior could ensue (McBride et al. 2007). Finally, the CHAMP Chicago research also indicated that caregivers benefited from the intervention, as their anxiety and depression measures showed a significant decrease from the pre-test to the post-test (Paikoff 1997).

The original CHAMP that began in Chicago morphed into the CHAMPNYC (Collaborative HIV Adolescent Mental Health Project – New York City), CHAMPWS-C (Collaborative HIV Adolescent Mental Health Project – West Side/Chicago), CHAMPSA (Collaborative HIV Adolescent Mental Health Project – South Africa), and CHAMPTandT (Collaborative HIV Adolescent Mental Health Project – Trinidad and Tobago) (McKay and Paikoff 2007). This metamorphosis did not change the core family-based HIV prevention principles of this evidence-based intervention. The basic goals of increasing family connectedness, family communication (i.e., frequency of communication about difficult topics), social skills training and practice of youth and caregivers, HIV transmission knowledge, etc. were preserved in each iteration of the CHAMP intervention. Differences in CHAMP multiple-family group manuals were based on language (e.g., the New York CHAMP manual was translated into Spanish) and cultural contexts (e.g., the CHAMPSA manual was adapted to fit Zulu culture). In addition, based on ethnographic assessments of the Zulu community, there were other adaptations in lessons in the manual. These modifications did not compromise the core principles necessary for family-based HIV prevention work, e.g., we added a lesson on bereavement owing to the large number of HIV deaths in South Africa.

The first international adaptation of the original CHAMP model (Paruk et al. 2005) was done in the semi-rural area of Durban, South Africa (Bell et al. 2007, 2008; Bhana et al. 2004). Due to the high rates of illiteracy of the target population, the intervention manual had to be illustrated (Petersen et al. 2006). The objective of the manual was to illustrate Bell's seven field principles of health behavior change:

- Rebuilding the village/constructing social fabric
- Providing access to modern and ancient technology
- Improving bonding, attachment, and connectedness dynamics
- Improving self-esteem – a sense of power, a sense of models, a sense of uniqueness, a sense
- Increasing social and emotional skills of target recipients

- Reestablishing the adult protective shield and monitoring
- Minimizing the residual effects of trauma (Bell et al. 2007, 2008)

Accordingly, a goal of the intervention was to "rebuild the village." Encouraging families to cultivate community/social fabric or "collective efficacy" (Sampson et al. 1997) accomplished this task. For example, family duties such as child rearing were supported by the social support CHAMPSA. Modern psychosocial technology (e.g., multiple-family group contexts) was used to deliver the intervention. The CHAMP intervention facilitated connectedness within the family (Bell 2001), i.e., positive parent–child interactions, and developed social and emotional skills related to parenting practices. Caregivers and youth were given models, such as how to communicate with "I messages," so that families could ensure good outcomes for their children. This enabled caregivers to develop a sense of power or self-efficacy in the rearing of their children. The CHAMPSA manual also encouraged families to provide an "adult protective shield" for their children by setting family rules, monitoring their whereabouts, and joining with neighbors to watch out for their children. Finally, the manual sought to relieve the participants' sense of "learned helplessness" from the HIV/AIDS epidemic in Durban, South Africa by teaching family members the "learned helpfulness" of being a major part of the solution to the epidemic. Subjects in the experimental condition had more knowledge about HIV/AIDS transmission and had less stigmatizing attitudes toward individuals with HIV/AIDS. Caregivers in the CHAMPSA prevention intervention significantly increased their monitoring of youth's activities and developed more family rules than those in the control group. The outcomes in experimental families illustrated increased frequency of care giving and comfort in communicating with youth about HIV/AIDS and other difficult subjects. Caregivers in the experimental condition reported less neighborhood disorganization and more social control and cohesion in their communities. Youth in the experimental CHAMPSA condition, who were 9–12 years old, had more knowledge about HIV/AIDS and had less stigmatizing attitudes toward individuals with HIV/AIDS than the control youth. Engaging indigenous community residents to recruit and retain experimental and control families and deliver the intervention resulted in a high retention rate. Similar to Chicago CHAMP, a significant number of families (94%) completed the entire CHAMPSA program. As the intervention began with young adolescents who had not made their sexual debut, CHAMPSA only has proximal outcomes. We have to wait for a longitudinal study to determine the long-term impact on sexual behavior and potential HIV infections.

2.6 Family-Based Teen Pregnancy Prevention Interventions

Another example of how family-based prevention interventions can change health behavior is in the area of teen pregnancy. As mentioned earlier, because different parts of the brain develop at different rates, teens are at risk for a variety of unhealthy sexual behaviors, such as early sexual debut and unsafe sex. Young pregnant teens are at risk for numerous health problems for their infants (e.g., preterm birth, intra-uterine growth retardation, and perinatal complications) (National Research Council and Institute of Medicine 2009). In addition, experience with teen pregnancy illustrates that pregnant teens are often "kicked out" of their family and society and shunned. Thus, they are often deprived of resources necessary to protect and nurture them and their infants. Although teenagers are heavily influenced by peers, their families continue to have influence on their behavior (Rai et al. 2003). Accordingly, family-based interventions have tried to decrease teenage pregnancy and the multiple, potential untoward consequences of having a child as a teen (see Guttmacher 2006). Furthermore, Bowlby (1969, 1973) and Ainsworth (1973) theorized that failure to form a secure attachment with caregivers during infancy has a strong influence on ability to form trusting relationships later in life. Thus, common sense dictates, if a teenage pregnancy is unavoidable, family-based interventions might help the teenage parents provide their infant with the attachment and connectedness necessary to form trusting relationships.

Teen pregnancies have been decreasing since 1991 (Guttmacher 2006). The National Research Council and Institute of Medicine (2009) notes that efficacious and effective family-based methods to prevent teenage pregnancy "remain elusive;" thus, the quality of this research needs strengthening. On the other hand, family-based interventions to increase maternal sensitivity and infant attachment are shown to be effective. A meta-analysis of 51 studies illustrates that interventions to increase maternal sensitivity were significantly and moderately effective ($p < 0.001$; effect size = 0.38) (Bakermans-Kranenburg et al. 2003). The meta-analysis by Bakermans-Kranenburg et al. (2003) of 23 studies illustrated that interventions to increase secure infant attachment had small effect sizes, but still important ($p < 0.05$; effect size = 0.20).

2.7 Family-Based Prevention Interventions Designed to Increase Connectedness and Attachment

As societies' understanding of the need for maternal sensitivity and fostering secure infant attachments has increased, more societal emphasis has been placed on this aspect of family life. Accordingly, there have been various widespread initiatives designed to increase maternal sensitivity and secure infant attachment. Nurse home visitation (Olds 2002), which teaches the social skill of parenting (i.e., understanding maternal sensitivity, attachment and connectedness, child development, etc.), has been repeatedly shown to foster pregnancies that have good outcomes. In addition to the parenting guidance designed to help children have nurturing early childhood environments, nurse home visitation programs also provide a number of other valuable family-based supports. Nurse home visitation programs provide social support, promotion of positive caregiver–child interactions, and direct social and health services (e.g., referrals to agencies for various services, including health and developmental screening) (Olds 2002). Sweet and Appelbaum (2004) conducted a meta-analysis of experimental and quasi-experimental evaluations of 60 home visiting programs. While it is clear that professional nurse home visitation has the best outcomes and effect size (compared to other mother/infant attachment approaches), programs to improve maternal sensitivity and secure infant attachment are still needed. (Zero to Three 2011). For example, "Zero To Three" offers a web-based, educational format to parents (Zero to Three 2011), and, although education, while essential, is not enough to significantly change behavior.

Early Head Start is designed to promote healthy prenatal outcomes by improving family functioning (Gray and Francis 2007). Early Head Start centers provide an excellent setting to implement family-based prevention interventions designed to increase connectedness and attachment between teen caregivers and infants (Stormshak et al. 2002). Started in 1994 and aimed at children 0–3, a major evaluation of "Early Head Start" by Love et al. (2005) found children in the program had significant improvements in cognitive and language development and social and emotional development. Compared to control children, "Early Head Start" children displayed higher parental emotional engagement, sustained attention with play objects, and were less aggressive. Compared to control parents, "Early Head Start" parents were more emotionally supportive, provided more language and learning, read to their children more and spanked less.

Finally, "Cradles to Classroom" (based on the philosophy of nurse home visitation) is a program that Paul Vallas, Chief Executive Officer, Chicago Public Schools, Philadelphia, and now New Orleans, has been implementing around the country with success (Bell et al. 2001; Lamberg 2003). This long-range prevention strategy teaches teenage mothers parenting skills needed to bond with and parent their babies and how to access community resources. Assuming a practical and resource-oriented philosophy, "Cradles to Classroom" provides counseling about domestic violence and access to prenatal, nutritional, medical, social, and childcare services. In 2002, of 495 seniors with babies, 100% graduated and 78% enrolled in a 2- or 4-year college and only five had a repeat pregnancy (Lamberg 2003).

Despite this success, when leadership changes, new programs are often initiated. Accordingly, the 2004 change in Chicago Public Schools leadership resulted in the initiation of the "Chicago KidStart Program" (a nurse home visitation program delivered by the Chicago Department of Public Health). This program services 17,000 young, at-risk mothers (Chicago KidStart 2008). As a subsystem of the "Chicago KidStart Program," "Cradle to Classroom," which serves more than 4,000 teen mothers, and the Ounce of Prevention Fund expanded pre-natal and post-natal services to asterisk teen mothers. One-on-one coaching (i.e., parent training on how to attach to their infants and guidance to understand child development) was provided to these mothers at three new sites in Chicago and will reach more than 300 mothers in the first year (Chicago KidStart 2008).

Clearly, the early theoretical propositions of Bowlby (1969, 1973) and Ainsworth (1973) (e.g., theories of attachment/separation) have been actualized in the academic study of Nurse Home Visitation by Olds (2002), and have been put into real world practice by "Zero to Three," "Early Head Start," and "Cradle to Classroom" programs.

2.8   Family-Based Child Abuse and Neglect
         Prevention Interventions

In 1999, the executive leadership team of Community Mental Health Council, Inc. got an opportunity to test the seven field principles through a large, naturalistic community-based demonstration project. Late that year, the Director of the Illinois Department of Children and Family Services (DCFS) informed us of a problem in McLean County. Early reports from McLean's DCFS office noted African-American children being removed from their families for abuse and neglect due to hotline calls was 35/1,000 (the statewide average was 4.3/1,000). Using a business model, CMHC's Executive Team strategically planned to apply Bell's seven field principles of health behavior change to this population-based problem (Redd et al. 2005). Two-year follow-up reports revealed that the number of African-American children being placed in foster care in McLean County had decreased to 11/1,000, while the hotline calls for abuse and neglect did not decrease. Furthermore, the rates of subsequent removal of children from families with unsubstantiated hotline calls were lower than the statewide average. Such efforts are important as they illustrate that theoretical paradigms, if implemented properly, have the potential to change individual outcomes in large population interventions. This project also spurred the development of innovative statistical methodology. This methodology gave some credence that the naturalistic prevention intervention that was implemented in McLean County was associated with few African-American children being removed from their families (Gibbons et al. 2007).

The McLean county intervention had the same core elements of community-based interventions found to be successful in a meta-analysis of 56 programs designed to promote family wellness and prevent child maltreatment (MacLeod and Nelson 2000). For instance, a "Family Advocates Program" achieved "rebuilding the village" by providing social support, parent training, childcare, community development, and in-home support programs for families that had been the focus of a DCFS hotline call (Redd et al. 2005). From their meta-analysis, MacLeod and Nelson (2000) concluded that most interventions that aim to promote family wellness and prevent child maltreatment are successful with an effect size of approximately 0.41.

2.9   Family-Based Aggression and Antisocial Behavior
         Prevention Interventions

There is extensive evidence that training interventions that emphasize behavioral parenting skills help families develop social and emotional skills. These skills are a potent preemptive tool in preventing youth from developing aggressive and antisocial behaviors (Mihalic et al. 2004; US DHHS 2001). Patterson's team has repeatedly shown that lack of parental monitoring, represented at its extreme by neglect and poor discipline methods and conflict about discipline, has been related to participation in delinquent and violent behavior for a range of populations (Patterson et al. 1989; Patterson and Stouthamer-Loeber 1984). Conversely, parenting with high levels of positive involvement with children and positive reinforcement of desirable behavior cultivates pro-social behavior. Similar to how the attachment theories of Bowlby (1969, 1973) and Ainsworth (1973) spawned interventions to improve attachment and bonding, Patterson et al.'s work (1989) has spawned numerous evidence-based interventions targeted at children in varying levels of development, e.g., the "Incredible Years" for young children (Webster-Stratton et al. 2001), "Strengthening Families Program" for early adolescence (Spoth et al. 2001), and "Multidimensional Treatment Foster Care" for adolescence (Chamberlain 1990; Chamberlain and Mihalic 1998). These programs teach and train parents to engage in behaviors that will reinforce positive connectedness between themselves and their children. The evidence is clear that parenting skills training to develop child management skills are efficacious (de Graaf et al. 2008; Kaminski et al. 2008).

2.10   Family-Based Substance Abuse Prevention Interventions

Ackard et al. (2006) note that adolescent perceptions of low parental caring, difficulty talking to their parents about problems, and overly valuing their friends' opinions for serious decisions were significantly associated with compromised behavioral and emotional health. Interventions aimed at improving the parent–child relationship may provide an avenue toward preventing health risk behaviors in youth. Brody et al. (2004, 2006a, b) have convincingly shown that their Strong African-American Families (SAAF) program increases protective factors preventing African-American adolescents from using drugs. SAAF, a family-based intervention positing "regulated, communicative parenting," causes changes in factors protecting youth from early alcohol use. Brody et al. (2004) proposed that parental variables (involvement-vigilance with children and their activities, racial socialization, communication about sex, and clear expectations for alcohol use) and youth variables (negative attitudes about early alcohol use and sexual activity, negative images of youth who drink, resistance efficacy, a goal-directed future orientation, and acceptance of parental influence) protect African-American youth from substance use/abuse. Brody et al. (2004) illustrate parents in the intervention group increases parental protective factors over a 7-month period. Brody's team performed a randomized prevention trial that included 667 African-American 11-year-old students and their caregivers (Brody et al. 2004, 2006a; Murry et al. 2005). According to adolescent reports, the 332 families who participated in SAAF, experienced increases over time in "regulated, communicative parenting." There were also increases in targeted parenting behaviors and lower rates of high-risk behavior initiation among youths (Brody et al. 2006a). In another study, Wills et al. (2007) tested a theoretical model of how ethnic pride and self-control are related to risk and protective factors. In this study the researchers interviewed a community sample of 670 African-American youth (mean age = 11.2 years) and measured cigarette smoking and alcohol use (lifetime to past month). The results of this study indicated that parenting was related to self-control and self-esteem, and racial socialization was related to ethnic pride. Self-control and self-esteem variables were related to levels of deviance-prone attitudes and to perceptions of those who engage or abstain from substance use. Thus, self-esteem and self-control are related to parenting approaches and have pathways to attitudes and social perceptions that are significant factors for predisposing to, or protecting against, early involvement in substance use. Further, in addition to preventing problems of substance abuse, SAAF has also been shown helpful in reducing conduct problems. Among youth who had more affiliations with deviance-prone peers, SAAF reduced the chances of engaging in conduct problems by 62% ($p < 0.01$) (Brody et al. 2008).

Family-based prevention interventions have also been show to prevent substance abuse in Hispanic adolescents. In addition to emphasizing improving family relationships (i.e., addressing family issues of conflict, inconsistent or inappropriate parenting, and parent–adolescent communication) which have been shown to prevent drug abuse in adolescents (Szapocznik and Murtines 1989), Structural Ecosystems Therapy (SET) also tackles familial interfaces with external systems (Szapocznik et al. 2004). SET emphasizes parental monitoring and supervision of peer activities and includes parental involvement in school. Thus, SET has demonstrated that the mere focus on family relationships is sufficient for reducing Hispanic adolescent drug use. Prevention interventions should also attend to exo-level structures (e.g., school) (Robbins et al. 2008).

2.11 Efforts to Move Research into Practice

Unfortunately, despite an increase in funding for children's mental health research, the US children's mental health infrastructure is not flourishing (Bell and McKay 2004; US DHHS 2000). While there have been several efforts at infusing modern technology into children's mental health systems (National Advisory Mental Health 1999; NECON 2005; President's New Freedom Commission on Mental Health 2003), these efforts have been stalled. In part, they have been stalled by a very strong anti-psychiatry push back (Bell 1996; Issac and Armat 1990) as well as an anti-government push back that did not want to see prevention programs from the government enter private lives (Paul 2008). Another reason such efforts are languishing is due to gaps in understanding how to transport, disseminate, and implement programs in various cultural and contextual settings while preserving sufficient program fidelity (National Research Council and Institute of Medicine 2009; Fixsen et al. 2005; Glasgow et al. 2003).

Bell (2008) points out that for an intervention to be culturally sensitive, it must have content that is welcoming to the target culture, contain issues of relevance to the culture, not be offensive, and be familiar to and endorsed by the target culture. However, if a given intervention has generic principles of health behavior change, such as aspects that create social fabric, generate connectedness, help develop social skills, build self-esteem, facilitate some social monitoring, and help minimize trauma (Bell et al. 2002), that intervention can usually be adapted to have an appropriate level of cultural sensitivity (Paruk et al. 2005; Bhana et al. 2004; Petersen et al. 2006; LaFromboise and Lewis 2008). In addition to the lack of knowledge of how to fit evidence-based interventions into culture and context, there are organizational dynamics (e.g., organizational culture that make it difficult to create change toward evidence-based practices in many service organizations) (Hoagwood et al. 2001; Kondrat et al. 2002; Redd et al. 2005; Rosenheck 2001).

There are several methods to help infuse science into service: (1) researcher-driven implementation, (2) adaptation of existing programs to the community done by researchers and community leaders, and (3) community-driven implementation. Unfortunately, very little braided state and Federal governmental support for focused family-based prevention infrastructure efforts (as opposed to scattered family-based prevention efforts) (e.g., occurring within education, juvenile justice, health and human services, foster care, law enforcement, mental health) are available (National Research Council and Institute of Medicine 2009).

2.11.1 Challenges for the Future

One of the National Institute of Mental Health's revised mission statement goals is to "Strengthen the Public Health Impact of NIMH-Supported Research" (US DHHS 2008). Accordingly, one of the major challenges for the future is to set up a monitoring system for NIMH grant funding awards that takes this goal seriously. One major method of accomplishing this goal is to ensure that adequate evaluation is done on family-based prevention interventions. In addition, there should be further development of the knowledge base that will support dissemination, adaptation, and implementation of evidence-based prevention interventions in various contexts and cultures. Many suggest that the cost effectiveness of family-based prevention interventions should be emphasized. This understanding will be an impetus to infuse research strategies designed to prevent mental and physical problems into practice. Time and experience have taught us to be less enamored by this strategy. Everyone knows it is cheaper to prevent a child from entering the criminal justice system by paying for the child's decent education. Despite the solidity of this cost-effective argument, the society continues to send more funds to juvenile justice systems than schools. One ostensible reason for this shortsighted behavior is that staff in juvenile justice systems and criminal justice facilities would rather be paid than send their revenues to schools. Accordingly, it is our view that until the science of prevention becomes so irrefutable that it becomes unethical not to spend money on youth's education, the criminal justice system will continue to profit from the nation's lack of prevention. After all, despite the cost-effective arguments of giving or not giving polio shots, it would be unethical not to prevent polio – using vaccines.

Finally, North America is in a "health care crisis" because we have an "illness care system," thus, our "illness care crisis." The only way to relieve ourselves of this challenge is to strengthen our mental health prevention and promotion practices. We need to use business models and technology to sell mental health prevention and promotion practices as we sell soap. We need to support more researcher-driven implementation, adaptation of existing programs to the community done by researchers and community leaders, and community-driven implementation. We can shorten the health disparities gap and resolve the "illness care crisis" by implementing the new NRC and IOM prevention report's recommendations (National Research Council and Institute of Medicine 2009). We are hopeful the new Obama White House will understand this necessity and move forward on this initiative with the same "Yes, we can" spirit of the most recent election.

References

Ainsworth MDS. The development of infant-mother attachment. In: Caldwell BM, Ricciuti HN, editors. Review of child development research, vol. 3. Chicago: University of Chicago Press; 1973. p. 1–95.

Ackard DM, Neumark-Sztainer D, Story M, Perry C. Parent-child connectedness and behavioral and emotional health among adolescents. American Journal of Preventive Medicine. 2006;30(1):59–66.

Bakermans-Kranenburg MJ, Van IJzendoorn MH, Juffer F. Less is more: meta-analyses of sensitivity and attachment interventions in early childhood. Psychol Bull. 2003;129:195–215.

Bannon WM, McKay MM. Addressing urban African American youth externalizing and social problem behavioral difficulties in a family oriented prevention project. In: McKay MM, Paikoff RL, editors. Community collaborative partnerships: the foundation for HIV prevention research efforts. Binghamton, NY: Haworth; 2007.

Baptiste DR, Bhana A, Petersen I, McKay M, Voisin D, Bell C, et al. Community collaborative youth-focused HIV/AIDS prevention in South Africa and Trinidad: preliminary findings. J Pediatr Psychol. 2006;31(9):905–16.

Barbarin O. Mental health screening of preschool children: validity and reliability of ABLE. Am J Orthopsychiatr. 2007;77(3):402–18.

Baumrind D. Effects of authoritative parental control on child behavior. Child Dev. 1966;37(4):887–907.

Bell CC, Bhana A, McKay MM, Petersen I. A commentary on the Triadic Theory of Influence as a guide for adapting HIV prevention programs for new contexts and populations: The CHAMP-South Africa story. In: McKay MM, Paikoff RI, editors. Community collaborative partnerships: The foundation for HIV prevention research efforts. Binghamton, NY: Haworth; 2007. p. 243–61.

Bell CC, Bhana A, Petersen I, McKay MM, Gibbons R, Bannon W, et al. Building protective factors to offset sexually risky behaviors among black South African youth: a randomized control trial. J Nat Med Assoc. 2008;100(8):936–44.

Bell CC. Cultivating resiliency in youth. J Adolesec Health. 2001;29:375–81.

Bell CC, Flay B, Paikoff R. Strategies for Health Behavioral Change. In: Chunn J, (ed.). The health behavioral change imperative: theory, education, and practice in diverse populations. New York: Kluwer Academic/Plenum Publishers; 2002. p.17–40.

Bell CC, Jenkins EJ. Traumatic stress and children. J Health Care Poor Underserved. 1991;2(1):175–88.

Bell CC, McKay MM. Constructing a children's mental health infrastructure using community psychiatry principles. J Legal Med. 2004;25(1):5–22.

Bell CC. Preventive strategies for dealing with violence among Blacks. Commun Mental Health J. 1987;23(3):217–28.

Bell CC. Should culture considerations influence early intervention? In: Ursano R, Blumenfield M, editors. Early psychological intervention following Mass Trauma: present and future directions. UK: Cambridge University Press; 2008. p. 127–48.

Bell CC. Taking issue: pimping the African-American community. Psychiatr Ser. 1996; 47(8):1025.

Bell CC, Vallas P, Gamm S, Jackson P. Strategies for the prevention of youth violence in chicago public schools. In: Shafii M, Shafii S, editors. School violence: contributing factors, management, and prevention. Washington, DC: American Psychiatric Press; 2001. p. 251–72.

Bhana A, Petersen I, Mason A, Mahintsho Z, Bell CC, McKay M. Children and youth at risk: adaptation and pilot study of the CHAMP (*Amaqhawe*) programme in South Africa. Afr J AIDS Res (AJAR). 2004;3(1):33–41.

Biglan A, Metzler CW, Wirt R, Ary D, Noell J, Ochs LL, et al. Social and behavioral factors associated with high-risk sexual behaviors among adolescents. J Behav Med. 1990;13:245–61.

Blanchard LT, Gurka MJ, Blackman JA. Emotional, developmental, and behavioral health of American children and their families: A report from the 2003 National Survey of Children's Health. Pediatrics. 2006;117:1202–12. Available via: http://www.pediatrics.org/cgi/content/full/117/6/e1202. Accessed 6 April 2011.

Bowlby J. Attachment and loss: Vol. 1. Attachment. New York: Basic Books; 1969.

Bowlby J. Attachment and loss: Vol. 2. Separation – anxiety and anger. New York: Basic Books; 1973.

Brody GH, Ge X, Conger R, Gibbons FX, Murry VM, Gerrard M, et al. The influence of neighborhood disadvantage, collective socialization, and parenting on African American children's affiliation with deviant peers. Child Dev. 2001;72(4):1231–46.

Brody GH, Dorsey S, Forehand R, Armistead L. Unique and protective contributions of parenting and classroom processes to the adjustment of African American children living in single-parent families. Child Dev. 2002;73(1):274–86.

Brody GH, Kim S, Murry VM, Brown AC. Longitudinal direct and indirect pathways linking older sibling competence to the development of younger sibling competence. Dev Psychol. 2003;39(3):618–28.

Brody GH, Murry VM, Gerrard M, Gibbons FX, Molgaard V, McNair L, et al. The Strong African American Families Program: translating research into prevention programming. Child Dev. 2004;75:900–17.

Brody GH, Murry VM, McNair L, Chen Y, Gibbons FX, Gerrard M, et al. Linking changes in parenting to parent child relationship quality and youth self control. J Res Adolesce. 2005;15:47–69.

Brody GH, Murry VM, Gerrard M, Gibbons FX, McNair L, Brown AC, et al. The Strong African American Families Program: prevention of high-risk behaviors and a test of a model of change. J Family Psychol. 2006a;20:1–11.

Brody GH, Murry VM, Kogan SM, Gerrard M, Gibbons FX, Brown AC, et al. The Strong African American Families Program: a cluster-randomized prevention trial of long-term effects and a mediational model. J Consult Clin Psychol. 2006b;74:356–66.

Brody GH, Kogan SM, Chen Y, Murry VM. Long-term effects of the Strong African American Families Program on youths' conduct disorders. J Adolesc Health. 2008;43:474–81.

Chamberlain P. Comparative evaluation of specialized foster care for seriously delinquent youths: a first step. Community Alternatives. Int J Family Care. 1990;2:21–36.

Chamberlain P, Mihalic SF. Blueprints for violence prevention, book eight: multidimensional treatment foster care. Boulder, CO: Center for the Study and Prevention of Violence; 1998.

Chicago: KidStart. Available via: http://www.chicagokidstart.org/General/kidstart/earlyLearning. htm. Cited 6 April 2011.

Costello EJ, Mustillo S, Erkanli A, Keeler G, Angold A. Prevalence and development of psychiatric disorders in childhood and adolescence. Arch Gen Psychiatr. 2003;60:837–44.

de Graaf I, Speetjens P, Smit F, de Wolff M, Tavecchio L. Effectiveness of the Triple P Positive Parenting Program on behavioral problems in children: a meta-analysis. Behav Modif. 2008;32(5):714–35.

Dey AN, Bloom B. Summary health statistics for U.S. children: National Health Interview Survey, 2003. National Center for Health Statistics. Vital Health Stat. 2004;10:1–78.

DiIorio C, McCarty F, Resnicow K, Lehr S, Denzmore P. REAL Men: a group-randomized trial of an HIV prevention intervention for adolescent boys. Am J Pub Health. 2007;97(6):1084–9.

Division of Adult and Community Health, National Center for Chronic Disease Prevention and Health Promotion. Adverse Childhood Experiences (ACE) Study (2008) Available via: http://www.cdc.gov/NCCDPHP/ACE/. Cited 6 April 2011.

Donenberg GR, Wilson HW, Emerson E, Bryant FB. Holding the line with a watchful eye: the impact of perceived parental permissiveness and parental monitoring on risky sexual behavior among adolescents in psychiatric care. AIDS Educ Prevent. 2002;14(2):138–57.

Donenberg GR, Bryant FB, Emerson E, Wilson HW, Pasch KE. Tracing the roots of early sexual debut among adolescents in psychiatric care. J Am Acad Child Adolesc Psychiatr. 2003;42(5):594–608.

Eaton DK, Kann L, Kinchen S, Ross J, Hawkins J, Harris WA, et al. Youth Risk Behavior Surveillance–United States, 2005. Atlanta, Ga: Centers for Disease Control and Prevention, 2006;55(SS05):1–108.

Farrington DP. Early predictors of adolescent aggression and adult violence. Violence and Victims. 1989;4:79–100.

Felitti VJ, Anda RF, Nordenberg D, Williamson DF, Spitz AM, Edwards V, et al. Relationship of Child Abuse and Household Dysfunction to Many of the Leading Causes of Death in Adults – The Adverse Childhood Experiences (ACE) Study. Am J Prev Med. 1998;14(4):245–58.

Fixsen DL, Naoom SF, Blasé KA, Friedman RM, Wallace F. Implementation Research: A Synthesis of the Literature. FHMI pub no 23. Tampa, Florida: University of South Florida, Louis de la Parte Florida Mental Health Institute, the National Implementation Research Network; 2005.

Flay BR, Graumlich S, Segawa E, Burns J, Amuwo S, Bell CC, et al. The ABAN AYA Youth Project: effects of comprehensive prevention programs on high-risk behaviors among inner city African American youth: a randomized trial. Arch Pediatr Adolesc Med. 2004;158(4):377–84.

Gray R, Francis E. The implications of US experiences with early childhood interventions for the UK Sure Start Programme. Child Care Health Development. 2007;33(6):655–63.

Gibbons RD, Hur K, Bhaumik DK, Bell CC. Profiling of county-level foster care placements using random-effects poisson regression models. Health Service Outcomes Res Methodol. 2007;7(3–4):97–108.

Glasgow RE, Lichtenstein E, Marcus AC. Why don't we see more translation of health promotion research to practice? Rethinking the efficacy-to-effectiveness transition. Am J Pub Health. 2003;93:1261–7.

Goldsmith SK, Pellmar TC, Kleinman AM, Bunney WE, editors. Reducing suicide: a national imperative. Washington, DC: National Academy Press; 2002.

Gorman-Smith D, Tolan PH, Zelli A, Huesmann LR. The relation of family functioning to violence among inner-city minority youths. J Family Psychol. 1996;10:115–29.

Guevara JP, Mandell DS, Rostain AL, Zhao H, Hadley TR. National estimates of health services expenditures for children with behavioral disorders: an analysis of the Medical Expenditure Panel Survey. Pediatrics. 2003;112:440–6.

Guttmacher Institute. Facts on American Teens' Sexual and Reproductive Health. New York: Guttmacher Institute, 2006. Available via: http://www.guttmacher.org/pubs/fb_ATSRH.pdf. Cited 6 April 2011.

Henggeler SW, Melton GB, Smith LA. Family preservation using multi systemic therapy: an effective alternative to incarcerating serious juvenile offenders. J Consult Clin Psychol. 1992;60:953–61.

Hoagwood K, Burns BJ, Kiser L, Ringeisen H, Schoenwald SK. Evidence-based practice in child and adolescent mental health services. Psychiatr Ser. 2001;52:1179–89.

Issac RJ, Armat UC. Madness in the streets: how psychiatry and the law abandoned the Mentally Ill. New York: Free Press; 1990.

Jaccard J, Dittus PJ, Gordon VV. Parent–adolescent congruency in reports of adolescents' sexual behavior and in communication about sexual behavior. Child Dev. 1998;69:247–61.

Jemmott JB, Jemmott LS, Braverman PK, Fong GT. HIV/STD risk reduction interventions for African American and Latino adolescent girls at an adolescent medicine clinic: a randomized controlled trial. Arch Pediatr Adolesc Med. 2005;159:440–9.

Jenkins EJ, Bell CC. Exposure and response to community violence among children and adolescents. In: Osofsky J, editor. Children in a violent society. New York: Guilford Press; 1997. p. 9–31.

Joe S, Baser RE, Breeden G, Neighbors HW, Jackson JS. Prevalence of and risk factors for lifetime suicide attempts among blacks in the United States. J Am Med Assoc. 2006;296:2112–23.

Kaminski JW, Valle LA, Filene JH, Boyle CL. A meta-analytic review of components associated with parent training program effectiveness. J Abnorm Child Psychol. 2008;36(4):567–89.

Kann L, Kinchen SA, Williams BI, Ross JG, Lowry R, Hill CV, et al. Youth Risk Behavior Surveillance – United States, 1997. State and Local YRBSS Coordinators. J School Health. 1998;68(9):355–69.

Kessler RC, Berglund P, Demler O, Jin R, Merikangas KR, Walters EE. Lifetime prevalence and age-of-onset distributions of DSM-IV disorders in the National Comorbidity Survey Replication. Arch Gen Psychiatr. 2005;62(6):593–602.

Kondrat ME, Greene GJ, Winbush GB. Using benchmarking research to locate agency best practices for African-American clients. Admin Policy Mental Health. 2002;29(6):495–518.

Krauss B, Goldstat L, Bula E. Parent-preadolescent communication about HIV in a high seroprevalence neighborhood. In: Sigman M (Chair), Mother-adolescent communication about sexuality and AIDS. Paper presented at symposium conducted at the Society for Research in Child Development Biennial Meeting, Washington, DC; 1997. unpublished.

LaFromboise TD, Lewis HA. The Zuni life skills development program: a school/community-based suicide prevention intervention. Suicide Life Threat Behav. 2008;38(3):343–53.

Lamberg L. Programs target youth violence prevention. J Am Med Assoc. 2003;290(5):585–6.

Lee, M.B., Lester, P., & Rotheram-Borus, J.J., The relationship between adjustment of mothers with HIV and their adolescent daughters. Clinical Child Psychology and Psychiatry. (2002); 7(1):171–84.

Love JM, Kisker EE, Ross CM, Constantine J, Boller K, Chazan-Cohen R, et al. The effectiveness of early head start for 3-year-old children and their parents: lessons for policy and programs. Dev Psychol. 2005;41(6):885–901.

MacLeod J, Nelson G. Programs for the promotion of family wellness and the prevention of child maltreatment: a meta-analytic review. Child Abuse Neglect. 2000;24(9):1127–49.

Madison S, McKay MM, Paikoff R, Bell CC. Basic research and community collaboration: necessary ingredients for the development of a family-based HIV prevention program. AIDS Educ Prevent. 2000;12(4):281–98.

Mash E. Child psychopathology: a developmental systems perspective. In: Mash EJ, Barkley RA, editors. Child psychopathology. 2nd ed. New York: The Guilford Press; 2003. p. 3–71.

McBride CK, Baptiste D, Paikoff RL, Madison-Boyd S, Coleman D, Bell CC. Family-Based HIV Preventive Intervention: Child Level Results from the CHAMP Family Program. In: McKay MM, Paikoff RL, editors. Community collaborative partnerships: the foundation for HIV prevention research efforts. Binghamton, NY: Haworth Press; 2007. p. 203–20.

McCormick A, McKay MM, Wilson M, McKinney L, Paikoff R, Bell C, et al. Involving families in an urban HIV prevention intervention: how community collaboration addresses barriers to participation. AIDS Educ Prevent. 2000;12(4):299–307.

McDermott PA, Weiss RV. A normative typology of healthy, subclinical, and clinical behavior styles among American children and adolescents. Psychol Assess. 1995;7:162–70.

McKay MM, Paikoff RL, editors. Community collaborative partnerships: the foundation for HIV prevention research efforts. Binghamton, NY: Haworth Press; 2007.

McKay MM, Chasse KT, Paikoff R, McKinney LD, Baptiste D, Coleman D, et al. Family-level impact of the CHAMP family program: a community collaborative effort to support urban families and reduce youth HIV risk exposure. Family Proc. 2004;43(1):79–93.

McKay MM, Block M, Mellins C, Traube DE. Adapting a family-based HIV prevention program for HIV-infected preadolescents and their families: Youth, families and health care providers coming together to address complex needs. In: McKay MM, Paikoff RI, editors. Community collaborative partnerships: the foundation for HIV prevention research efforts. Binghamton, NY: Haworth Press; 2007a. p. 349–72.

McKay MM, Hibbert R, Lawrence R, Miranda A, Paikoff R, Bell CC, et al. Creating mechanisms for meaningful collaboration between members of Urban communities and university-based HIV prevention researchers. In: McKay MM, Paikoff RL, editors. Community collaborative partnerships: The foundation for HIV prevention research efforts. Binghamton, NY: Haworth Press; 2007b. p. 147–68.

Mihalic S, Fagan A, Irwin K, Ballard D, Elliott D. Blueprints for Violence Prevention. Washington, DC: Office of Juvenile Justice and Delinquency Prevention, 2004. NCJ 204274.

Murry VM, Brody GH, McNair LD, Luo Z, Gibbons FX, Gerrard M, et al. Parental involvement promotes rural African American youths' self-pride and sexual self-concepts. J Marriage Family. 2005;67(3):627–42.

National Advisory Mental Health Council. Bridging Science and Service: A Report by the National Advisory Mental Health Council's Clinical Treatment and Services Research Workgroup. NIH pub no 99–4353. Rockville, MD, National Institute of Mental Health; 1999.

National Research Council and Institute of Medicine. Preventing mental, emotional, and behavioral disorders among young people: progress and possibilities. Washington, DC: National Research Council; 2009.

NECON (The New England Coalition for Health Promotion and Disease Prevention). Prevention Works – Proceedings of a New England Regional Conference on Evidence-Based Programs for the Promotion of Mental Health and Prevention of Mental and Substance Abuse Disorders. Providence, RI: New England Coalition for Health Promotion and Disease Prevention (NECON), 2005. Available via: www.neconinfo.org/04-26-2004_Proceedings.pdf. Cited 6 April 2011.

Office of Applied Studies. National Survey on Drug Use and Health. Washington, DC: US Department of Health and Human Services Substance Abuse and Mental Health Services Administration, 2003. Web site. Available via: www.oas.samhsa.gov/nhsda/2k3nsduh/2k3Results.htm. Cited 7 April 2011.

Olds DL. Prenatal and infancy home visiting by nurses: from randomized trials to community replication. Prevent Sci. 2002;3(3):153–72.

Paikoff RL, Early heterosexual debut: Situations of sexual possibility. American Journal of Orthopsychiatry. 1995;65(3):389–401.

Paikoff RL. Adapting developmental research to intervention design: applying developmental psychology to an AIDS prevention model for urban African American Youth. J Negro Educ. 1997;65(1):44–59.

Paikoff RL, Traube DE, McKay MM. Overview of community collaborative partnerships and empirical findings: The Foundation for Youth HIV Prevention. In: McKay MM, Paikoff RL, editors. Community collaborative partnerships: The foundation for HIV prevention research effort. Binghamton, NY: Haworth Press; 2007. p. 3–26.

Paruk Z, Petersen I, Bhana A, Bell C, McKay M. Containment and contagion: how to strengthen families to support youth HIV prevention in South Africa. Afr J AIDS Res. 2005;4(1):57–63.

Patterson GR, Stouthamer-Loeber M. The correlation of family management practices and delinquency. Child Dev. 1984;55(4):1299–307.

Patterson GR, DeBaryshe BD, Ramsey E. A developmental perspective on antisocial behavior. Am Psychol. 1989;44(2):329–35.

Paul R Don't Let Congress Fund Orwellian Psychiatric Screening of Kids. Texas Straight Talk, 2008. Available via: http://www.ronpaullibrary.org/document.php?id=394. Cited 27 November 2008.

Pequegnat W, Bray J. Families and HIV/AIDS: introduction to the special sections. J Family Psychol. 1997;11(1):3–10.

Pequegnat W, Stover E. Behavioral prevention is today's AIDS vaccine! AIDS. 2000;14 Suppl 2:S1–7.

Pequegnat W, Szapocznik J. Working with families in the era of HIV/AIDS. Thousand Oaks, CA: Sage Publications; 2000.

Petersen I, Mason A, Bhana A, Bell C, McKay M. Mediating social representations using targeted micro media in the form a cartoon narrative in the context of HIV/AIDS: The AmaQhawe Family Project (CHAMP) in South Africa. Journal of Health Psychology. 2006;11(2):197–208.

Prado G, Pantin H, Schwartz SJ, Feaster D, Huang S, Sullivan S, et al. A randomized controlled trial of a parent-centered intervention in preventing substance use and HIV risk behaviors in Hispanic adolescents. J Consult Clin Psychol. 2007;75(6):914–26.

President's New Freedom Commission on Mental Health. Achieving the Promise: Transforming Mental Health Care in America (DHHS Publication No. SMA-03-3832). Rockville, MD: Substance Abuse and Mental Health Services Administration, 2003. Available via: http://www.mentalhealthcommission.gov. Cited 6 April 2011.

Rai AA, Stanton B, Wu Y, Li X, Galbraith J, Cottrell L, et al. Relative influences of perceived parental monitoring and perceived peer involvement on adolescent risk behaviors: an analysis of six cross-sectional data sets. J Adolesc Health. 2003;33:108–18.

Redd J, Suggs H, Gibbons R, Muhammad L, McDonald J, Bell CC. A plan to strengthen systems and reduce the number of African-American children in child welfare. Illinois Child Welfare. 2005;2(1 and 2):34–46.

Resnick M, Bearman P, Blum R, Bauman KE, Harris KM, Jones J, et al. Protecting adolescents from harm: findings from the National Longitudinal Study on Adolescent Health. J Am Med Assoc. 1997;278:823–32.

Robbins MA, Szapocznik J, Dillon FR, Turner CW, Mitrani VB, Feaster DJ. The efficacy of structural ecosystems therapy with drug-abusing/dependent African American and Hispanic American adolescents. J Family Psychol. 2008;22(1):51–61.

Rosenheck RA. Organizational process: a missing link between research and practice. Psychiatr Ser. 2001;52:1607–12.

Sampson RJ, Raudenbush SW, Earls F. Neighborhoods and violent crime: a multilevel study of collective efficacy. Science. 1997;277:918–24.

Schor EL. Family pediatrics: Report of the American Academy of Pediatrics Task Force on the Family. Pediatrics. 2003;111:1541–71.

Spoth R, Redmond C, Shin C. Randomized trial of brief family interventions for general populations: adolescent substance use outcomes 4 years following baseline. J Consult Clin Psychol. 2001;69:627–42.

Stormshak EA, Kaminski RA, Goodman MR. Enhancing the parenting skills of Head Start families during the transition to kindergarten. Prevent Sci. 2002;3(3):223–34.

Sweet MA, Appelbaum MI. Is home visiting an effective strategy? A meta-analytic review of home visiting programs for families with young children. Child Dev. 2004;75(5):1435–56.

Szapocznik J, Feaster DJ, Mitrani VB, Prado G, Smith L, Robinson-Batista C, et al. Structural ecosystems therapy for HIV-seropositive African American women: effects on psychological distress, family hassles and family support. J Consult Clin Psychol. 2004;72(2):288–303.

Szapocznik J, Murtines WM. Breakthroughs in family therapy with drug abusing problem youth. New York: Springer; 1989.

Tolan PH, Lorion RP. Multivariate approaches to the identification of delinquency-proneness in males. Am J Commun Psychol. 1988;16:547–61.

US Department of Health and Human Services (US DHHS). Mental Health: A Report of the Surgeon General–Executive Summary. Rockville, MD: US DHHS; 1999.

US DHHS. Healthy people 2010. Washington, DC: US DHHS; 2000.

US DHHS. National Institute of Mental Health Strategic Plan. Washington, DC: National Institutes of Health NIH Publication No. 08–6368; 2008.

US DHHS. Youth Violence: A Report of the Surgeon General. Rockville, Maryland: US DHHS; 2001.

US Public Health Service. Report of the Surgeon General's Conference on Children's Mental Health: A National Action Agenda. Washington, DC: US DHHS; 2000.

US Surgeon. General Surgeon General's Workshop on Making Prevention of Child Maltreatment a National Priority: Implementating Innovations of a Public Health Approach, 2005. Available via: http://www.surgeongeneral.gov/topics/childmaltreatment/. Cited 6 April 2011.

Webster-Stratton C, Mihalic S, Fagan A, Arnold D, Taylor T, Tingley C. The incredible years series. In: Elliott DS, editor. Blueprints for violence prevention: Book 11. Boulder, CO: Center for the Study and Prevention of Violence, Institute of Behavioral Science, University of Colorado at Boulder; 2001.

Wills TA, Gibbons FX, Gerrard M, Murry VM, Brody GH. Family communication and religiosity related to substance use and sexual behavior in early adolescence: a test for pathways through self-control and prototype perceptions. Psychol Addict Behav. 2003;17(4):312–23.

Wills TA, Murry VM, Brody GH, Gibbons FX, Gerrard M, Walker C, et al. Ethnic pride and self-control related to protective and risk factors: test of the theoretical model for the strong African American families program. Health Psychol. 2007;26(1):50–9.

Wilson HW, Donenberg G. Quality of parent communication about sex and its relationship to risky behavior among youth in psychiatric care: a pilot study. J Child Psychol Psychiatr. 2004;45(2): 387–95.

Yang H, Stanton B, Li X, Cottrel L, Galbraith J, Kaljee L. Dynamic association between parental monitoring and communication and adolescent risk involvement among African–American adolescents. J Natl Med Assoc. 2007;99(5):517–24.

Zero to Three. Zero to Three, 2011. http://www.zerotothree.org. Accessed 6 April 2011.

Chapter 3
The Role of Settings in Family Based Prevention of HIV/STDs

Scott C. Brown, Kathryn Flavin, Sheila Kaupert, Maria Tapia, Guillermo Prado, Ikkei Hirama, Gabriel Lopez, Nicole Cano, and Hilda Pantin

Abstract This chapter provides a broad overview of the role of setting in family based prevention. This chapter has several related goals: First, we provide a brief overview of the ecodevelopmental model. Second, we explore the existing empirical literature providing evidence to support how specific settings may present risk or protection for HIV/STDs for individuals within a family, using the framework of the ecodevelopmental model. The settings to be explored in this chapter include the home, school, neighborhood, church, and substance abuse treatment settings. Finally, for each setting we provide examples illustrating which aspects of settings may be most important for conducting HIV/STD family based preventive interventions.

3.1 Introduction

This chapter examines the role of settings and contextual factors in family based prevention for HIV and other sexually transmitted diseases (STDs). Both the role of risk and/or protective factors of settings on individuals in a family, and the potential impact of family based preventive interventions on settings are discussed (e.g., Perrino et al. 2000; Pantin et al. 2003, 2009; Prado et al. 2007; McBride-Murry et al. 2011). More specifically, the focus is on those settings most applicable to adolescents – an age group at high risk of developing HIV/STD risk behaviors (Centers for Disease Control and Prevention (CDC) 2007; DiClemente et al. 2004; Jemmott et al. 2005, 2010; Perrino et al. 2000).

There is consensus (Lescano et al. 2009; Coatsworth et al. 2002; Poundstone et al. 2004) that individuals do not operate in isolation with regard to risk or protection for certain health outcomes, including acquiring HIV/STDs. Rather, individuals are embedded within various settings (e.g., home, school, neighborhood,

W. Pequegnat and C.C. Bell (eds.), *Family and HIV/AIDS: Cultural and Contextual Issues in Prevention and Treatment*, DOI 10.1007/978-1-4614-0439-2_3, © Springer Science+Business Media, LLC 2012

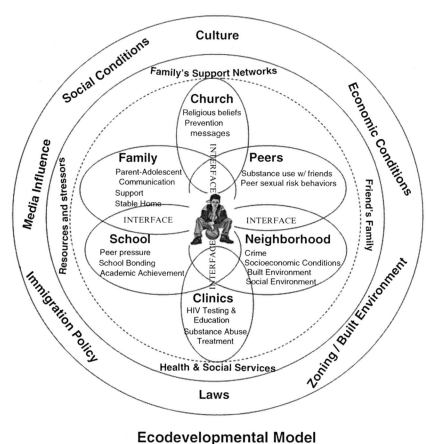

Fig. 3.1 Ecodevelopmental model of the relationship of settings to adolescents' HIV/STD risk

church, substance abuse treatment clinic) within which individuals interact, to influence behaviors and health over time (see Fig. 3.1). The ecodevelopmental model (Pantin et al. 2004) provides a framework for understanding these contexts and their associated risk and/or protection for behaviors which may lead to HIV/STDs. For the purpose of this chapter, HIV/STD risk encompasses a number of related behaviors (Santelli et al. 2000; Hallfors et al. 2007), which include alcohol use/abuse (Murphy et al. 2009; Rashad and Kaestner 2004), drug use/abuse (Sorensen et al. 2007; Morrill et al. 2001), conduct problems (Bachanas et al. 2002), school dropout (Edgardh 2002), having antisocial friends (who engage in unsafe sex, delinquency, or substance use) (Doljanac and Zimmerman 1998; McMahon 2000), early onset of sexual behavior (Kotchick et al. 2001; Boyer et al. 2000), risky sexual behavior (Bachanas et al. 2002; Kotchick et al. 2001), and a history of HIV or other STDs (Fleming and Wasserheit 1999).

This chapter has several related goals. First, we provide a brief overview of the ecodevelopmental model. Second, we explore the existing empirical literature providing evidence to support how specific settings may present risk or protection for HIV/STDs for individuals within a family, using the framework of the ecodevelopmental model. The settings to be explored in this chapter include the home, school, neighborhood, church, and substance abuse treatment settings. Finally, for each setting we provide examples illustrating which aspects of settings may be most important for conducting HIV/STD family based preventive interventions.

3.2   Ecodevelopmental Model

A range of factors in an individual's social ecology determine the individual's likelihood of engaging in unsafe sexual behavior, alcohol use, drug use, and related behaviors, which can lead to an increased risk for and HIV/STDs (Kotchick et al. 2001; Miller et al. 2000). Ecodevelopmental theory emphasizes the impacts of social contextual influences on the individual's behaviors and health over time by integrating social–ecological and developmental theories. The first element is comprised of the multiple social contexts which influence adolescent development, structured along four levels: (1) microsystems (contexts in which the adolescent participates directly); (2) mesosystems (interactions among important members of the different contexts in which the adolescent participates directly); (3) exosystems (contexts that indirectly affect members of the individual's life); and (4) macrosystems (the broad social and philosophical ideals that define a particular culture).

The second element, the developmental perspective, is applied to individuals and their social context. Both individuals and their contexts develop and change throughout the life span and are subject to broad social and historical influences. The third element, social interactions, involves the risks and protective processes that are manifested in the patterns of relationships among individuals within and across the different contextual levels of the social ecology.

Ecodevelopmental theory (e.g., Pantin et al. 2004; Szapocznik and Coatsworth 1999) postulates that the processes that may either increase risk for or protect against HIV/STDs are located at varying distances from the individual. For example, at the microsystem level, there are proximal factors such as parent–adolescent communication in a family/home setting and peer dynamics in a school or neighborhood setting. These communications have direct effects on adolescents. At the mesosystem level (represented in Fig. 3.1 by the overlapping of the "petals" in the center of the diagram) there are factors such as teachers' communications with parents (reflecting an interaction between the family and school) as well as parents' monitoring of their children's friends (reflecting interactions between the family and peers), both of which may influence adolescents' HIV/STD risk behaviors. At the exosystem level, factors such as the amount of social support that a parent receives, or friends' interactions with their family members may indirectly influence an adolescents' risk through their impact on important members of the adolescent's life (parents and peers). Finally, at the macrosystem level, the individual is influenced by factors such as media and social norms. These risk factors do not operate in isolation; they interact with one another and can amplify effects. Thus, an understanding of factors in the macrosystem is essential to address the multiple risk and protective processes. When supported by a strong evidence base, this framework can be used to develop interventions to reduce and prevent HIV risk behaviors.

3.3   Settings or Physical and Social Environments

This section focuses on the microsystem level (i.e., those factors that affect the individual family members directly). These factors include the physical environment which refers to the structural aspects of an individual's surroundings that are made by human beings (e.g., aspects of a neighborhood, such as the design of buildings, blocks, and neighborhoods). Settings are places where activities occur in a physical environment; some structures are built for that purpose and others are retrofitted to permit those activities. Depending on the design of the built environment, different types of social interactions may occur that elicit more risky behaviors. The settings that we are focusing on are homes, schools, neighborhoods, churches, and substance abuse treatment clinics (Srinivasan et al. 2003).

Certain characteristics of the built environment have been associated with opportunities for physical activity (e.g., walking, jogging, and cycling), such as stores near homes, accessible parks, and walking and bicycle paths that are well maintained rather than deteriorating (IOM/TRB 2005). Having places to walk has been linked to greater physical activity among residents, including adolescents (IOM/TRB 2005; Saelens et al. 2003; Frank et al. 2007), as well as facilitating supportive social processes in the neighborhood (Leyden 2003).

Emerging evidence suggests that certain built environment characteristics linked to physical activity may be related to drug and alcohol use (Collingwood et al. 2000; Collins et al. 2005; Raj et al. 2009). For example, residents living in neighborhoods characterized by "poorer" aesthetic qualities and dilapidation (e.g., buildings with peeling paint, broken windows, and stairway problems) are more likely to report heavy drinking than residents living in more well-maintained built environments (Bernstein et al. 2007). A further study found that the association between income inequality and rate of drug overdose mortality in New York City was mediated by the quality of the built environment in the neighborhood (Nandi et al. 2006). Physical activity may also potentially serve as a pathway to reductions in some sexual risk-tasking behaviors (Miller et al. 2002); however, further research is needed.

One possible interpretation of this pattern of findings is that a deteriorating built environment may be equated with perceived danger, which may deter individuals from engaging in pedestrian activity in the area surrounding their homes (Hembree et al. 2005). This may lead to less social interaction and a reduced sense of social cohesion among residents, or lack of informal social control regarding deviant behaviors (Sampson et al. 1997), which in turn may increase HIV/STD risk at the neighborhood level (Collins et al. 2005; Raj et al. 2009).

Accumulating evidence has also identified an association between the built environment and STDs. Cohen et al. (2000) examined the relationship between gonorrhea levels and the aesthetics of the built environment, such as dilapidated buildings and boarded-up housing. A "broken windows" index (summing properties of structural or cosmetic damage, street litter, and graffiti) was used to measure neighborhood deterioration; high "broken-windows scores" were associated with higher levels of gonorrhea. This broken-windows index was found to account for more variance in gonorrhea levels than did other sociodemographic factors (e.g., income, unemployment, low education). The investigators suggest that a deteriorating built environment with a high broken-windows index may be a marker for a neighborhood where adherence to rules and regulations is low and deviant behaviors are ignored by residents. In such neighborhood environments, there may be little or no surveillance of truancy, vandalism, or illegal behaviors. Furthermore, boarded-up or vacant structures may create an environment where youth go unsupervised, leaving greater opportunities to participate in risky behaviors (see also Nandi et al. 2006).

Other built environment characteristics – such as mixed land use – may play a protective role against HIV/STD risk behaviors, by providing destinations for walking as well as monitoring of the neighborhood (e.g., by storekeepers, people at home during the day, postal delivery persons, police) (Jacobs 1992). For example, Ford and Beveridge (2004) reported that neighborhoods with the highest levels of visible drug sales had significantly less mixed use than those with lower levels of visible drug sales. Similarly, Szapocznik et al. (2006) reported that children's school conduct problems, within a single low-SES neighborhood, were significantly worse for children living on a residential-only block, compared to children living on a mixed-use block. An implication of this work is that a more walkable environment is more likely to be associated with positive community social processes and more monitoring of the neighborhood for problem behaviors (e.g., collective efficacy) (Kim and Kaplan 2004; Leyden 2003; Sampson et al. 1997).

Another aspect of the built environment which has been examined in relation to HIV/STD risk behavior is the presence/absence of alcohol outlets, which may increase availability of alcohol in the neighborhood and possibly drug use paraphernalia (e.g., tobacco rolling papers that can be used for marijuana; clear tubing used to make crack cocaine pipes) and hence increase the likelihood of risk behaviors (Cohen et al. 2006). In addition, alcohol outlets may provide a "hang-out" where people may gather for drinking and using and exchanging drugs, which in turn may increase their risk for HIV/STDs (Mena et al. 2008; Raj et al. 2009).

Of course, it is necessary to rule out the corollary of that interpretation that people with dysfunctional behaviors may end up in poor housing developments. Collective efficacy, defined as social cohesion among neighbors combined with their willingness to intervene on behalf of the common good, is linked to reduced violence. This hypothesis was tested in a 1995 survey of 8,782 residents of 343 neighborhoods in Chicago, Illinois. When SES and quality of built environment were controlled for statistically, in neighborhoods where there was strong collective efficacy, violence was well regulated by the residents (e.g., Sampson and Raudenbush 1999). (For a more detailed discussion of collective efficacy, see Sect. 3.3.3).

3.3.1 Home and Housing Stability

A substantial body of evidence suggests that the presence or absence of a stable home and more specifically, homelessness may be an important risk and/or protective factor in relation to HIV risk behaviors. Homeless persons are more likely than others to engage in multiple behaviors associated with increased risk of acquiring or transmitting HIV, including substance use, injection drug use (IDU) and needle sharing, risky sexual practices, such as having multiple sexual partners, and exchanging sex for money, drugs, or a place to stay (Wolitski et al. 2007). Additionally, HIV rates are 3–9 times higher in homeless persons compared to those in stable housing. Moreover, homeless individuals are also more likely than individuals in stable housing to have high HIV viral load levels, which increases the likelihood of HIV transmission to others during risky sexual or drug use behaviors (Kidder et al. 2008).

HIV/STD risks may loom particularly large for adolescents, given nationally representative data suggesting that 7.6% of adolescents were homeless at some point in the previous year (Solorio et al. 2008). Homeless adolescents are known to engage in risky sexual behaviors that increase their risk for HIV/STDs, including entering the street economy using survival sex and daily sex work as a primary means of acquiring money for food or shelter (Clatts et al. 2005). Moreover, some homeless adolescents may be at additional risk for HIV/STDs due to their history of early sexual debut, substance abuse, and dropping out of school, as well as lack of connectedness to trusted adults and family (Clatts et al. 2005; Solorio et al. 2008).

Other studies suggest that homeless adolescents who relocate to increasingly stable housing situations, especially in family settings, are less likely to engage in HIV-related risk behaviors, given that family settings tend to provide the opportunity for adult monitoring of peer relationships, educational, and social activities. Milburn et al. (2006) compared HIV/STD risk behaviors in newly homeless adolescents versus experienced homeless adolescents (those living away from home for more than 6 months). Results suggested that the longer adolescents remained away from home, the more likely they were to engage in risky sexual behavior. Additionally, the more chronically homeless adolescents had higher rates of drug use and alcohol use (Rosenthal et al. 2007). These findings support the need for interventions to return homeless adolescents to stable homes and families as soon as possible. Such interventions may have a significant impact on HIV/STD infection rates. In the next section, we review the evidence pertaining to whether family based HIV preventive interventions that address homelessness are effective in reducing HIV/STD risk for adolescent members of a family.

3.3.1.1   Examples of HIV Family Based Preventive Interventions Targeting Homelessness

Ecologically Based Family Therapy (EBFT) (Slesnick and Prestopnik 2005) is a family based intervention for youth (ages 12–17) in shelters and their parents. This program aims to improve youth substance use and other risk behaviors as well as HIV knowledge, family functioning, and psychological functioning. For youth who have maintained contact with their families after leaving home, their continuing family ties are used to motivate both parents and children to shift their interactions and problematic actions. EBFT builds upon family preservation and multisystemic interventions that address the numerous influences on youths' behaviors. Fifteen individual and family sessions are conducted. The family sessions target dysfunctional interactions that help initiate and sustain problem behaviors. Reductions in substance use are also addressed. EBFT has been shown to be efficacious in reducing youth substance use, improvement in family functioning, and knowledge of HIV. The reductions in dysfunctional interactions among family members may also lead to a return to the home for some youth over time (Milburn 2007).

3.3.1.2   Summary of Research on Homelessness and HIV/Risk

Research suggests that conditions leading to homelessness, coupled with the many challenges of being homeless, result in a substantially higher risk of behaviors related to HIV/STD transmission, including substance use, multiple sex partners, and unprotected sex (see Wolitski et al. 2007 for a review). There is a need for interventions that prevent homelessness by early intervention to remedy conditions that may lead to youths running away from home (such as addressing dysfunctional family interactions, e.g., Slesnick and Prestopnik 2005) and returning homeless youth to stable homes (Milburn 2007), as a means of reducing HIV/STD risk (see Rosenthal et al. 2007).

3.3.2   School

School settings are important for understanding the social and structural factors that confer risk and/or protection for development of adolescents' HIV/STD-related behaviors. Children and adolescents spend much of their day in school where they are exposed to positive role models, such as counselors, teachers, and coaches. On the other hand, schools may also expose adolescents to antisocial peers who engage in a number of related problem behaviors, including substance use and unsafe sexual behavior, all of which may increase HIV/STD risk (e.g., Capaldi et al. 2002; Clark and Loheac 2007; Harper et al. 2008; Jones et al. 2003).

Several behaviors in school setting have been linked to either concurrent or future HIV/STD risk in adolescents. For example, lack of interest in school may indicate increased risk for substance abuse and unsafe sexual behavior (e.g., Simons-Morton et al. 1999; Vazsonyi and Flannery 1997). Additionally, academic failure and school conduct problems have both been linked to substance abuse, unsafe sex, and other behaviors that put the adolescent at risk for HIV/STDs (Gruber and Machamer 2000; Hops et al. 1999; Manlove 1998). Moreover, once adolescents drop out of school, their risk for substance use and unsafe sexual behavior may increase dramatically (Ellickson et al. 1998; Guagliardo et al. 1998; Hallfors et al. 2007).

One of the most important influences on behaviors related to HIV/STD risk in the school setting is the influence of peers. Adolescents are vulnerable to the pressures exuded by their peer groups, and those pressures may be amplified in the school setting where adolescents spend much of their time, at a point in the life course that may be considered a particularly sensitive window for exposure to adopting risky behaviors (e.g., Clark and Loheac 2007). While having a network of friends in the school setting is a crucial component to healthy adolescent development, an adolescent's peers have a major influence on many potentially risky behaviors such as substance use, sexual behavior, negative attitudes toward school, and delinquent behavior (Harper et al. 2008). Pressure by friends and influence from antisocial peers engaging in problem behaviors has been linked to HIV/STD risk behaviors of drunkenness and unsafe sexual behavior (Clark and Loheac 2007; Harper and Robinson 1999). However, parents continue to play a major role in the sexual development of their children during adolescence (Stanton et al. 2002; Dancy et al. 2006).

Other studies have focused on school connectedness as a protective factor against HIV/STD risk behaviors. School connectedness is defined as the feeling of closeness to school personnel and the school environment (Bonny et al. 2000). School connectedness may provide an environment within which an adolescent feels cared for and connected to school personnel and peers, which in turn may reduce the likelihood that the adolescent will use substances or initiate sexual activity at an early age (McNeely et al. 2002). The Centers for Disease Control (2009) has acknowledged school connectedness as a protective factor against the development of these risks (including alcohol and drug use, violence and gang involvement, and early sexual initiation) (e.g., McNeely et al. 2002; Taylor-Seehafer and Rew 2000) and provides various science-based recommendations for increasing school connectedness. These recommendations include creating decision-making processes that facilitate engagement, academic achievement, and staff empowerment; providing education and opportunities to enable families to be actively involved; and providing students with the academic, emotional, and social skills necessary to be actively engaged in school (Centers for Disease Control 2009).

Schools have also been shown to provide an effective setting for implementing intervention programs aimed at promoting healthy behaviors and preventing risk for HIV/STDs. A recent systematic review analyzed the impact of curriculum-based sex and HIV education programs on sexual behaviors and mediating factors among youth under 25 years anywhere in the world (Kirby et al. 2007). Two-thirds of the 83 programs reviewed significantly improved one or more sexual behaviors, which suggest that programs were effective in delaying or decreasing sexual behaviors and/or in increasing condom or contraceptive use. This review (Kirby et al. 2007) cited 17 characteristics that make for effective curricula, including using a logic model approach to develop the curriculum; addressing multiple risk and protective factors; designing activities consistent with community values and resources; and actively involving youth through lessons. Programs that incorporated these characteristics were more likely to change behavior positively, and skill-based programs were more effective at changing behavior than knowledge-based programs. Such programs may provide an important positive context in which to implement family based HIV/STD preventive interventions, given the importance of establishing consistent prevention messages across multiple settings that impact the adolescent family member (Dittus et al. 2004).

3.3.2.1 Examples of HIV Family Based Preventive Interventions Embedded in School Settings

Safer Choices (Coyle et al. 1999) is a 2-year, school-based HIV, other-STD, and pregnancy-prevention program for high school youth. The program seeks to modify several factors related to sexual risk-taking behavior, such as increasing knowledge of HIV/STDs; enhancing students' belief in their abilities to refuse sexual intercourse or unprotected sexual intercourse, and to use a condom; and improving communication with parents. This multicomponent intervention focuses on curriculum and staff development, peer resources and school environment, parent education, and school-community linkages. Safer Choices was found to be effective in increasing the extent to which students talked with parents regarding ways to prevent HIV/STDs, including abstinence and condom use. Intervention students reported significantly greater increases in adolescent–parent communication than did comparison students.

Another HIV/STD preventive intervention in the school setting involves the *Familias Unidas* intervention (in English, "United Families") (Prado et al. 2007). This is a family based intervention which aims to prevent substance use and unsafe sexual behavior in Hispanic adolescents, by targeting positive parenting and parent–adolescent communication about substance use, unsafe sex, and other HIV/STD risks (Pantin et al. 2004). Adolescents' participation in intervention activities is limited to family visits and parent–adolescent discussion circles in the schools. Facilitators meet separately with each parent and adolescent dyad and conduct exercises to help parents to reinforce skills learned by their adolescents in group sessions. Results suggest that there were significantly greater improvements in illicit drug use, incidence of STDs, protected sex, and family functioning through 36-month follow-up in the *Familias Unidas* intervention condition, as compared to a control condition which presented HIV/STD prevention messages *without* addressing family functioning (Prado et al. 2007).

3.3.2.2 Summary of the School Setting and HIV/STD Risk

Although certain negative school environments may increase risk for HIV/STDs in adolescents, schools with protective policies that promote high levels of school connectedness as well as HIV/STD prevention curricula may be protective against the development of risky behaviors such as unsafe sexual behavior (Centers for

Disease Control 2009; Kirby et al. 2007). Moreover, embedding family based interventions in the schools may be an effective means of reducing HIV/STD risk, by bolstering parent–child communication processes and parent/teacher collaboration in monitoring of children, and by educating parents about HIV/STD risk factors and thus facilitating more consistent HIV/STD preventive messages across settings (Coyle et al. 1999).

3.3.3   Neighborhood

There are multiple environmental factors that characterize neighborhoods as settings. This discussion will focus on the following factors in relation to risk and/or protection for HIV/STD-related behaviors: (1) neighborhood socioeconomic conditions; (2) neighborhood crime; (3) neighborhood social and physical environments (with a focus on collective efficacy).

3.3.3.1   Neighborhood Socioeconomic Conditions

Evidence suggests that neighborhood socioeconomic conditions, which refer broadly to the social and economic resources available at the community level (including access to money and education in one's neighborhood), may be an important predictor of sexual risk-taking behaviors among adolescents. Moreover, disadvantaged neighborhoods (e.g., those characterized by high poverty, low residential stability, and single parenthood) (Leventhal and Brooks-Gunn 2000) have been shown to put an adolescent at greater risk.

A nationally representative longitudinal study in the USA investigated the effects of neighborhood socioeconomic conditions on measures of adolescent premarital sexual activity (the frequency of intercourse, number of sexual partners, and odds of engaging in unprotected intercourse) (Baumer and South 2001). The researchers followed a population-based sample of 7- to 11-year-old children over a 9-year period. Neighborhood socioeconomic disadvantage was the strongest predictor of the frequency of sexual intercourse compared to other variables such as race, gender, and home ownership. Moreover, after holding all other variables constant, participants residing in the most disadvantaged neighborhoods were 39% more likely to have multiple sex partners, and 2.5 times more likely to engage in unprotected sexual intercourse compared to those participants in the least disadvantaged neighborhoods. A later study by Dupéré et al. (2008) built upon these earlier findings by revealing a positive correlation between neighborhood poverty level and risk for early sexual activity among 12- to 15-year-old females with a history of conduct problems. It should be noted that other factors may play a role. For example, females with a history of conduct problems may be more likely to affiliate with deviant, older males. This phenomenon may be more problematic in low-SES neighborhoods where they may be high crime, few opportunities for employment, and low collective efficacy or monitoring of adolescents' activities by adults (Sampson et al. 1997, 1999).

Any attempt to decrease the occurrence of HIV/STD risk behaviors must address additional problems that may co-occur in resource-poor communities, such as high crime, low collective efficacy, and/or undesirable built (physical) environmental characteristics, any one of which may contribute to HIV/STD risk for individuals in a family. The following subsections will address each of these additional facets of neighborhoods in relation to HIV/STD risk.

3.3.3.2 Neighborhood Crime

Several studies have attempted to address the role of neighborhood crime in the chain of causality for HIV/STD risk. For example, neighborhood crime has been found to be related to the presence of visible drug sales and drug use at the neighborhood level (Ford and Beveridge 2006). Possible interpretations of this finding are either that crime encourages drug dealing or else that the presence of drug dealing in a neighborhood attracts other types of criminal behavior. Both drug dealing and other types of crime may signify a degree of social disorder and a lack of social control (Ford and Beveridge 2006), which may lead to an increased risk for the development of risk behaviors in adolescents (see Sect. 3.3.3).

The presence of gangs, organized groups with a criminal affiliation, is an additional contextual influence that tends to increase crime and violence in a neighborhood (Herrenkohl et al. 2000; Rosenfeld et al. 1999), which in turn may be related to increases in HIV/STD risk behaviors (Lane et al. 2004; Seal et al. 2003). Gangs are particularly influential to adolescents, who are at a developmental stage where they may be especially vulnerable to peer influence (Gifford-Smith et al. 2005; Henry et al. 2001) and who may join a gang in a search of establishing an identity apart from parents or other authority figures (Henry et al. 2001). Gang presence has been shown to increase adolescent likelihood of participating in risky sexual behavior (Walker-Barnes and Mason 2004). Relative to those not involved in gangs, gang members have been shown to exhibit earlier age of sexual debut, higher rates of sexual activity, sex while under the influence of drugs or alcohol, and lower rates of condom use (Brooks et al. 2009; Voisin et al. 2004; Wingood et al. 2002).

A longitudinal study using an ethnically diverse sample of 300 ninth-grade students suggests that parenting variables (i.e., behavioral control, psychological control, parent–adolescent conflict, and warmth) may moderate the relationship between gang involvement and problem behavior (Walker-Barnes and Mason 2004). Thus, structural interventions using a multilevel approach to address neighborhood crime and gang involvement – including embedding family based prevention within communities at high risk for crime and gang activity – may be a potentially effective means of preventing HIV/STD-related behaviors, given the likelihood of a multifaceted etiology being at play with regards to HIV/STD risk in crime-ridden communities.

3.3.3.3   Neighborhood Social and Physical Environment

Protection or risk for HIV/STDs in the neighborhood social environment may be understood through collective efficacy. Collective efficacy is a construct that refers to social cohesion among neighbors and their willingness to intervene on each other's behalf (including supervision of each other's children; Sampson et al. 1997, 1999). An initial study in this area examined the relationship between collective efficacy and variations in violence across 343 neighborhood clusters in the city of Chicago (Sampson et al. 1997). Sampson et al. (1997) found an association between collective efficacy and variations in violence between neighborhoods, when controlling for individual characteristics, measurement error, and prior violence. Moreover, both race and concentrated poverty were significantly associated with collective efficacy. However, with race removed as a confounding factor (e.g., limiting the analysis to African American neighborhoods), collective efficacy continued to explain variations in neighborhood violence. Further analysis suggested that collective efficacy may be viewed as partially mediating the association between these neighborhood socioeconomic characteristics and violence. However, there was substantial variation in collective efficacy among low-SES neighborhoods, suggesting that high levels of collective efficacy may be protective against risky adolescent behaviors even among low-SES neighborhoods. Follow-up analyses suggested that, even accounting for differences in physical characteristics of neighborhoods (e.g., graffiti; litter), collective efficacy accounted for substantial variation in neighborhood level violence (Sampson and Raudenbush 1999). A third study found that collective efficacy was related to collaboration of neighbors in parenting of children, including monitoring of children in the neighborhood (Sampson et al. 1999). These findings suggest that crime and other dangerous activity in the neighborhood may create an environment of fear, detracting from the sense of collective efficacy by neighbors, including monitoring of adolescent activities which may put the adolescent at risk for HIV/STDs (Sampson et al. 1997, 1999).

Recent studies have indicated that neighborhood collective efficacy may reduce the likelihood of high-risk sexual behavior among adolescents. For instance, collective efficacy has been linked to age of initiation of first sexual intercourse among urban adolescents in Chicago (Browning et al. 2005). Findings suggest that adolescents residing in neighborhoods low in collective efficacy were 64% more likely to experience sexual onset by age 16 compared to adolescents residing in neighborhoods high in collective efficacy. Follow-up research suggests that low levels of neighborhood collective efficacy are associated with an increased number of sexual partners (Browning et al. 2008), which may in turn increase HIV/STD risk (Rosenberg et al. 1999). Thus, family based prevention interventions which foster collective efficacy at the neighborhood level may serve as a mechanism for reducing HIV/STD risk for individuals in a family.

3.3.3.4   Example of HIV/STD Family Based Preventive
Interventions in Neighborhood Settings

The Collaborative HIV Adolescent Mental Health Program (CHAMP) intervention has emphasized the role of family in HIV prevention and targets preadolescents (fourth and fifth grade), in an effort to reach youth before they transition to adolescence (McKay et al. 2004). The CHAMP program was implemented in the USA (Chicago: McKay et al. 2000; McKay and Paikoff 2007; New York: McKay et al. 2007) and adapted for sites in Trinidad and Tobago (Baptiste et al. 2007) and South Africa (Bell et al. 2008). CHAMP highlights the role of community involvement and cultural sensitivity in implementation of its curriculum. Community members play a role in the direction, facilitation, and evaluation of the program. The intervention is then administered to small groups of families and their "preadolescent" by trained program leaders. Group workshops are designed to increase HIV knowledge, increase family communication skills, increase parental monitoring, decrease neighborhood disorganization, and increase social cohesion and control (Bell et al. 2008). CHAMP participants in the USA showed improvements in family functioning and comfort in parent–child communication, which are thought to be protective factors against adolescent HIV risk (McKay et al. 2004). Similarly, CHAMP participants in the South Africa study had significantly more knowledge regarding HIV transmission at postintervention and greater caregiver communication comfort and frequency in discussing sensitive topics, compared to a nonintervention control group (Baptiste et al. 2006; Bell et al. 2008). This study was also successful in strengthening primary support networks (i.e., the caregiver or parent–child relationship; Bell et al. 2008). Strong primary support networks are essential for social capital which can lead to larger social networks (Carpiano 2006). Social networks are the basis for the development of more socially cohesive communities which, in turn, harbor a greater collective efficacy, creating safer environments and strengthening the "community protective shield" for youths (Bell et al. 2008).

3.3.3.5   Summary of Neighborhood Characteristics and HIV/STD Risk

Epidemiologic studies suggest that multiple neighborhood characteristics (e.g., poor socioeconomic conditions, high crime, and undesirable built environment characteristics such as dilapidated buildings and alcohol outlets) may increase HIV/STD risk behaviors. On the other hand, neighborhoods high in collective efficacy and desirable physical environments (e.g., shops near homes, few liquor stores, well-kept homes and apartments) may be protective against these risk behaviors. Intervention studies suggest that collaboration with community-based partners may be an effective means of disseminating HIV preventive messages and fostering collaboration among community members in monitoring of adolescents' activities, particularly in low-SES, crime-ridden neighborhoods.

3.3.4   Church or Faith-Based Organization

A small body of work has considered the role that local faith-based organizations may play in preventing some HIV/STD risk behaviors. Studies have largely been conducted with African Americans, a group disproportionately affected by

HIV/AIDS, and one which has traditionally maintained strong ties to their church or other faith-based organizations.

Research suggests that religious involvement, at least for adolescent females (e.g., McCree et al. 2003; Rostosky et al. 2004) serves as a possible protective process through which local faith-based organizations may impact HIV/STD risk. Religious involvement includes church attendance, talking to a religious leader, praying, or talking to others about spiritual concerns. McCree et al. (2003) conducted a systematic literature review on religious involvement and HIV/STD risk, and found that for African American adolescent females, reports of higher religious involvement were associated with later sexual initiation, higher rates of condom use, and higher rates of self-efficacy in speaking with sexual partners about HIV/STDs. Results, however, were mixed regarding the role of religious involvement, including church attendance for male adolescents (Rostosky et al. 2004). Moreover, evidence was limited about whether the relationship of religious involvement to HIV/STD risk behaviors varied by race/ethnicity.

There are several compelling reasons to examine the church or other local faith-based organizations as potential settings for interventions. The church is usually a respected institution in the neighborhood; it has a captive audience; it may already offer youth developmental programs; and research indicates that religious faith and moral sense may play a protective role for youth (Francis and Liverpool 2009). While the church may be an ideal setting for preventive interventions, this setting has traditionally been a venue where discussion of sexual behavior is avoided, and the stigma surrounding HIV and related risk and/or protective behaviors (drug use, sexual behavior, and condom use) has presented challenges to implementing HIV/STD preventive programs within the church. Leaders may also be reluctant to discuss sensitive topics such as anal or oral sex, bisexuality, or homosexuality. Additionally, leaders may wish to emphasize abstinence rather than sex education. Nevertheless, recent studies have shown that members and leaders of faith-based organizations are generally receptive to more open communication about sexual topics and specifically HIV/STD prevention within their faith-based organization (Cornelius et al. 2008; Francis et al. 2009).

A recent review of the literature describing faith-based HIV/STD programs identified four formal faith-based/public health collaboration programs among African American populations designed to prevent HIV/AIDS risk behaviors (Francis and Liverpool 2009). Two of the four faith-based programs reviewed focused on adolescents: These two programs presented HIV/substance abuse prevention messages to adolescents, combined with culturally sensitive faith-based messages, and both programs were found to be effective in reducing substance use and increasing HIV/AIDS knowledge in adolescents (Mertz 1997; Marcus et al. 2004). In their summary of these interventions, Francis and Liverpool (2009) conclude that faith-based leaders and public health professionals must be able to compromise over what leaders will and will not discuss, and what information public health professionals deem necessary to present. For example, to decrease faith-based leaders' discomfort in discussion of sexually related topics, it may be necessary to partner with other organizations that provide HIV prevention for adolescents (i.e., Planned Parenthood and community organizations such as the Religious Coalition for Reproductive Choice). However, research on diverse communities and the specific processes through which faith-based organizations may impact HIV/STD risk (e.g., church attendance), and for whom, require further explication (Rostosky et al. 2004).

3.3.4.1 Example of HIV Family Based Preventive Interventions Embedded in Faith-Based Settings

One example of a faith-based organization is a church-based sexuality program focused on increasing the level of communication about various sexual topics between adolescents and their parents (Green and Sollie 1989). This program is based on the notion that communication is essential for increasing responsible sexual behavior and decision making, and that when parents serve as the major source of sexual information for adolescents, these adolescents are less sexually active, have fewer sexual partners, and are more consistent and effective contraceptive users. Moreover, Green and Sollie (1989) argue that a church-based sex education program offers the advantages of providing more comprehensive sex education, in that a framework is established for examining personal values and discussing personal responsibility and controversial issues. This program involves adolescents' participation in a 10-hour weekend program, which presents a view of sexuality that is positive and affirming. Results revealed a significant increase in self-disclosure to parents on sexual topics in the intervention condition, as compared to a no-intervention control condition. Thus, preliminary evidence suggests that, at least in the short term, a church-based sex education program may increase adolescent–parent communication regarding sexual topics (see also Infectious Disease 2009; Jackson 2009).

3.3.4.2 Summary of Research on Churches/Faith-Based Organizations and HIV/STD Risk

Epidemiologic studies suggest that religious involvement may serve as a possible protective process through which faith-based organizations may reduce HIV/STD risk, particularly among African American adolescent females (Francis and Liverpool 2009). It may be necessary to collaborate with other secular agencies to provide additional resources and address sensitive issues. Additionally, limited evidence on embedding family based HIV/STD preventive interventions within a faith-based setting suggests that this may be an effective approach for reducing HIV/STD risk, by disseminating consistent HIV/STD prevention messages and supporting parent–adolescent communication (Green and Sollie 1989).

3.3.5 Substance Abuse Treatment

Substance use has been shown to impair individual judgment and decision-making, which can lead to unprotected sexual activity and other risk behaviors (Collins et al. 2005; National Institute on Drug Abuse NIDA 2006; Raj et al. 2009). It follows that people who have sex with injection drug users, and children whose mothers have acquired HIV through needle sharing are at higher risk for infection (NIDA Report Series/HIV-AIDS 2006). Multiple studies corroborate that any drug use – not just injection drug use – can significantly put a person at risk for HIV/STD infection (e.g., Ferrando 2001; Koblin et al. 2006). Studies suggest that the prevalence rates of sexual risk behaviors for adolescents who abuse alcohol and/or illicit drugs tend to be higher than adolescents without a history of substance use (Mena et al. 2008).

A study of 407 crack cocaine users in three drug treatment clinics found that such populations are more likely to engage in oral sex, have increased infection markers for some STDs, and have an increased number of sexual partners in the last 4 weeks (Ross et al. 2002). Similarly, injection drug users (IDUs) who do not receive treatment are six times more likely to acquire HIV than those who enter and remain in treatment (Centers for Disease Control and Prevention 2002). Substance abuse treatment clinics may be important settings for the delivery of HIV/STD prevention interventions because it provides access to high-risk populations.

Current interventions in substance use treatment settings offer drug users valuable medical and social services that have effectively proven to reduce the number of new infections (McCusker et al. 1998; Rhodes and Creson 1998; Sorensen and Copeland 2000). Various publications support the claim that interventions to prevent HIV/STDs in individuals in drug abuse treatment are highly effective (e.g., McCusker et al. 1998; Rhodes and Creson 1998; Sorensen and Copeland 2000). One study of injection drug users found that those in methadone maintenance treatment (MMT) injected less and borrowed syringes less frequently (Stark et al. 1996; see also Greenfield et al. 1995). More recently, a randomized study of women from 12 drug treatment programs, with one or more unprotected vaginal or anal sex occasions with a male partner in the past 6 months, reported that those women receiving treatment showed significant decreases in risky sexual behaviors (Tross et al. 2008).

A fairly large proportion of American adolescents are at risk for using drugs or alcohol and/or engaging in unsafe sex (Eaton et al. 2006). Adolescents may be especially vulnerable to substance use, because they are at a developmental stage where they may be more willing to experiment with new behaviors (Kalant 2004). Research suggests that substance abuse treatment is more effective when the adolescent's family members are involved (Mena et al. 2008; Stanton and Shadish 1997; Szapocznik and Williams 2000). This is in contrast to traditional individual-based approaches that focus on the individual adolescent, and exclude ecosystems, such as the family (Smith et al. 1980). Parents' experiences in talking about HIV/STDs with their substance-abusing adolescents can be difficult in that the relationship may be strained and communication dysfunctional (Santisteban et al. 2003), even prior to their children entering substance abuse treatment. Thus, it may be important to engage in family based interventions to improve parent–child communication and other aspects of family functioning as a critical component of interventions for adolescents in substance abuse treatment programs (see, e.g., Santisteban et al. 2006).

3.3.5.1 Examples of Family Based HIV Preventive Interventions in Substance Abuse Treatment

Marvel et al. (2009) reported initial findings for a new, family based HIV/STD prevention model, which embeds HIV/STD-focused multifamily groups within an existing adolescent drug abuse evidence-based treatment: Multidimensional family therapy (MDFT) is a short-term, multicomponent, family based outpatient treatment for adolescent substance use, involving family therapy to change parenting behaviors and family interactions, as well as case management among the various systems impacting the adolescent (e.g., substance abuse treatment clinic, juvenile justice system, and family). MDFT was previously shown to be efficacious in improving family functioning and in reducing drug abuse in substance-using adolescents (e.g., Liddle et al. 2001, 2004). Marvel et al. (2009) extended standard MDFT by adding a HIV/STD risk-reduction module (MDFT-HIV/STD) focusing on reducing sexual risk-taking behaviors, which was administered to substance-abusing, juvenile-justice-involved adolescents and their parents. Preliminary outcomes for the HIV/STD intervention (MDFT-HIV/STD) are promising. Adolescents randomly assigned to MDFT reported more open conversations with their sex partners about HIV/AIDS and safer-sex practices than participants who received treatment as usual. In addition, adolescents in MDFT reported a greater increase in protected sex acts and MDFT participants' risks for STD exposure decreased more rapidly than adolescents receiving treatment as usual (see also Henderson et al. 2009).

3.3.5.2 Summary of Research on Substance Abuse Treatment Settings and HIV/STD Risk

Epidemiologic studies suggest that substance abuse treatment may be an important means of reducing HIV/STD risk behaviors, including but not limited to drug and alcohol use/abuse (Mena et al. 2008; Tross et al. 2008). In addition, incorporation of an HIV/STD prevention component in substance abuse treatment settings, particularly in conjunction with family based prevention and multisettings approaches (e.g., case management across juvenile justice and treatment settings) may be an effective means of reducing HIV/STD risk (Marvel et al. 2009).

3.4 Conclusions and Recommendations

This chapter has reviewed a number of settings that may impact family based HIV/STD preventive interventions, with a specific focus on adolescents. This was described within the framework of the ecodevelopmental model (e.g., Szapocznik and Coatsworth 1999). The focus was primarily on settings at the microsystem level – those contexts in which the adolescent is directly involved – and evidence was provided on how these settings may confer risk and/or protection for risk behaviors which may be relevant to family based interventions for preventing HIV/STDs. The settings reviewed include the home, school, neighborhood, church, and substance abuse treatment clinics. Consistent with ecodevelopmental theory, the evidence presented suggests that all of these systems are important for conferring risk and/or protection for adolescents' HIV/STD-related behaviors. Additionally, the available research suggests that risk may be compounded across multiple settings, and therefore the more of these systems are engaged in family based HIV/STD prevention interventions, the more adolescents' risk for HIV/STDs will be reduced (e.g., Bell et al. 2008; Marvel et al. 2009; Prado et al. 2007). Some main points of research in this area are as follows:

- Housing instability, and in particular homelessness, may put the adolescent at increased risk for HIV/STD risk behaviors. However, interventions that address homelessness, such as repairing family relationships, may be a means of returning youth to stable homes and reducing HIV/STD risk (e.g., Slesnick and Prestopnik 2005).
- Aspects of the school environment may confer either risk and/or protection for HIV/STDs: On the one hand, negative peer influence may increase substance use, unsafe sex, and risk for HIV/STDs. On the other hand, school connectedness may reduce/prevent initiation of HIV/STD risk behaviors. Emerging evidence suggests that embedding parent education and addressing family functioning in a school HIV/STD prevention programs may be effective in improving parent–adolescent communication as well as reducing HIV/STD risk behaviors (Coyle et al. 1999; Prado et al. 2007).
- Several aspects of the neighborhood environment may increase HIV/STD risk behaviors (e.g., low-collective efficacy; low SES; crime). Moreover, features of the neighborhood built environment such as dilapidated buildings and lack of desirable businesses near homes may reduce monitoring of the street as well as providing a "hang-out" spot for HIV/STD-related behaviors. Collaborating with community partners in HIV/STD prevention may be an effective means of facilitating parent/adolescent communication of HIV/STD preventive messages as well as creating a social "net" to collaborate in monitoring of adolescents' activities and hence reduce HIV/STD risk (Bell et al. 2008).
- The local church may be an effective means of reducing risky behaviors related to HIV/STDs; however, faith-based officials may not be receptive to discussing certain topics with youth. Nonetheless, limited evidence suggests that embedding family based prevention within faith-based settings may reduce HIV/STD risk, by increasing adolescents' self-disclosure to parents regarding sexual topics (Green and Sollie 1989).
- Substance abuse treatment is a critical setting for conducting HIV/STD prevention, given the relatively high risk for HIV/STD-related behaviors in a substance-abusing population (NIDA 2006). Preliminary evidence suggests that embedding a family based HIV/STD prevention module in a substance abuse treatment setting may be effective in improving family functioning and parental monitoring of adolescents, which in turn may reduce adolescent substance use and unsafe sexual behaviors (e.g., Marvel et al. 2009).

References

Bachanas PJ, Morris MK, Lewis-Gess JK, Sarett-Cuasay EJ, Flores AL, Siri KS, et al. Psychological adjustment, substance abuse, HIV knowledge, and risky sexual behavior in at-risk minority females: developmental differences during adolescence. J Pediatr Psychol. 2002;27:373–84.

Baptiste DR, Bhana A, Petersen I, McKay M, Voisin CB, et al. Community collaborative youth-focused HIV/AIDS prevention in South Africa and Trinidad: preliminary findings. J Pediatr Psychol. 2006;31(9):905–16.

Baptiste DR, Voisin DR, Smithgall C, Martinez DD, Henderson G. Preventing HIV/AIDS among Trinidad and Tobago teens using a family-based program. Soc Work Ment Health. 2007; 5(3 and 4):333–54.

Baumer EP, South SJ. Community effects on youth sexual activity. J Marriage Fam. 2001;63(2):540–54.

Bell CC, Bhana A, Petersen I, McKay MM, Gibbons R, Bannon W, et al. Building protective factors to offset sexually risky behaviors among black youths: a randomized control trial. J Natl Med Assoc. 2008;100:936–44.

Bernstein KT, Galea S, Ahern J, Tracy M, Vlahov D. The built environment and alcohol consumption in urban neighborhoods. Drug Alcohol Depend. 2007;91:244–52.

Bonny AE, Britto MT, Klostermann BK, Hornung RW, Slap GB. School disconnectedness: identifying adolescents at risk. Pediatrics. 2000;106(5):1017–21.

Boyer C, Shafer M, Wibbelsman CJ, Seeberg D, Teitle E, Lovell N, et al. Associations of sociodemographic, psychosocial, and behavioral factors with sexual risk and sexually transmitted diseases in teen clinic patients. J Adolesc Health. 2000;27(2):102–11.

Brooks RA, Lee S, Stover G, Barkley TW. Condom attitudes, perceived vulnerability, and sexual risk behaviors of young Latino male urban street gang members: implications for HIV prevention. AIDS Educ Prevent. 2009;21(5):80.

Browning CR, Leventhal T, Brooks-Gunn J. Sexual initiation in early adolescents: the nexus of parental and community control. Am Soc Rev. 2005;70:758–78.

Browning CR, Burrington LA, Leventhal T, Brooks-Gunn J. Neighborhood structural inequality, collective efficacy, and sexual risk behavior among urban youth. J Health Soc Behav. 2008;49(3):269–85.

Capaldi DM, Stoolmiller M, Clark S, Owen DL. Heterosexual risk behaviors in at-risk young men from early adolescence to young adulthood prevalence, prediction and association with STD contraction. Dev Psychol. 2002;38:394–406.

Carpiano RM. Toward a neighborhood resource-based theory of social capital for health: can Bourdieu and sociology help? Soc Sci Med. 2006;62:165–75.

Centers for Disease Control (2009) Strategies for Increasing Protective Factors Among Youth. Available via: http://www.cdc.gov/HealthyYouth/AdolescentHealth/connectedness.htm. Cited 5 May 2010.

Centers for Disease Control and Prevention (CDC) 2007 Youth Risk Behavior Survey. Available via: http://www.cdc.gov/HealthyYouth/yrbs/index.htm. Cited 1 February 2009.

Centers for Disease Control and Prevention (February, 2002) Substance abuse treatment for injection drug users: a strategy with many benefits. Available via: http://www.cdc.gov/idu/facts/TreatmentFin.pdf. Cited 5 May 2010.

Clark AE, Loheac Y. "It wasn't me, it was them!": social influence in risky behavior by adolescents. J Health Econ. 2007;26(4):763–84.

Clatts MC, Goldsamt L, Yi H, Gwadz MV. Homelessness and drug abuse among young men who have sex with men in New York City: a preliminary epidemiological trajectory. J Adolesc. 2005;28(2):201–14.

Coatsworth JD, Pantin H, Szapocznik J. Familias Unidas: a family-centered ecodevelopmental intervention to reduce risk for problem behavior among Hispanic adolescents. Clin Child Family Psychol Rev. 2002;5(2):113–32.

Cohen D, Spear S, Scribner R, Kissinger P, Mason K, Wildgen J. "Broken windows" and the risk of gonorrhea. Am J Public Health. 2000;90(2):230–6.

Cohen DA, Ghosh-Dastidar B, Scribner R, Miu A, Scott M, Robinson P, et al. Alcohol outlets, gonorrhea, and the Los Angeles civil unrest: a longitudinal analysis. Soc Sci Med. 2006;62(12):3062–71.

Collingwood TR, Sunderlin J, Reynolds R, Kohl HW. Physical training as a substance abuse prevention intervention for youth. J Drug Educ. 2000;30(4):435–51.

Collins RL, Ellickson PL, Orlando M, Klein DJ. Isolating the nexus of substance use, violence and sexual risk for HIV infection among young adults in the United States. AIDS Behav. 2005;9(1):73–87.

Cornelius JB, LeGrand S, Jemmott L. African American grandparents' and adolescent grandchildren's sexuality communication. J Fam Nurs. 2008;14:333–46.

Coyle K, Basen-Engquist K, Kirby D, Parcel G, Banspach S, Harrist R, et al. Short-term impact of safer choices: a multicomponent, school-based HIV, other STD, and pregnancy prevention program. J School Health. 1999;69(5):181–8.

Dancy BL, Crittenden KS, Talashek ML. Mothers' effectiveness as HIV risk reduction educators for adolescent daughters. J Health Care Poor Underserved. 2006;17(1):218–39.

DiClemente RJ, Wingood GM, Harrington KF, Lang DL, Davies SL, Hook E, et al. Efficacy of an HIV prevention intervention for African American adolescent girls: a randomized controlled trial. J Am Med Assoc. 2004;292(2):171–9.

Dittus P, Miller KS, Kotchick BA, Forehand R. Why parents matter!: the conceptual basis for a community-based HIV prevention program for the parents of African American youth. J Child Fam Stud. 2004;13:5–20.

Doljanac RF, Zimmerman MA. Psychosocial factors and high-risk sexual behavior: race difference among urban adolescents. J Behav Med. 1998;21:451–67.

Dupéré V, Lacourse É, Willms JD, Leventhal T, Tremblay RE. Neighborhood poverty and early transition to sexual activity in young adolescents: a developmental ecological approach. Child Dev. 2008;79(5):1463–76.

Eaton D, Kann L, Kinchen S, Ross J, Hawkins J, Harris W, et al. Youth Risk Behavior Surveillance – United States 2005. Mort Morb Weekly Report. 2006;55:SS-5.

Edgardh K. Adolescent sexual health in Sweden. Sexually Transmit Infect. 2002;78:352–6.

Ellickson P, Bui K, Bell R, McGuigan KA. Does early drug use increase the risk of dropping out of high school? J Drug Issues. 1998;28:357–80.

Ferrando SJ. Substance abuse and HIV infection. Psychiatr Annals. 2001;31(1):57–62.

Fleming DT, Wasserheit JN. From epidemiological synergy to public health policy and practice: the contribution of other sexually transmitted diseases to sexual transmission of HIV infection. Sex Transm Infect. 1999;75:3–17.

Ford JM, Beveridge AA. "Bad" neighborhoods, fast food, "sleazy" businesses, and drug dealers: relations between the location of licit and illicit businesses in the urban environment. J Drug Issues. 2004;34:51–76.

Ford JM, Beveridge AA. Neighborhood crime victimization, drug use and drug sales: results from the "Fighting Back" evaluation. J Drug Issues. 2006;36(2):393–416.

Francis SA, Liverpool J. A review of faith-based HIV prevention programs. J Relig Health. 2009;48:6–15.

Francis SA, Lam WK, Cance JD, Hogan VK. What's the 411? Assessing the feasibility of providing African American adolescents with HIV/AIDS prevention education in a faith-based setting. J Relig Health. 2009;48:164–77.

Frank L, Kerr J, Chapman J, Sallis J. Urban form relationships with walk trip frequency and distance among youth. Am J Health Promot. 2007;21(4 Supplement):305–11.

Gifford-Smith M, Dodge KA, Dishion TJ, McCord J. Peer influence in children and adolescents: crossing the bridge from developmental to intervention science. J Abnorm Child Psychol. 2005;33:255–65.

Green S, Sollie DL. Long-term effects of a church-based sex education program on adolescent communication. Fam Relat. 1989;38:152–6.

Greenfield L, Bigelow GE, Brooner RK. Validity of intravenous drug abusers' self-reported changes in HIV high-risk drug use behaviors. J Drug Alcohol Depend. 1995;39(2):91–8.

Gruber E, Machamer AM. Risk of school failure as an early indicator of other health risk behaviour in American high school students. Health Risk Soc. 2000;2:59–68.

Guagliardo M, Huang Z, Hicks J, D'Angelo L. Increased drug use among old-for-grade and dropout urban adolescents. Am J Prevent Med. 1998;15:42–8.

Hallfors DD, Iritani BJ, Miller WC, Bauer DJ. Sexual and drug behavior patterns and HIV/STD racial disparities: the need for new directions. Am J Public Health. 2007;97(1):1–8.

Harper GW, Robinson WL. Pathways to risk among inner-city African American adolescent females: the influence of gang membership. Am J Commun Psychol. 1999;27:383–404.

Harper GW, Davidson J, Hosek SG. Influence of gang membership on negative affect, substance use, and antisocial behavior among homeless African American male youth. Am J Men's Health. 2008;2:229.

Hembree C, Galea S, Ahern J, Tracy M, Markham Piper T, Miller J, et al. The urban built environment and overdose mortality in New York neighborhoods. Health and Place. 2005;11:147–56.

Henderson CE, Rowe CL, Dakof GA, Hawes SW, Liddle HA. Parenting practices as mediators of treatment effects in an early-intervention trial of multidimensional family therapy. Am J Drug Alcohol Abuse. 2009;35:220–6.

Henry DB, Tolan PH, Gorman-Smith D. Longitudinal family and peer group effects on violence and nonviolent delinquency. J Clin Child Psychol. 2001;30:172–86.

Herrenkohl T, Maguin E, Hill KG, Hawkins JD, Abbott RD, Catalano RF. Developmental risk factors for youth violence. J Adolesc Health. 2000;26:176–86.

Hops H, Davis B, Lewis LM. The development of alcohol and other substance use: a gender study of family and peer context. J Studies Alcohol. 1999;13:22–31.

Infectious Disease News (2009, August 28) Churches may have a role in HIV prevention in Black community. Available via: http://www.infectiousdiseasenews.com/articles/43247.aspx. Cited 1 May 2010.

Institute of Medicine/Transportation Research Board (IOM/TRB). (2005). *Does the built environment influence physical activity? Examining the evidence.* Washington, DC: Institute of Medicine and Transportation Research Board of the National Academies. Report No. 282.

Jackson N (2009, August 23–26), *Church-based parent-child HIV prevention project. #C03-1.* Presented at: 2009 National HIV Prevention Conference, Atlanta, Georgia.

Jacobs J (1992) The Death and Life of Great American Cities. New York, NY: Vintage Books. (Original work published in 1961).

Jemmott JB, Jemmott LS, Braverman PK, Fong GT. HIV/STD risk reduction interventions for African American and Latino adolescent girls at an adolescent medicine clinic. Arch Pediatr Adolesc Med. 2005;159:440–9.

Jemmott JB, Jemmott LS, Fong GT. Efficacy of a theory-based abstinence-only intervention over 24 months: a randomized controlled trial with young adolescents. Arch Pediatr Adolesc Med. 2010;164(2):152–9.

Jones DJ, Beach SR, Forehand R, Foster SE. Self-reported health in HIV-positive African American women: the role of family stress and depressive symptoms. J Behav Med. 2003;26(6):577–99.

Kalant H. Adverse effects of cannabis on health: an update of the literature since 1996. Prog Neuro-Psychopharmacol Biol Psychiatr. 2004;28:849–63.

Kidder D, Wolitski RJ, Pals S, Campsmith M. Housing status and HIV risk behaviors among homeless and housed persons with HIV. J Acquir Immune Defic Syndr. 2008;49(4):451–5.

Kim J, Kaplan R. Physical and psychological factors in sense of community: new Urbanist Kentlands and nearby Orchard Village. Environ Behav. 2004;36(3):313–40.

Kirby DB, Laris BA, Rolleri LA. Sex and HIV education programs: their impact on sexual behaviors of young people throughout the world. J Adolesc Health. 2007;40(3):206–17.

Koblin BA, Husnik MJ, Colfax G, Huan Y, Madison M, Mayer K, et al. Risk factors for HIV infection among men who have sex with men. AIDS. 2006;20(5):731–9.

Kotchick BA, Shaffer A, Miller KS, Forehand R. Adolescent sexual risk behavior: a multi-system perspective. Clin Psychol Rev. 2001;21(4):493–519.

Lane SD, Rubinstein RA, Keefe RH, Webster N, Cibula DA, Rosenthal A, et al. Structural violence and racial disparity in HIV transmission. J Health Care Poor Underserved. 2004;15(3):319–35.

Lescano CM, Brown LK, Raffaelli M, Lima L. Cultural factors and family-based HIV prevention intervention for Latino youth. J Pediatr Psychol. 2009;34(10):1041–52.

Leventhal T, Brooks-Gunn J. The neighborhoods they live in: the effects of neighborhood residence on child and adolescent outcomes. Psychol Bull. 2000;126(2):309–37.

Leyden KM. Social capital and the built environment: the importance of walkable neighborhoods. Am J Public Health. 2003;93:1546–51.

Liddle HA, Dakof GA, Parker K, Diamond GS, Barrett K, Tejeda M. Multidimensional family therapy for adolescent drug abuse: results of a randomized clinical trial. Am J Drug Alcohol Abuse. 2001;27(4):651–88.

Liddle HA, Rowe CL, Dakof GA, Ungaro RA, Henderson CE. Early intervention for adolescent substance abuse: pretreatment to posttreatment outcomes of a randomized clinical trial comparing multidimensional family therapy and peer group treatment. J Psychoact Drugs. 2004;36(1):49–63.

Manlove J. The influence of high school dropout and school disengagement on the risk of school-age pregnancy. J Res Adolesc. 1998;8:187–220.

Marcus MT, Walker T, Swint J, Smith BP, Brown C, Busen N, et al. Community-based participatory research to prevent substance abuse and HIV/AIDS in African-American adolescents. J Interprof Care. 2004;18:347–59.

Marvel F, Rowe C, Colon-Perez L, DiClemente R, Liddle HA. Multidimensional family therapy HIV/STD risk-reduction intervention: an integrative family-based model for drug involved juvenile offenders. Fam Process. 2009;48(1):69–83.

McBride-Murry V, Berkel C, Pantin H, Prado G. Family-Based HIV Prevention with African American and Hispanic Youth. In: Pequegnat W, Bell CC, editors. Families and HIV/AIDS: cultural and contextual issues in prevention and treatment. New York: Springer; 2011.

McCree DH, Wingood GM, DiClemente R, Davies S, Harrington KF. Religiosity and risky sexual behavior in African-American adolescent females. J Adolesc Health. 2003;33:2–8.

McCusker J, Willis G, Vickers-Lahti M, Lewis B. Readmissions to drug abuse treatment and HIV risk behaviors. Am J Drug Alcohol Abuse. 1998;24(4):523–40.

McKay MM, Paikoff RL. Community Collaborative Partnerships: The Foundation for HIV Prevention Research Efforts. Binghamton, NY: The Haworth Press; 2007.

McKay MM, Baptiste D, Coleman D, Madison S, Paikoff R, Scott R. Preventing HIV Risk Exposure in Urban communities: The CHAMP Family Program. In: Pequegnat W, Szapocznik J, editors. Working with Families in the Era of HIV/AIDS. Thousand Oaks, CA: Sage Publications; 2000. p. 67–88.

McKay MM, Chasse KT, Paikoff R, McKinney L, Baptiste D, Coleman D, et al. Family-level impact of the CHAMP family program: a community collaborative effort to support urban families and reduce youth HIV risk exposure. Fam Process. 2004;43:79–93.

McKay M, Block M, Mellins C, Traube DE, Brackis-Cott E, Minott D, et al. Adapting a family-based HIV prevention program for HIV-infected preadolescents and their families – Youth, families and health care providers coming together to address complex needs. Soc Work Mental Health. 2007;5(3):335–78. doi:10.1300/J200v05n03_06.

McMahon PM. The public health approach to the prevention of sexual violence. Sexual abuse. J Res Treat. 2000;12(1):27–36.

McNeely CA, Nonnemaker JM, Blum RW. Promoting school connectedness: evidence from the national longitudinal study of adolescent health. J School Health. 2002;72(4):138–46.

Mena MP, Dillon F, Mason CA, Santisteban DA. Communication about sexually-related topics among Hispanic substance-abusing adolescents and their parents. J Drug Issues, Special Issue: Explaining Contempor Hispanic Drug Use/Abuse: Issues Challeng. 2008;38:215–34.

Mertz J. The role of churches in helping adolescents prevent HIV/AIDS. J HIV/AIDS Prevent Educ Adolesc Children. 1997;1:45–55.

Milburn NG (2007, May) Project STRIVE. Paper presented at the meeting of the Society for Prevention Research, Washington, DC.

Milburn NG, Rotheram-Borus MJ, Rice E, Mallet S, Rosenthal D. Cross-national variations in behavioral profiles among homeless youth. Am J Commun Psychol. 2006;37(1–2):63–76.

Miller KS, Forehand R, Kotchick BA. Adolescent sexual behavior in two ethnic minority groups: a multisystem perspective. Adolescence. 2000;35:313–33.

Miller KE, Barnes GM, Melnick MJ, Sabo DF, Farrell MP. Gender and racial/ethnic differences in predicting adolescent sexual risk: athletic participation versus exercise. J Health Soc Behav. 2002;43:436–50.

Morrill AC, Kasten L, Urato M, Larson MJ. Abuse, addiction, and depression as pathways to sexual risk in women and men with a substance abuse. J Subst Abuse. 2001;13:169–84.

Murphy DA, Brecht ML, Herbeck DM, Huang D. Trajectories of HIV risk behavior from age 15 to 25 in the national longitudinal survey of youth sample. J Youth Adolesc. 2009;38(9):1226–39.

Nandi A, Galea S, Ahern J, Bucciarelli A, Vlahov D, Tardiff K. What explains the association between neighborhood-level income inequality and the risk of fatal overdose in New York City? Soc Sci Med. 2006;63(3):662–74.

National Institute on Drug Abuse (NIDA) (2006) (March). *Research Report Series: HIV-AIDS* (NIH Publication No. 06–5760). Bethesda, Maryland: NIH. Available via: http://www.drugabuse. gov/PDF/RRhiv.pdf. Cited 6 May 2010.

Pantin H, Coatsworth JD, Feaster DJ, Newman FL, Briones E, Prado G, et al. Familias Unidas: the efficacy of an intervention to promote parental investment in Hispanic immigrant families. Prevent Sci. 2003;4(3):189–201.

Pantin H, Schwartz SJ, Sullivan S, Prado G, Szapocznik J. Ecodevelopmental HIV prevention program for Hispanic adolescents. Am J Orthopsychiatr. 2004;74(4):545–58.

Pantin H, Prado G, Lopez B, Huang S, Tapia MI, Schwartz SJ, et al. A randomized controlled trial of Familias Unidas for Hispanic adolescents with behavior problems. Psychosomat Med. 2009;71(9):987–95.

Perrino T, Gonzalez-Soldevilla A, Pantin H, Szapocznik J. The role of families in adolescent HIV prevention: a review. Clin Child Family Psychol Rev. 2000;3(2):81–96.

Poundstone KE, Strathdee SA, Celentano DD. The social epidemiology of human immunodeficiency virus/acquired immunodeficiency syndrome. Epidemiol Rev. 2004;26:22–35.

Prado G, Pantin H, Briones E, Schwartz SJ, Feaster D, Huang S, et al. A randomized controlled trial of a parent-centered intervention in preventing substance use and HIV risk behaviors in Hispanic adolescents. J Consult Clin Psychol. 2007;75(6):914–26.

Raj A, Reed E, Santana MC, Walley AY, Welles SL, Horsburgh CR, et al. The associations of binge alcohol use with HIV/STI risk and diagnosis among heterosexual African American men. Drug Alcohol Depend. 2009;101(1–2):101–6.

Rashad I, Kaestner R. Teenage sex, drugs and alcohol use: problems identifying the cause of risky behaviors. J Health Econ. 2004;23(3):493–503.

Rhodes HM, Creson D. Retention, HIV risk, and illicit drug use during treatment: methadone dose and visit frequency. Am J Public Health. 1998;88(1):34–9.

Rosenberg MD, Gurvey JE, Adler N, Dunlop MBV, Ellen JM. Concurrent sex partners and risk for sexually transmitted diseases among adolescents. Sex Transm Dis. 1999;26(4):208–12.

Rosenfeld R, Bray TM, Egley A. Facilitating violence: a comparison of gang-motivated, gang-affiliated, and non-gang youth homicides. J Quantitative Criminol. 1999;15:495–516.

Rosenthal D, Rotheram-Borus MJ, Batterham P, Mallett S, Rice E, Milburn NG. Housing stability over two years and HIV risk among newly homeless youth. AIDS Behav. 2007;11(6):831–41.

Ross M, Hwang L, Zack C, Bull L, Williams ML. Sexual risk behaviours and STIs in drug abuse treatment populations whose drug of choice is crack cocaine. Int J STD AIDS. 2002;13(11):769–74.

Rostosky SS, Wilcox BL, Wright MLC, Randall BA. The impact of religiosity on adolescent sexual behavior: a review of the evidence. J Adolesc Res. 2004;19(6):677–97.

Saelens BE, Sallis JF, Frank LD. Environmental correlates of walking and cycling: findings from the transportation, urban design, and planning literatures. Ann Behav Med. 2003;25(2):80–91.

Sampson RJ, Raudenbush SW. Systematic social observation of public spaces: a new look at disorder in urban neighborhoods. Am J Sociol. 1999;105(3):603–51.

Sampson RJ, Raudenbush SW, Earls F. Neighborhoods and violent crime: a multilevel study of collective efficacy. Science. 1997;277:918–24.

Sampson RJ, Morenoff JD, Earls F. Beyond social capital: spatial dynamics of collective efficacy for children. Am Soc Rev. 1999;64:633–60.

Santelli JS, Lowry R, Brener ND, Robin L. The association of sexual behaviors with socioeconomic status, family structure, and race/ethnicity among US adolescents. Am J Public Health. 2000;90(10):1582–8.

Santisteban DA, Coatsworth JD, Perez-Vidal A, Kurtines WM, Schwartz SJ, LaPerriere A, et al. The efficacy of brief strategic/structural family therapy in modifying behavior problems and an exploration of the mediating role that family functioning plays in behavior change. J Fam Psychol. 2003;17:121–33.

Santisteban DA, Suarez-Morales L, Robbins MS, Szapocznik J. Brief strategic family therapy: lessons learned in efficacy research and challenges to blending research and practice. Fam Process. 2006;45:259–71.

Seal DW, Margolis AD, Sosman J, Kacanek D, Binson D, and Project START Study Group (2003) HIV and STD risk behavior among 18- to 25-year-old men released from US prisons: Provider perspectives. AIDS Behav, 7(2):131–141.

Simons-Morton BG, Crump AD, Haynie DL, Saylor KE. Student school bonding and adolescent problem behavior. Health Educ Res. 1999;14:99–107.

Slesnick N, Prestopnik JL. Ecologically based family therapy outcome with substance abusing runaway adolescents. J Adolesc. 2005;28(2):277–98.

Smith ML, Glass GV, Miller TI. The benefits of psychotherapy. Baltimore, MD: Johns Hopkins University Press; 1980.

Solorio MR, Rosenthal D, Milburn NG, Weiss RE, Batterham PJ, Gandara M, et al. Predictors of sexual risk behaviors among newly homeless youth: a longitudinal study. J Adolesc Health. 2008;42(4):401–9.

Sorensen JL, Copeland AL. Drug abuse treatment as an HIV prevention strategy: a review. J Drug Alcohol Depend. 2000;59(1):17–31.

Sorensen JL, Brown L, Calsyn D, Tross S, Booth RE, Song Y, et al. AIDS research in the NIDA Clinical Trials Network: emerging results. Drug Alcohol Depend. 2007;89:310–3.

Srinivasan S, O'Fallon LR, Dearry A. Creating health communities, healthy homes, healthy people: initiating a research agenda on the built environment and public health. Am J Public Health. 2003;93(9):1446–50.

Stanton MD, Shadish WR. Outcome, attrition, and family-couples treatment for drug abuse: a meta-analysis and review of the controlled comparative studies. Psychol Bull. 1997;122(2):170–91.

Stanton B, Li X, Pack R, Cottrell L, Harris C, Burns JM. Longitudinal influence of perceptions of peer and parental factors on African American adolescent risk involvement. J Urban Health. 2002;79(4):536–48.

Stark K, Müller R, Bienzle U, Guggenmoos-Holzmann I. Methadone maintenance treatment and HIV risk-taking behavior among injecting drug users in Berlin. J Epidemiol Commun Health. 1996;50(5):534–7.

Szapocznik J, Coatsworth JD. An ecodevelopmental framework for organizing the influences on drug abuse: a developmental model of risk and protection. In: Glantz MD, Hartel CR, editors. Drug abuse: origins and interventions (pp. 331–366). Washington, DC: American Psychological Association; 1999.

Szapocznik J, Williams RA. Brief strategic family therapy: twenty-five years of interplay among theory, research and practice in adolescent behavior problems and drug abuse. Clin Fam Psychol Rev. 2000;3(2):117–34.

Szapocznik J, Lombard J, Martinez F, Mason CA, Gorman-Smith D, Plater-Zyberk E, et al. The impact of the built environment on children's school conduct grades: the role of diversity of use in a Hispanic neighborhood. Am J Commun Psychol. 2006;38:299–310.

Taylor-Seehafer M, Rew L. Risky sexual behavior among adolescent women. Soc Pediatr Nurses. 2000;5(1):15–25.

Tross S, Campbell AN, Cohen LR, Calsyn D, Pavlicova M, Miele GM, et al. Effectiveness of HIV/STD sexual risk reduction groups for women in substance abuse treatment programs: results of a NIDA Clinical Trials Network trial. J Acquir Immune Defic Syndr. 2008;48(5):581–9.

Vazsonyi AT, Flannery DJ. Early adolescent delinquent behaviors: associations with family and school domains. J Early Adolesc. 1997;17:271–93.

Voisin DR, Salazar LF, Crosby R, DiClemente RJ, Yarder WL, Staples-Horne M. The association between gang involvement and sexual behaviours among detained adolescent males. Sex Transm Infect. 2004;80(6):440–2.

Walker-Barnes CJ, Mason CA. Delinquency and substance use among gang-involved youth: the moderating role of parenting practices. Am J Commun Psychol. 2004;34(3–4):235–50.

Wingood GM, DiClemente RJ, Harrington K, Davies SL, Hook EW. Gang involvement and the health of African American female adolescents. Pediatrics. 2002;110(5):57.

Wolitski RJ, Kidder DP, Fenton KA. HIV, homelessness, and public health: critical issues and a call for increased action. AIDS Behav. 2007;11(2):167–71.

Part II
Role of Families
in Prevention and Care

Chapter 4
Parents as HIV/AIDS Educators

Beatrice J. Krauss and Kim S. Miller

Abstract Parents and caregivers play a special role in HIV prevention efforts for youth. Parents are able to reach youth early and in a non-controversial way. Parents can engage in continuous discussions about sex and sexuality, HIV, substance use, and sexual risk prevention. Having frequent contact with their children allows them to provide sequential and time-sensitive information that is immediately responsive to the child's questions and anticipated needs. Parents and caregivers help youth shape and form healthy attitudes and behaviors, and support youth with supervision, positive reinforcement and skills building. Given the proper tools to harness their parenting and communication skills, parents and caregivers are a force to be reckoned with. There is a growing literature that highlights the important role parents and caregivers play in addressing teen substance use and sexual risk behavior; however, evidence-based interventions to strengthen parents' role in HIV prevention or even in reproductive health promotion are rare and not widely disseminated. This chapter describes two evidence-based interventions, *Parents Matter!* and the *Parent/ Preadolescent Training for HIV (PATH) Prevention*. Both are based on research addressing the need to intervene early, child–parent communication, and risk reduction science and strategies. Data on outcomes and description of the dissemination of these interventions are presented. Among the intriguing findings are that both projects were easily accepted by communities, both led to reported risk reduction or intention to reduce risk, and that improved communication may have generalized to create positive outcomes for risks other than those associated with HIV. Each intervention has found new audiences, through formal and informal pathways. A continuing challenge is to maintain and update interventions as new risks emerge and as new populations are at risk as the HIV epidemic changes.

W. Pequegnat and C.C. Bell (eds.), *Family and HIV/AIDS: Cultural and Contextual Issues in Prevention and Treatment*, DOI 10.1007/978-1-4614-0439-2_4, © Springer Science+Business Media, LLC 2012

4.1 Introduction

Media, parents, peers, health professionals, and schools are important sources of HIV prevention information and education. If addressed in a culturally and developmentally sensitive fashion, prevention of HIV and its consequences may require all of those resources (DiClemente et al. 2007). This chapter will discuss the special role of parents in HIV prevention. By "parents," we mean anyone – mothers, fathers, grandparents, stepparents, foster parents, legal guardians – in the parenting role.

Recent national data suggest that parents in 90.57% of over 38 million US households with children under 18 are raising their children, that is, children by birth, marriage, or adoption (United States Census Bureau 2009).[1] Although household composition varies by income and ethnicity, the majority of all parenting households are dual-parent (69.11%). Among single parent households (30.89% of parenting households), mothers account for approximately three in four (76.72%) and fathers account for approximately one in four (23.28%). US households also include over 2 million grandparents (70.4% of whom are married) who are responsible for their grandchildren's care. Young men and women, therefore, are being supervised and spoken to by both male and female "parents." Thus, as other chapters in this book will stress, advice to "parents" should be tailored to ensure appropriate HIV prevention is communicated across genders and across generations of adult caregivers.

4.2 Scope of the Problem: The Need to Strengthen Parents as Health Educators

Parents are the primary health educators of their children. They not only provide information and care, but also are charged with transmitting values and expectations that will guide their children's behavior. Relative to other information sources, parents have opportunities to engage their children in dialogues about HIV/sexually transmitted infection (STI) prevention, substance use, and sexuality-related issues. Because the discussions can be continuous (i.e., not one-time events), sequential (i.e., building one upon the next as the child's development and experiences change), and time-sensitive (i.e., information is immediately responsive to the child's questions and anticipated needs rather than programmed, such as in a school curriculum), parents have the potential to be particularly effective.

Parents have opportunities to have their prevention messages be personal, relevant, and understandable. Parents are aware of their children's biographies: physical,

---

[1] The US census defines households raising their "own children" by birth, marriage, or adoption as family, and others as "non-family," including extended family who have not adopted. The National Institute of Mental Health Consortium of Family Researchers, in contrast, has consistently defined the family as a network of mutual commitment.

cognitive, and emotional development; social context; and social experience. A classroom of 12 year olds, for example, might include a broad range of students from sexually naïve to sophisticated, physically pre-pubertal to post-pubertal, socially confident to shy, and with a broad range of hypothetical thinking, planning, and decision-making skills (Kirby and DiClemente 1994). One set of messages may not be effective for all members of a group. In contrast, parents can tailor their health messages and guidance to each child in their family and address "common pathways" (e.g., responsible sexual and substance use behaviors) that influence multiple health outcomes (e.g., substance abuse, teen pregnancy, and STIs including HIV) (Eaton et al. 2008; Forhan 2008; New York City Department of Health and Mental Hygiene 2008).

Parents can initiate guidance and instruction early. Parents provide supervision, information, and skill-building early in the life course, long before establishment of risk beliefs (e.g., the right time to have first intercourse), and behaviors. The sexual trajectories of youth begin well before onset of intercourse as do the friendship choices and experimental behaviors that may precede problem substance use (Butler et al. 2006; Hawkins et al. 1985; Zimmer-Gembeck and Helfand 2008). They are able to prepare youth in advance to anticipate, understand, avoid, negotiate, or leave risk situations and to build skills that lead their children toward healthy behaviors.

4.2.1 Parents Can Be Effective

Most reviews of the literature on teen substance use or sexual behavior cite parent and family dynamics – conversations and communication about sex and drugs, warmth and connectedness, monitoring of youth activities, availability for advice – as protective of risks. Recent empirical studies continue to find family factors significant, especially in the prediction of early risk behavior (DiClemente et al. 2006; DiClemente et al. 2007; DiIorio et al. 2003; Kirby 2007; Longmore et al. 2001; Pluhar and Kuriloff 2004; Ryan et al. 2007; Vakalahi 2001; Zimmer-Gembeck and Helfand 2008). New studies have clarified that parent–child communications occurring prior to risk behaviors (on time), rather than as a probable reaction to risk behaviors that have already occurred (off time), are predictive of positive health outcomes (Clawson and Reese-Weber 2003; Miller et al. 1998c). Other researchers (Eisenberg et al. 2006) have suggested that parents too often wait until they perceive that their children are in romantic relationships before talking about sex and sex-related issues.

Reviews recommend "beginning earlier" than current school programs to establish habits, values, and expectations that promote healthy sexual development and health (e.g., Dittus et al. 2004; Kirby 2007). In fact, the need for parents to provide HIV education is underscored by the dearth of HIV education in schools. Only 15.4% of US schools in 2006 required elementary school teachers to deliver HIV prevention education. This education included how HIV is transmitted (14.8%), how HIV affects the body (12.2%), compassion for persons living with HIV (11.0%), signs and symptoms of HIV or AIDS (9.6%), how to find information about HIV services including testing (7.6%), or how HIV is diagnosed or treated (6.4%) (Kann et al. 2007). Comparable figures for middle schools range between 71.6% (how HIV is transmitted) and 50.9% (how HIV is diagnosed or treated). Yet, school-age youth are curious about these issues and an even broader range of HIV-related topics (Krauss 1997), including interpretation of neighborhood or family events (some of which would raise confidentiality concerns in the classroom or require extensive processing of events).

In the absence of information and discussion, youth say they experience a high degree of unrealistic HIV-related worry (Brown et al. 1990, 1994; Holcomb 1990; Krauss 1997; Krauss et al. 2006a), often manifested in worry that someone they know has HIV and has not told them or someone they know will become infected.

If parents are trained to educate youth using skill, self-efficacy, and information-building interventions, two generations are exposed to risk reduction and compassion toward those with HIV: parents as teachers and youth as learners (Krauss 1997; Krauss et al. 2000; Wilder and Watt 2002).

Nonetheless, clusters of sexual and drug risks persist (Eaton et al. 2008) and STIs and HIV have not abated among youth, particularly youth of color (Centers for Disease Control 2008a, b; Forhan 2008). For instance, 73% of sixth graders, in a primarily African American and Hispanic sample, had engaged in at least one precoital behavior (O'Donnell et al. 2006). Recent data suggest a substantial minority of seventh graders in at least one US region have experienced oral (7.9%), anal (6.5%), or vaginal–penile intercourse (12.0%) (Markham et al. 2009). Findings suggest that preadolescence is a critical period of sexual development, and that these sexual experiences signal the beginning of a sexual trajectory toward higher-risk sexual behaviors. Evidence-based interventions to strengthen parents' role in HIV prevention or even in reproductive health promotion are rare (Kirby 2007), and, to date, not widely disseminated (see Chaps. 1, 2, 4, 5, 6, 12, 13, 14).

In early 2009, only one of the 19 Diffusion of Effective Behavioral Interventions (DEBIs) programs listed as part of the Centers for Disease Control and Prevention's Centers for Disease Control and Prevention (CDC) efforts to promote adoption of scientifically sound and efficacious HIV prevention interventions had a specific, parent-focused component (Focus On Youth + Impact, Stanton et al. 2004; Wu et al. 2003). Only one other program (REAL Men; Dilorio et al. 2007) had entered the 2008 compendium of nearly 60 interventions with promising evidence for HIV prevention (http://www.cdc.gov/hiv/topics/research/prs/promising-evidence-interventions.htm, accessed November 2010). Yet, for more than a decade, multiple researchers have been at work on interventions that help strengthen parenting skills and parent–child communication effectiveness, enlist parents to prevent HIV, or help parents to strengthen coping in HIV-affected families (see, for example, Bauman et al. 2000; Dilorio et al. 2000; Dittus et al. 2004; Forehand et al. 2007; Jemmott et al. 2000; Krauss et al. 2000; McKay et al. 2000; Mitrani et al. 2000;

Pequegnat and Szapocznik 2000; Prado et al. 2007; Rapkin et al. 2000; Rotheran-Borus and Lightfoot 2000; Wingood and DiClemente 2000). Many of these programs have demonstrated the importance of the role of parents in their children's healthy sexual development.

4.3 Parents as Health Educators

Parents are the first and most consistently present physical and mental health educators of their children. Parents' influence is home-based, rather than institutionally based. Parents can address the health needs of young children prior to entering school and older youth, 18–24, who reside inside or outside of the home. Their role is active and comprehensive. They make environments safe; establish early health habits; provide home-based health assessment and care; negotiate informal and formal care systems; carry out the directives of formal health care providers; assist their children in processing health information from multiple sources and channels – schools, peers, media, and health providers alike; model for their children how to care for themselves and others; and support behaviors, values, and expectations that are associated with lifelong health consequences (Blane et al. 1996; Eaton et al. 2008; Hogan 2001; McWright 2002; Wang et al. 2007; Wilder and Watt 2002).

Parents provide a consistent presence across important transitions – childhood, preadolescence, adolescence, and young adulthood (Graber et al. 1996; Holmbeck 1996).They may direct youth in their choice of friends (Conger et al. 1989; Crystal et al. 2005; Hawkins et al. 1985; Kandel 1985) and provide a buffer for negative peer influences (Collins et al. 2000; Whitaker and Miller 2000). The developmental psychologist Eleanor Maccoby (1980) has argued that parents "burn-in" attitudes and values that guide later behavior through their emotionally charged relationships with their children, which increases their effectiveness as socialization agents over that of peers and institutions. Indeed, research with young adults indicates that they received and can articulate verbal and non-verbal messages about sexuality conveyed by their parents to them when they were children (Darling and Hicks 1982; Heisler 2005).

Research demonstrates that adolescent risk behavior varies depending on the timing, frequency, and quality of parent–adolescent communication. Effective communication on sexual risk behaviors is associated with decreased sexual risk-taking behavior among adolescents (DiClemente et al. 2006; Dittus et al. 1999; Dutra et al. 1999; Karofsky et al. 2000; Kotchick et al. 1999; Leland and Barth 1993), including increased partner communication (Whitaker et al. 1999), increased condom use, and reduced rates of teen pregnancy and STIs among adolescent females (DiClemente et al. 2002, 2006). Parent communication is most effective when discussions occur prior to sexual debut (Miller et al. 1998a, b, c). Similarly, reports of past month alcohol use, binge alcohol use, and illicit drug use were all significantly less prevalent among youth who reported talking to at least one parent about the dangers of tobacco, alcohol, or drug use in the past year (Substance Abuse and Mental Health Services Administration [SAMHSA] 2004) than among those who reported not talking to a parent.

4.3.1 Parents as Educators/Communicators About Sex, Drugs, and HIV

A distinction has been made between education – transmission of knowledge and information – and communication, which can involve more complex two-way discussions where joint construction of meaning may take place (Warren 1995). We prefer a distinction between (1) communication and (2) guidance. Communication can involve one- or two-way discussions, which are educative or non-educative. In guidance, parents set down limits within which a range of youth behavior is permissible. These limits may be conveyed clearly or not, verbally or non-verbally, and with or without an underlying rationale. They may be narrow or broad, negotiated or imposed, strictly or loosely enforced, and may apply to one, some, or all household members, varying by gender and as age and roles change. Either communication or guidance can be stylistically warm and open; either can acknowledge or ignore changes in youth culture and youth circumstances (Krauss et al. 2006a, b).

4.3.2 Prevalence of Conversations

The majority of parents do communicate with their preadolescent and adolescent children about sex, drugs, and HIV. DiIorio and colleagues (2003) indicate in their review of the literature that 72–98% of parents report having had sex, sexuality, and sexual issue-related conversations during their child's life, with the majority of studies reviewed concerning youth ages 11–18. When the topic is drugs, national surveys of youth suggest about 59% of youth report having had a conversation with one or both parents about preventing alcohol, tobacco, or other substance use during the past year (SAMHSA 2004). For both sex and drugs, parental report of conversation frequency is often higher than youth report. At least one investigator (Krauss 1997) has found that there was concordance between parent and child recall, if the talk was addressed to a specific child, or if the talk was "private," with only the parent and one child present. Parents are consistently named among the top ten sources for HIV education by youth, increasingly edged out by media, electronic (e.g., cell phone), and internet sources over history (Fishbein 2009; Sprecher et al. 2008; Strasburger et al. 2008) and by peers as youth mature (DiIorio et al. 2003). Theory examining peer and parental influence suggests that parents retain influence to the extent that they meet their children's needs – that is, in regard to HIV, provide their children with adequate answers, skills, and guidance regarding their child's HIV-related questions and concerns. Peers' influence ascends in areas in which parents will not or cannot meet their children's informational, social, or practical needs (Floyd and South 1972; Wang et al. 2007). However, a national survey of youth suggests parents, especially mothers, are the *first* source of information that youth turn to in addressing their health concerns and needs (Ackard and Neumark-Sztainer 2001).

4.3.3 Frequency of Conversations

Parental conversations about sex-related issues are often characterized in the literature as infrequent (Fisher 2004) when compared to conversations on other topics such as school (Krauss et al. 2002), but when sex is discussed HIV-related topics are near the top of the list in frequency (Miller et al. 1998b, c). Drugs are at the top of the list when either HIV is discussed or fathers are involved in discussions about HIV-related risk (Freidin et al. 2005; Wyckoff et al. 2008). In research in housing projects in New York City, randomly sampled 10–13-year-old youth estimated that their parents who were trained spoke to them about 3 min every 5 days about HIV-related topics, including sexual risk, drug risk, HIV, and people with HIV (Krauss et al. 2002). This frequency was much lower than communications about other topics, such as school, sports, and relatives. If the youth's estimate about HIV is accurate, parents annually exceed the median number of hours per year devoted to HIV, other STI prevention, and pregnancy prevention in elementary schools with required health instruction on these topics (Kann et al. 2007). In 4 years, parents exceed the 14 h of intervention recommended by experienced intervention researchers (National Institutes of Health 1997). As Martino and colleagues (2008) have suggested, frequency of communication may be important in establishing openness and closeness, because repeated conversations about the same topics allow understanding to evolve and deepen.

4.3.4 Confidence in Ability to Communicate and Quality of Conversations

Parents may be unprepared (Eisenberg et al. 2004) or feel unprepared for their role as educators and communicators in preventing HIV. In fact, parents' concerns about their ability to communicate on HIV-related topics are similar to the concerns of their children (Krauss 1997; Krauss et al. 1997) (see Table 4.1).

Other researchers have suggested that parents are worried about (1) when to have conversations about sexual topics, (2) whether discussions about sex or drugs will encourage risk behavior, and (3) whether communication about sex or drugs will be understood. Researchers also indicate that parental messages are often general (Angera et al. 2008; Fisher 2004; Heisler 2005; Lefkowitz et al. 2000; Sprecher et al. 2008), and that the specific topics covered in parent–child conversations may be

Table 4.1 Concerns of parents and youth

Parents worry that if they talk about sex, drugs and HIV with their kids…	Youth are concerned…
My information is not accurate. I will give them the wrong information	They [parents] are not up to date
I will get too emotional. I will be embarrassed	They will get too emotional
I will find out something about my child that I don't want to know	If I ask about it, they will accuse me of doing it
I will find out about all the risks there are out there now	They'll start talking about what it was like when they were growing up. They won't understand what I face
	My parents can't keep a secret. Everyone will know what we talked about
	[For boys] I am already supposed to know

dependent on the context of the discussion. In a high HIV seroprevalence community, Krauss and collaborators (1997, 2002) found that the prototypic parent–child HIV-related conversation often began with children's queries about what they had seen or heard and ended with parents terminating the discussion. Parents and 10–13-year-old children report the prototypic conversation had the following format:

Child: Request for explanation (Our neighbor has AIDS. What is AIDS?)
Parent: Admonition followed by negative consequence (Don't do sex or you'll die.)
Child: Reassurance of the parent (I won't.)

A few parents had effective conversations. They were specific, responsive to what the child had asked, put information in the context of the child's life, had accurate information, concretely talked or instructed about positive actions that the child could take, and shared and clarified emotions. These conversations were remembered if directed to only one child at a time in a private setting (Krauss et al. 1997, 2002). These conversations significantly predicted children's HIV-related knowledge and understanding 6 months later, whether delivered by mothers or fathers (see Chaps. 5 and 6).

Quality of conversation is related not only to content (e.g., accuracy, developmental, and contextual appropriateness), but also to style. Parent–adolescent communication that is open, receptive, and comfortable is related to less sexual experience and less risky behavior among adolescents (Dutra et al. 1999; Kotchick et al. 1999; Miller et al. 1998a, b, c; Whitaker et al. 1999). For example, discussions with mothers about sex and HIV-related issues are associated with more consistent condom use when mothers are perceived as skilled, open, and comfortable during such discussions (Whitaker et al. 1999). Parents' communication style may also be a factor in whether the message is internalized by the child (Miller et al. 1998a, b, c) and whether information is retained. Confirming understanding can only occur within interactive communication. When parents employ open and interactive communication styles, their children demonstrate greater sexuality knowledge about

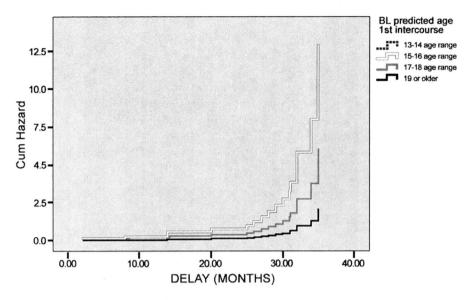

Fig. 4.1 Predicted age of first intercourse by youth ages 10–13 is predictive of delay of first inter-course for youth sexually active before 15. Please note, the data for the 13–14 age range was infrequent and overlaps with other groups and is thus less visible

HIV (Lefkowitz et al. 2000). This conversational style (e.g., in depth, accurate, warm, open, interactive, and early in life) and the skills that underpin it, can be taught (Forehand et al. 2007; Krauss et al. 2008).

4.3.5   Timing of Conversations

There are at least four reasons for parents to begin discussions about sex, drugs, and health with their children early in the life course: (1) HIV-related health risks span the age range (e.g., a toddler can learn to non-verbally or verbally ask a parent or adult to pick up a sharp object or clean up blood; parents can be observant of toddlers, their activities and surroundings; Hagan et al. 2008); (2) early age-appropriate conversations lay the groundwork for later discussions about issues related to sex and substance use that may require more detail and more depth; (3) data suggests that a substantial minor-ity of US youth (7.1%) are sexually active before age 13, and 34.8% are sexually active by ninth grade, with rates varying by gender, geography, and ethnicity (Eaton et al. 2008); and (4) values and expectations about the appropriate timing for sexual and drug risk may already be in place by preadolescence. Longitudinal data suggest these values and expectations significantly predict later risk behavior (Krauss et al. 2008). This tra-jectory is illustrated by the following Cox proportional hazards' regressions model for delay of first intercourse among youth who had intercourse before age 15 (see Fig. 4.1). The graph illustrates that youth (age 10–13) are accurate in predicting when they will make their sexual debut (e.g., have their first experience of intercourse).

Predicted age of first intercourse remained significant in the model ($p=0.017$), even when age at baseline ($p=0.029$) and age of first partner (<0.001) are in the equation. Parent training in the PATH program ($p=0.047$) continued to contribute significantly to the model (see Sect. 4.4).

A small, but growing, body of research corroborates the finding that youth can fairly accurately predict one or more years in advance when they will have their first sexual intercourse (Forste and Haas 2002; Miller et al. 1997; Whitaker et al. 2000). "Anticipators" are youth who believe that they will have intercourse within the next year, while "delayers" believe they will not (Miller et al. 1997). Being an "anticipator" or "delayer" has, in turn, been associated with family characteristics (e.g., mother having given birth as a teen, looser ties to family, perceived approval of premarital sex, parent education), underscoring the usefulness of categories meaningfully describing adolescent patterns of sexual experience. In a secondary analysis of national longitudinal data, Zimmer-Gembeck and Helfand (2008) have found predictors differ for early, middle, and late adolescent initiators of sexual intercourse, some of which vary also by gender and ethnicity. Little is known about emerging sexuality among preadolescents, particularly those under the age of 10 (however, see Butler et al. 2006; McBride et al. 2003). In general, the literature suggests that boys begin their sexual trajectory earlier than girls (Butler et al. 2006), and more preadolescent boys intend to engage in sexual behaviors in the future and have engaged in more sexual behaviors than girls (Browning et al. 2004; Kinsman 1998; McBride et al. 2003; O'Donnell et al. 2006; Rose et al. 2005). Timely preparation of youth for their first sexual experiences has important potential consequences. Miller and colleagues (1998a, b, c) found that behavior at sexual debut is an important determinant of subsequent behavior, where condom use at first penile–vaginal intercourse is associated with a 20-fold increase in rates of continued regular condom use.

4.3.6 Targets for Conversations

Reviews of communication about sex (DiIorio et al. 2003) note that mothers direct more communication to their children than fathers, and that daughters are the recipient of more communication than sons. The content of the communication also appears to differ; daughters receive more messages about responsibility for setting limits and the potential negative consequences of sex. National surveys also indicate more young women report conversations about alcohol and substance use than young men (61.3% vs. 56.5%, SAMHSA 2004). Youth 12–15 years old are more likely to report conversations with parents than youth who are 16 or 17. Some recent data from a neighborhood where HIV is prevalent, however, suggest that communication does not differ by the genders represented in parent–child dyads (Freidin et al. 2005). Fathers and mothers talk to their sons and daughters about the same amount of time about sex, HIV transmission, people living with HIV, and other HIV-related concerns; the only difference is that fathers tend to discuss drugs more. The data originated with 375 parent–child pairs randomly sampled from public housing in a neighborhood with a 10% prevalence of HIV positive adults. These pairs were quota-sampled to obtain equal numbers of father–daughters, father–sons, mother–daughters and mother–sons. The imperatives to educate and protect youth may have over-ridden the traditional role concerns ("It's the mother's job" to address health) and the accompanying discomfort for being "out-of-role" often cited to account for gender disparities in communication (Wyckoff et al. 2008).

4.3.7 Parental Monitoring, Guidance, and Discipline

Supervisory and disciplinary practices are among the most powerful tools parents have to encourage their children to refrain from or reduce sexual and drug risk behaviors (Kirby 2007; Hawkins et al. 1985; Rai et al. 2003). The most "robust" is parental monitoring (i.e., knowing where your children are and what they are doing) (DiClemente et al. 2006). However, it is the youth's perception of parental monitoring, rather than the parents' report of it, that is most frequently included in measurement and is largely responsible for the consistent significant effects. New theorizing about monitoring emphasizes youth's comfort in "reporting in" as being as important as parents' queries and desire to have the report (Kerr and Stattin 2000). DiClemente and colleagues (2002) have suggested that monitoring is a parental strategy to foster responsibility and demonstrate concern. Krauss and colleagues (2006a) found youth reciprocated this concern and also wished reassurances about their parents' activities and safety. The most effective monitoring begins early and is supported by the community (Miller et al. 2007; Sampson et al. 1997, 1999). Similar to communication, monitoring is more often reported by girls while boys may be more likely to experience the punishments of coercive control (e.g., yelling).

Form of discipline (e.g., coercive, authoritative), family support (e.g., encouraging, praising), orderliness of the household (e.g., clear and consistent rules), and household composition (e.g., more than one adult available for supervision) have all been implicated in youth's sexual and drug risk (Longmore et al. 2001). Some research suggests the parents' or siblings' risk behaviors may be a factor in youth's sex and drug use behaviors. However, it seems it is not parent/sibling risk, per se, but how a disruptive or permissive household allows or supports youth risk. Paikoff (1995) has written extensively on "sexual possibility situations" (i.e., youth left alone without supervision). In fact, Wilder and Watt (2002), in their analysis of national survey data, found that unrelated parental health risks (e.g., smoking, not using seat belts, drinking) had "substantial and independent effects" on children's sexual risk behavior.

Community support that reinforces the parental role can be important in communities with few resources. The research findings focused on parents have caveats because they do not address the dangers that youth face in neighborhoods where violence or risk behaviors are prevalent (Sampson et al. 1997, 1999). What may be considered controlling or over-involved behaviors in other circumstances may be appropriate and protective in such environments and with troubled youth (Donenberg et al. 2002; Fletcher et al. 2004; Miller et al. 2007; Toulou-Shams et al. 2006).

4.4 Research Innovations to Address Parent-Based HIV Intervention

We now describe two interventions with demonstrated efficacy that encompass some of the points that we have made about the role of parents. They deliver HIV prevention interventions primarily through parents to preadolescent children and, thus, often prior to the onset of risk behavior. They demonstrate that parents are in a unique and powerful position to deliver HIV/AIDS education to their children. The factors outlined above – parent communication quality and quantity, monitoring, and supervision – are addressed, and no presumption is made that only mothers will participate. Other interventions aimed at adolescents or preadolescents are described by Pedlow and Carey (2004) and Pequegnat and Szapocznik (2000), and other chapters in this volume.

4.4.1 Parents Matter!

The Parents Matter! Program (PMP) (Dittus et al. 2004) is an evidence-based (Forehand et al. 2007), parent-focused intervention funded by the Centers for Disease Control and Prevention (CDC) to promote positive parenting and effective parent–child communication about sexuality and sexual risk reduction for parents and guardians of 9–12 year olds. PMP can address pre-risk behaviors in a non-controversial way and help youth acquire the necessary skills to develop healthy behaviors and make positive life choices. PMP recognizes that many parents and guardians may need support to convey values and expectations about sexual behavior and communicate important HIV, STI, and pregnancy prevention messages to their children. The ultimate goal of PMP is to reduce sexual risk behaviors among youth, including delaying the onset of sexual debut, by giving parents and guardians tools to deliver sexuality and sexual risk reduction prevention to their children. PMP is delivered in five 2.5-h sessions over a 5-week period. Sessions include activities for: (1) increasing parents' awareness of the sexual risks many teens face today; (2) encouraging general parenting practices (e.g., relationship building, monitoring) that increase the likelihood that children will avoid risky sexual behaviors; and (3) improving parents' ability to communicate with their children about sexuality and sexual risk reduction. For more information on the specific content of the intervention sessions see Long and colleagues (2004). As Table 4.2 illustrates, each PMP session has a specific focus and measurable participant objective.

4.4.1.1 PMP Program Efficacy

Results from a randomized controlled trial conducted in two African American communities demonstrate the effectiveness of PMP (Forehand et al. 2007). At the 1-year follow-up, parents who participated in the enhanced intervention (five sessions) and

Table 4.2 PMP curriculum

Session number	Session name	Purpose of the session
1	Why do parents matter?	Provide participants with an understanding of the purpose and goals of the intervention
		Provide basic information on child development and what children need to achieve their life goals
		Provide information on preadolescent and adolescent development
		Emphasize the influence that parents have on their child's health and decision making
		Provide information on the pressures that children face in today's society and what parents can do to help their children confront these issues
		Establish group cohesion and a desire to continue in the program
2	Parenting Positively	Improve parent–child communication skills
		Teach group members effective parenting practices
3	Parents are educators	Provide general sexual education information
		Increase parents understanding of adolescent sexual behavior
		Increase parents' awareness of the need for parents to be sex educators
		Increase parents understanding of sexual issues and what it means to be sexually healthy
4	I think I can, I know I can	Increase parents comfort/skills in discussing sex with their child
		Provide parents with tools for talking about sex with their child. PMP does not tell parents what to say
		Provide parents with an opportunity to role play their parent–child communication skills
5	Moving forward	Continue improving parents' comfort in discussing sex with their child
		Provide parents with an opportunity to work on their communication skills with their child
		Help parents provide guidance to their children about peer pressure
		Review and summarize the major points in the intervention

their preadolescents both reported higher levels of sexuality communication and parental comfort and confidence to communicate about sexuality compared to those in the brief (one session) and control (health information) interventions. Preadolescents whose parents attended all five sessions of the enhanced intervention were less likely to report engaging in sexual risk at the 1-year follow-up as compared to those whose parents attended the control (relative risk, 0.65; 95% confidence interval, 0.41–1.03) and brief interventions (relative risk, 0.62; 95% confidence interval, 0.40–0.97). Additional analyses are examining a range of parent and youth outcomes, including adolescent's sexual attitudes, norms, intentions, and sexual risk reduction self-efficacy, and parent's communication and monitoring efficacy.

4.4.2 The Parent/Preadolescent Training for HIV

Another intervention that addresses parent–child communication is PATH. PATH used elicitation techniques and parent and child community advisors to adapt Cornell's "Talking with Kids about AIDS" curriculum (Tiffany et al. 1993a, b) for a high HIV seroprevalence, multicultural, inner-city community. During the process of adaptation, the team made the following changes: (1) strengthened the emphasis on the parent's communication to their preadolescent child about HIV, unplanned pregnancy, substance use, hepatitis, and risk reduction; (2) deepened youth and parent understanding of each other's views about risks/dangers in the neighborhood; (3) reinforced the representation of gender/relationship issues throughout the curriculum; (4) added a curricular unit on safe and sensitive socializing with persons living with HIV; (5) added a parent–child session, in which each parent answered his/her child's risk or HIV-related questions using PATH training materials and other resources; (6) added a booster session where parents jointly problem-solved about "real-life" challenges; and (7) at parents' and youths' request, added two sessions about the transition to adolescence, each emphasizing mutual caring through household rules and organization that are protective of parent and child safety.

During the process of training, parents met in interactive sessions co-facilitated by male and female pairs who modeled respectful gender interaction. The six-session 15-h curriculum is described in detail in Krauss and colleagues (2000). Beginning with 375 PATH youth and parent pairs, over 240 have been followed for up to 7 years.

4.4.2.1 PATH Efficacy

PATH is unique in using random dwelling unit sampling and quota sampling to obtain nearly equivalent numbers of father–daughter, father–son, mother–daughter, and mother–son pairs. It also uses a random invitation to treatment design (Campbell and Krauss 1991), which, when combined with random recruitment, controls for many self-selection biases (e.g., voluntarism, interest, recent worrisome events). The comparison arm of PATH was the community standard colorful materials in English and Spanish, provided by Centers for Disease Control, New York State and New York City Departments of Health, which covered every aspect of the parent group intervention.

PATH is associated with delay of first intercourse for both young men and women among those initiating intercourse before age 15, and with increased consistent condom use intentions for all youth (Krauss et al. 2008). For the entire sample, both parents and children, there was increased comfort in interacting with persons with HIV, a reduction in their stigmatization (Krauss et al. 2006a), increases in HIV-related knowledge, and decreases in unrealistic HIV-related worry (Krauss et al. 2002). PATH identified the characteristics of effective conversations. In this highly affected community and with an emphasis on positive relationships between genders, PATH found few statistically significant parent or child gender effects for any of these outcomes (Krauss et al. 2008). Male and female youth both delayed intercourse, increased knowledge, reduced worry, and became more comfortable with persons with HIV, regardless of the gender of their parent participating in PATH. One of the few differences was that fathers tended to talk more about drugs than mothers.

Colleagues adopting PATH for a Hispanic population in Miami (Prado et al. 2007) have also found PATH protective of smoking and illegal substance use (see Chap. 12 for a fuller discussion).

4.5 Efforts to Move Research into Practice

Offering strong evidence-based HIV prevention programs is not sufficient. For these programs to make an impact on HIV they need to reach parents of the most affected youth populations, and parents must attend the programs and adopt the protective strategies. Thus, the success lies not just in the provision of HIV prevention programming, but also in the type of programs we offer and the way we involve and engage the target community in the process.

4.5.1 Operational Research Phase of the PMP Program

Resource constraints may make it difficult for parents to attend multi-session interventions. This, however, was not the experience when conducting a randomized controlled trial of PMP. Demographic data collected at enrollment show that the 378 parents in PMP intervention arm had time and resource constraints. Despite these constraints, of the 378 parents eligible for PMP participation, 90% ($n=339$) attended one or more PMP intervention session. Of the 339 participating in the intervention, 86% ($n=293$) attended four or more sessions and 67% ($n=227$) attended all five sessions. Program participant data at post-intervention assessment ($n=313-315$ due to missing data) revealed that 97% ($n=304$) of participants had a "very positive" overall experience in the PMP. When asked "how important do you think the information and skills covered in the Parents Matter Program are to families like yours?" 94% ($n=295$) found the program information and skills "very important." The program's high retention rates and reported relevancy suggest that if programming is provided that resonates with the needs and experiences of parents in high HIV-risk communities, it is feasible to implement such programs.

Although randomized, controlled trials provide critical information on the efficacy of prevention programs, the programs are implemented under ideal circumstances with support from the research team. To determine how the results of PMPs randomized controlled trial translated to program implementation under typical programmatic circumstances, Centers for Disease Control and Prevention (CDC) conducted an operational research project in 15 sites throughout the US and Puerto Rico (Miller et al. 2010). The project was conducted with community- and faith-based organizations, health departments, and schools to assess their ability to implement PMP, the relevancy of the program and program materials, and the organizational, facilitator, and parental satisfaction with the program.

The results of the Centers for Disease Control and Prevention (CDC) demonstration project demonstrate the ability to transfer an evidence-based pre-risk prevention program from a research setting to real-world community sites. Training, program materials, and technical assistance were provided to sites as they worked to implement the program in their communities in need of prevention programs. Data analyzed from site, organization, facilitator, and parent level all demonstrate that the program is relevant, useful, and feasible. Programs like PMP that address the needs and desires of the target population and employ practical solutions (e.g., offering programs after work hours, having programs located close to home, and offering childcare and homework help) can engage parents, including those with children who may soon be at high risk for unwanted pregnancy, STIs, and HIV. Families matter has been adapted and is currently being implemented in seven African countries. As of November 2010, non-governmental organizations are implementing FMP in seven out of eight provinces in Kenya and have reached over 95,000 families (Poulsen et al. 2010; Vandenhoudt et al. 2010).

4.5.2 Operational Research Phase of the PATH Program

From recruitment through participation, PATH was accepted by the community. Interventions often depend on voluntarism, that is, families stepping forward to participate. Sometimes these "volunteer" participants are those most interested rather than those most in need. In contrast, PATH recruited randomly door-to-door. Over 76% of eligible parent–child pairs recruited in this manner signed informed consent and completed baseline measures. Predictors of study entry included distance from the intervention site (1/2 mile or less) and parents' assessment of their child's ability to protect themselves against HIV. Those who disagreed with the statement that their children knew enough about HIV to avoid infection were the most likely to accept the offer of participation (80.5% vs. 71.3% of parents who thought their children knew enough). At every choice point, the random invitation design allowed the PATH research team to analyze and verify that PATH was serving those who felt most needy (e.g., those insecure about their children's HIV knowledge). Once in the study and in the interactive training, over 93% of parents completed at least four out of the total six sessions of "basic training," parent–child session, and booster. Exit data, 7 years later, indicate that many of the activities are a part of the parental repertoire of the trained parents and memorable to the youth.

4.5.2.1 PATH Dissemination

Dissemination began with training other research teams to implement PATH in Miami, Mexico, and Mumbai. However, requests for the "destigmatization" module as a free-standing intervention led to adaptation of "pieces" of the intervention. Requests were received for "destigmatization" training of hospital staff, clinic staff at residential housing, and individuals who would be cleaning the houses of persons with HIV. Centered in New York City, this work on destigmatization led to a World AIDS Day talk at the United Nations on reducing stigma, inclusion on the topic in an expert panel, and to revision of the World Programme of Action for Youth's goals and targets for HIV and youth (Krauss 2008), ultimately included in the United Nation's Millennial Development Goals for HIV.

Because PATH research had documented recollections of conversations by youth, PATH assisted with the update of the New York City Public Schools' K-12 HIV curriculum (Krauss 2007; New York City Department of Education 2009). The PATH team continues to pursue traditional venues, including publications and funding for further implementation. However, out of all of PATH activities, work with the schools and the United Nations has the potential for the most far-reaching impact. Experience with institutionalization of delivery and with policy change has led the PATH team to think about new ways of adapting interventions and of disseminating them once they have an evidence base.

4.6 Challenges for the Future

Dissemination of effective parental interventions remains a challenge, not only because there is no easy bridge between research and practice (and from practice to research), but also because HIV is a dynamic epidemic. Training should include methods for update by reinforcing parents' roles as lifelong learners, creating communication routes for new findings, and accommodating to new local circumstances (e.g., new trends in substance use, new ways of sexual debut). A new generation of parents, exposed to comprehensive family life and sex education, will emerge, but even then they will need to be supported as "things change."

The current and future generations of parents include fathers (DiIorio et al. 2003; Peterson 2007). They are an underutilized resource for intervention. Both mothers and fathers rise to the challenge if they perceive their children are at risk.

Training needs to lead to "deep" understanding. Children ask the most interesting questions: "Why do people use drugs?" "What does HIV do to the body?" Youth will turn elsewhere for answers if parents, clinics, or schools cannot provide satisfactory explanations. These sources often give contradictory messages or have competing agendas. Consistent communication about responsible sexual and substance use behavior can impact not only HIV, but outcomes as diverse as intimate partner violence, early pregnancy, and accidents, to name a few. Finally, early education sets down the template for discussion between parents and children on sensitive topics. For example, PATH results were improved in Miami when combined with an early parenting program (Prado et al. 2007). This ability to discuss sensitive topics can generalize to later relationships and can result in greater respect between genders.

More concretely, findings suggest that sexual thoughts, intentions, and precoital behaviors are precursors to intercourse debut; preadolescence is a critical period when youth begin to view sexuality in a self-relevant way (Butler et al. 2006; O'Sullivan and Brooks-Gunn 2005). In order to effectively intervene before sexual risk behaviors take hold, parents must be equipped with the tools to have early and effective communications with, and supervisory techniques for, their children. Research shows that it is easier to prevent risk behaviors before their onset than to change established behavioral patterns once they occur (Botvin et al. 1990). Parents can be HIV/AIDS educators!

References

Ackard DM, Neumark-Sztainer D. Health care information sources for adolescents: age and gender differences on use, concerns, and needs. J Adolesc Health. 2001;29:170–6.

Angera JJ, Brookins-Fisher J, Inungu JN. An investigation of parent/child communication about sexuality. Am J Sex Edu. 2008;32(2):165–81.

Bauman LJ, Draimin B, Levine C, Hudis J. Who will care for me? Planning the future care and custody of children orphaned by HIV/AIDS. In: Pequegnat W, Szapocznik J, editors. Working with children in the era of HIV/AIDS. Thousand Oaks, CA: Sage; 2000. p. 189–212.

Blane D, Brunner E, Wilkinson R, editors. Health and social organization: towards a health policy for the twenty-first century. New York: Routledge; 1996.

Botvin GJ, Baker E, Dusenbury L, Tortu S, Botvin EM. Preventing adolescent drug abuse through a multimodal cognitive-behavioral approach: results of a 3-year study. J Consult Clin Psychol. 1990;58:437–46.

Brown LK, Nassau JH, Vincent BJ. Differences in AIDS knowledge and attitudes by grade level. J Health Educ. 1990;60(6):270–5.

Brown LK, Reynolds LA, Brenman AJ. Out of focus: children's conceptions of AIDS. J Health Educ. 1994;25(4):204–8.

Browning CR, Leventhal T, Brooks-Gunn J. Neighborhood context and racial differences in early adolescent sexual activity. Demography. 2004;41(4):697–720.

Butler T, Miller K, Holtgrave D, Forehand R, Long N. Stages of sexual readiness and six-month stage progression among African American pre-teens. J Sex Res. 2006;43(4):378–86.

Campbell DT. Regression artifacts in time-series and longitudinal data. Eval Prog Plann. 1996;19(4):377–89.

Campbell DT, Krauss B. Speculations on quasi-experimental designs for AIDS research. Eval Pract. 1991;15(3):291–8. Duplicated paper for the July 1991 Rockville, MD Conference on AIDS survey research methodology, Ronald Kessler, Organizer. Cited in Campbell DT (1994). Retrospective and prospective on program impact assessment.

Centers for Disease Control and Prevention (CDC). Subpopulation estimates from the HIV incidence surveillance System – United States, 2006. MMWR Morb Mortal Wkly Rep. 2008a;57(36):985–9, Atlanta, GA: CDC.

Centers for Disease Control and Prevention. Slide set: HIV/AIDS surveillance in adolescents and young adults (through 2006). [PowerPoint slides]. Available via Centers for Disease Control and Prevention Web site: http://www.cdc.gov/hiv/topics/surveillance/resources/slides/adolescents/index.htm (2008b). Cited 1 Jan 2010.

Clawson CL, Reese-Weber M. The amount and timing of parent adolescent sexual communication as predictors of late adolescent sexual risk taking behaviors. J Sex Res. 2003;40:256–65.

Collins WA, Maccoby EE, Steinberg L, Hetherington EM, Bornstein MH. Contemporary research on parenting: the case for nature and nurture. Am Psychol. 2000;55:218–32.

Conger R, Lorenz F, Simons R, Whitbeck L. Value socialization and peer group affiliation among early adolescents. J Early Adolesc. 1989;9(4):436–53.

Darling CA, Hicks MW. Recycling parental sexual messages. J Sex Marital Ther. 1982;9(3):233–43.

DiClemente RJ, Crosby RA, Wingood GM. Enhancing STD/HIV prevention among adolescents: the importance of parental monitoring. Minerva Pediatr. 2002;54:171–7.

DiClemente RJ, Crosby RA, Salazar LF. Family influences on adolescents' sexual health: synthesis of the research and implications for clinical practice. Curr Pediatr Rev. 2006;2:369–73.

DiClemente RJ, Salazar LF, Crosby RA. A review of STD/HIV preventive interventions for adolescents: sustaining effects using an ecological approach. J Pediatr Psychol. 2007;32(8):888–906.

DiIorio C, Pluhar E, Belcher L. Parent-child communication about sexuality: a review of the literature from 1980–2002. J HIV/AIDS Prev Educ Adolesc Child. 2003;5(3/4):7–32.

DiIorio C, Resnicow K, Denzmore P, Rogers-Tillman G, Wang DT, Dudley WN, et al. Keeping it R.E.A.L! A mother-adolescent HIV prevention program. In: Pequegnat W, Szapocznik J, editors. Working with children in the era of HIV/AIDS. Thousand Oaks, CA: Sage; 2000. p. 113–54.

DiIorio C, McCarty F, Resnicow K, Lehr S, Denzmore P. REAL men: a group-randomized trial of an HIV prevention intervention for adolescent boys. Am J Public Health. 2007;97:1084–9.

Dittus PJ, Jaccard J, Gordon VV. Direct and nondirect communication of maternal beliefs to adolescents: adolescent motivation for premarital sexual activity. J Appl Soc Psychol. 1999;29:1927–63.

Dittus PJ, Miller KS, Kotchick BA, Forehand R. Why parents matter: the conceptual basis for a community-based HIV prevention program for parents of African American youth. J Child Fam Stud. 2004;13(1):5–20.

Donenberg GR, Wilson HW, Emerson E, Bryant FB. Holding the line with a watchful eye: the impact of perceived parental permissiveness and parental monitoring on risky sexual behavior among adolescents in psychiatric care. AIDS Educ Prev. 2002;14(2):138–57.

Dutra R, Miller KS, Forehand R. The process and content of sexual communication with adolescents in two-parent families: associations with sexual risk-taking behavior. AIDS Behav. 1999;3(1):59–66.

Eaton DK, Kann LJ, Kinchen S, Shanklin S, Ross J, Hawkins J, et al. Youth risk behavior surveillance – United States, 2007. MMRW Surveill Summ. 2008;57(4):1–130.

Eisenberg ME, Bearinger LH, Sleving RE, Swain C, Resnick MD. Parents' beliefs about condoms and oral contraceptives: are they medically accurate? Perspect Sex Reprod Health. 2004;36(2):50–7.

Eisenberg ME, Sieving RE, Bearinger LH, Swain C, Resnick MD. Parents' communication with adolescents about sexual behavior: a missed opportunity for prevention? J Youth Adolesc. 2006;35:893–902.

Fishbein M. Toward an understanding of the media's influence on adolescent sexual behavior. Presented in Grand Rounds at the HIV center for clinical and behavioral studies, Columbia University, New York, NY; 2009 Feb.

Fisher TD. Family foundations of sexuality. In: Harvey JH, Wenzel A, Sprecher S, editors. The handbook of sexuality in close relationships. Mahwah, NJ: Lawrence Erlbaum; 2004. p. 385–409.

Fletcher AC, Steinberg L, Williams-Wheeler M. Parental influences on adolescent problem behavior: revisiting Stattin and Kerr. Child Dev. 2004;75(3):781–96.

Floyd HH, South DR. Dilemma of youth: the choice of parents or peers as a frame of reference for behavior. J Marriage Fam. 1972;34(4):627–34.

Forehand R, Armistead L, Long N, Wyckoff SC, Kotchick BA, Whitaker D, et al. Efficacy of a family-based, youth sexual risk prevention program for parents of African American pre-adolescents. Arch Pediatr Adolesc Med. 2007;161(12):1123–9.

Forhan S. Prevalence of sexually transmitted infections and bacterial vaginosis among female adolescents in the United States: data from the National Health and Nutrition Examination Survey (NHANES) 2003–2004. Presented at the 2008 National STD prevention Conference, Chicago, IL; 2008 Mar.

Forste R, Haas DW. The transition of adolescent males to first sexual intercourse: anticipated or delayed? Perspect Sex Reprod Health. 2002;34(4):184–90.

Freidin E, Hodorek S, Krauss B, Godfrey C. What they walked away with: what children say they learn from HIV-related conversations with their parents. Poster presented at the national institute of mental health international research conference on the role of families in preventing and adapting to HIV/AIDS, Brooklyn, NY; 2005 July.

Graber JA, Brooks-Gunn J, Peterson AC, editors. Transitions through adolescence: interpersonal domains and context. Mahwah, NJ: Lawrence Erlbaum; 1996.

Hagan JF, Shaw JS, Duncan P, editors. Bright futures: guidelines for health supervision of infants, children, and adolescents. 3rd ed. Elk Grove Village, IL: American Academy of Pediatrics; 2008.

Hawkins JD, Lishner DM, Catalano RF. Childhood predictors and the prevention of adolescent substance abuse. In: Jones CL, Battjes RJ, editors. Etiology of drug abuse: implications for prevention. Rockville, MD: National Institute on Drug Abuse [NIDA]; 1985. p. 75–125, NIDA Research Monograph 56.

Heisler JM. Family communication about sex: parents and college-aged offspring recall discussion topics, satisfaction, and parental involvement. J Fam Commun. 2005;5(4):295–312.

Hogan MJ. Parents and other adults: models and monitors of healthy media habits. In: Singer D, Singer J, editors. Handbook of children and the media. Thousand Oaks, CA: Sage; 2001. p. 663–79.

Holcomb TF. Fourth grader's attitudes towards AIDS issues: a concern for the elementary school counselor. Elem School Guid Couns. 1990;25:83–90.

Holmbeck GN. A model of family relational transformations during the transition to adolescence: parent-adolescent conflict and adaptation. In: Graber JA, Brooks-Gunn J, Peterson AC, editors. Transitions through adolescence: interpersonal domains and context. Mahwah, NJ: Lawrence Erlbaum; 1996. p. 167–99.

Jemmott LS, Outlaw FH, Jemmott III JB, Brown EJ, Howard M, Hopkins B. Strengthening the bond: the mother-son health promotion program. In: Pequegnat W, Szapocznik J, editors. Working with children in the era of HIV/AIDS. Thousand Oaks, CA: Sage; 2000. p. 155–88.

Kandel DB. On processes of peer influences in adolescent drug use: a developmental perspective. Adv Alcohol Subst Abuse. 1985;4(3–4):139–63.

Kann L, Telijohann SK, Wooley SF. Health education: results from the school health policies and programs study 2006. J School Health. 2007;77(8):408–34.

Karofsky PS, Zeng L, Kosorok MR. Relationship between adolescent-parental communication and initiation of first intercourse by adolescents. J Adolesc Health. 2000;28:41–5.

Kerr M, Stattin H. What parents know, how they know it, and several forms of adolescent adjustment: further support for a reinterpretation of monitoring. Dev Psychol. 2000;36:366–80.

Kinsman SB. Early sexual initiation: the role of peer norms. Pediatrics. 1998;102(5):1185–92.

Kirby, D. and DiClemente, R. J. School-based interventions to prevent unprotected sex and HIV among adolescents. In R.J. DiClemente, R. J. and J.L. Peterson (Eds). *Preventing AIDS: Theories and Methods of Behavioral Interventions* (pp. 117–139). New York, NY: Plenum Press, 1994.

Kirby D. School-based interventions to prevent unprotected sex and HIV among adolescents. In: DiClemente R, Person J, editors. Preventing AIDS: theories and methods of behavioral interventions. New York: Plenum Press; 2000. p. 83–102.

Kirby D. Emerging Answers 2007: research findings on programs to reduce teen pregnancy and sexually transmitted diseases. Washington, DC: The National Campaign to Prevent Teen and Unplanned Pregnancy; 2007.

Kotchick BA, Dorsey S, Miller KS, Forehand R. Adolescent sexual risk taking behavior in single-parent ethnic minority families. J Fam Psychol. 1999;13(1):93–102.

Knoester, C., Haynie, D. L, & Stephens, CM (2006). Parenting practices and adolescents' friendship networks. Journal of Marriage and Family, 68, 1247–1260.

Krauss B. HIV education for teens and preteens in a high-seroprevalence inner-city neighborhood. Fam Soc. 1997;78(6):579–91.

Krauss B. Youth and the global HIV/AIDS epidemic: considerations for goals and targets. Expert group meeting on goals and targets for the World Programme of Action for Youth: Youth in civil society and youth and their well-being, invited presentation. United Nations Headquarters, New York, NY; 2008, May.

Krauss B. Summary of the Center for Community and Urban Health's technical assistance to, and research foundations for the New York City Department of Education for the Center's Summer 2004 revision of the New York City Public School's K-12 HIV curriculum. Presentation to the Sex Education Alliance of New York City, New York, NY; 2007 May.

Krauss B, Goldsamt L, Bula E. Parent-preadolescent communication about HIV in a high seroprevalence neighborhood. In: Sigman M (Chair), Mother-adolescent communication about sexuality and AIDS. Symposium conducted at the Society for Research in Child Development Biennial Meeting, Washington DC; 1997 April.

Krauss BJ, Godfrey C, Yee DS, Goldsamt L, Tiffany J, Almeyda L, et al. Saving our children from a silent epidemic: the PATH program for parents and pre-adolescents. In: Pequegnat W, Szapocznik J, editors. Working with families in the era of HIV/AIDS. Thousand Oaks, CA: Sage; 2000. p. 89–112.

Krauss B, Godfrey C, O'Day J, Pride J, Donaire M. Now I can learn about HIV – effects of a parent training on children's practical HIV knowledge and HIV worries: a randomized trial in an HIV-affected neighborhood [Abstract]. XIV-th World AIDS Conference, Conference Record, Vol. 2, 170; 2002 July.

Krauss B, Godfrey C, O'Day J, Freidin E. Hugging my uncle: the impact of a parent training on children's comfort interacting with persons with HIV. J Pediatr Psychol. 2006a;31(9):891–904.

Krauss B, O'Day J, Godfrey C, Rente K, Freidin L, Bratt E, et al. Who wins in the status games? Violence, sexual violence and an emerging single standard among adolescent women. Ann N Y Acad Sci. 2006b;1087(November):56–73.

Krauss BJ, Hodorek S, McGinniss S, O'Day J. Mothers, fathers, daughters and sons: long term gender-fair risk and stigma reduction outcomes of a family- and community-based intervention for young adolescents [Abstract]. XVII-th International AIDS Conference, Conference Record, Vol. 2, 155; 2008 Aug.

Lefkowitz ES, Romo LF, Corona R, Au TK, Sigman M. How Latino American and European adolescents discuss conflicts, sexuality, and AIDS with their mothers. Dev Psychol. 2000;36:315–25.

Leland N, Barth R. Characteristics of adolescents who have attempted to avoid HIV and who have communicated with parents about sex. J Adolesc Res. 1993;8:58–76.

Long N, Austin BJ, Gound MM, Kelly AO, Gardner AA, Dunn R, et al. The parents matter! Program interventions: content and the facilitation process. J Child Fam Stud. 2004;13(1):47–69.

Longmore MA, Manning WD, Giordano PC. Preadolescent parenting strategies and teens' dating and sexual initiation: a longitudinal analysis. J Marriage Fam. 2001;63(2):322–35.

Maccoby EE. Social development: psychological growth and the parent child relationship. New York: Harcourt Brace Janovich; 1980.

Markham CM, Perkins MF, Addy RC, Baumler ER, Tortolero SR. Patterns of vaginal, oral, and anal intercourse in an urban seventh-grade population. J School Health. 2009;79(4):193–200.

Martino SC, Elliott MN, Corona R, Kanouse DE, Schuster MA. Beyond the "big talk": the roles of breadth and repetition in parent-adolescent communication about sexual topics. Pediatrics. 2008;121(3):e612–8.

McBride CK, Paikoff RL, Holmbeck GN. Individual and familial influences on the onset of sexual intercourse among urban African American adolescents. J Consult Clin Psychol. 2003; 71(1):159–67.

McKay M, Baptiste D, Coleman D, Madison S, Paikoff R, Scott R. Preventing HIV risk exposure in urban communities: the CHAMP family program. In: Pequegnat W, Szapocznik J, editors. Working with children in the era of HIV/AIDS. Thousand Oaks, CA: Sage; 2000. p. 67–88.

McWright L. African American grandmothers' and grandfathers' influence in the socialization of children. In: McAdoo HP, editor. Black children: social, educational and parental environments. Thousand Oaks, CA: Sage; 2002. p. 27–44.

Miller KS, Clark LF, Wendell DA, Levin ML, Gray-Ray P, Velez CN, et al. Adolescent heterosexual experience: a new typology. J Adolesc Health. 1997;20:179–86.

Miller BC, Norton MC, Fan X, Christopherson CR. Pubertal development, parental communication, and sexual values in relation to adolescent sexual behaviors. J Early Adolesc. 1998a;18: 27–52.

Miller KS, Kotchick BA, Dorsey S, Forehand R, Ham AY. Family communication about sex: what are parents saying and are their adolescents listening? Fam Plann Perspect. 1998b;30(5): 218–35.

Miller KS, Levin ML, Whitaker DJ, Xu X. Patterns of condom use among adolescents: the impact of mother-adolescent communication. Am J Public Health. 1998c;88(10):1542–15444.

Miller S, McKay M, Baptiste D. Social support for African American low income parents: the influence of preadolescents' risk behavior and support role on parental monitoring and child outcomes. Soc Work Ment Health. 2007;5(1/2):121–47.

Miller KS, Maxwell KD, Fasula AM, Parker JT, Zackery S, Wyckoff SC. Pre-risk HIV prevention paradigm shift: the feasibility and acceptability of the parents matter! Program in HIV risk communities. Public Health Rep. 2010;125 Suppl 1:38–46.

Mitrani VB, Szapocznik J, Batista CR. Structural ecosystems therapy with HIV and African-American women. In: Pequegnat W, Szapocznik J, editors. Working with children in the era of HIV/AIDS. Thousand Oaks, CA: Sage; 2000. p. 67–88.

National Institutes of Health. Consensus development conference statement: interventions to prevent HIV risk behavior. Rockville, MD: National Institutes of Health; 1997.

New York City Department of Education. HIV/AIDS curriculum. Available via: http://schools.nyc.gov/Academics/FitnessandHealth/StandardsCurriculum/HIVAIDScurriculum (2009). Cited 14 Apr 2009.

New York City Department of Health and Mental Hygiene. NYC youth risk behavior survey. Available via: http://www.nyc.gov/html/doh/html/episrv/episrvyouthriskbehavior.shtml (2008). Cited 24 June 2009.

O'Donnell L, Stueve A, Wilson-Simmons R, Dash K, Agronick G, Jean Baptiste V. Heterosexual risk behaviors among urban young adolescents. J Early Adolesc. 2006;26(1):87–109.

O'Sullivan L, Brooks-Gunn J. The timing of changes in girls' sexual cognitions and behaviors in early adolescence: a prospective cohort study. J Adolesc Health. 2005;37:211–9.

Paikoff RL. Early heterosexual debut: situations of sexual possibility. Am J Orthopsychiatry. 1995;65(3):389–401.

Pedlow CT, Carey MP. Developmentally appropriate sexual risk reduction interventions for adolescents: rationale, review of interventions, and recommendations for research and practice. Ann Behav Med. 2004;27(3):172–84.

Pequegnat W, Szapocznik J, editors. Working with children in the era of HIV/AIDS. Thousand Oaks, CA: Sage; 2000.

Peterson SH. The importance of fathers: contextualizing sexual risk-taking in "low risk" African American adolescent girls. J Hum Behav Soc Environ New Perspect. 2007;15(2/3):329–46.

Pluhar EI, Kuriloff P. What really matters in family communication about sexuality? A qualitative analysis of affect and style among African American mothers and adolescent daughters. Sex Educ. 2004;4:303–21.

Poulsen MN, Vandenhoudt H, Wyckoff SC, Obongo C, Ochura J, Njiki G, et al. Cultural adaptation of a US evidence-based parenting intervention for rural Western Kenya: from parents matter! To families matter! AIDS Educ Prev. 2010;22(4):273–85.

Prado G, Pantin H, Schwartz SJ, Feaster D, Huang S, Sullivan S, et al. A randomized controlled trial of a parent-centered intervention in preventing substance use and HIV risk behaviors in Hispanic adolescents. J Consult Clin Psychol. 2007;75(6):914–26.

Rai AA, Stanton B, Wu Y, Li X, Galbraith J, Cottrell L, et al. Relative influences of perceived parental monitoring and perceived peer involvement on adolescent risk behaviors: an analysis of six cross-sectional data sets. J Adolesc Health. 2003;33(2):108–18.

Rapkin BD, Bennett J, Murphy P, Munoz M. The family health program: strengthening problem solving in families affected by AIDS to mobilize systems of support and care. In: Pequegnat W, Szapocznik J, editors. Working with children in the era of HIV/AIDS. Thousand Oaks, CA: Sage; 2000. p. 243–80.

Rose A, Koo HP, Bhaskar B, Anderson K, White G, Jenkins RR. The influence of primary caregivers on the sexual behavior of early adolescents. J Adolesc Health. 2005;37:135–44.

Rotheran-Borus MJ, Lightfoot M. Helping adolescents and parents with AIDS to cope effectively with daily life. In: Pequegnat W, Szapocznik J, editors. Working with children in the era of HIV/AIDS. Thousand Oaks, CA: Sage; 2000. p. 213–42.

Ryan S, Franzetta K, Manlove J, Holcombe E. Adolescents' discussions about contraception or STDs with partners before first sex. Perspect Sex Reprod Health. 2007;39(3):149–57.

Sampson RJ, Raudenbush SW, Earls F. Neighborhoods and violent crime: A multilevel study of collective efficacy. Science. 1997;277:918–924.

Sampson, Robert J., Jeffrey D. Morenoff, and Felton Earls. 1999. "Beyond Social Capital: Spatial Dynamics of Collective Efficacy for Children." American Sociological Review 64:633–660.

Sprecher S, Harris G, Meyers A. Perceptions of sources of sex education and targets of sex communication: sociodemographic and cohort effects. J Sex Res. 2008;45(1):17–26.

Stanton B, Cole M, Galbraith J, Li X, Pendleton S, Cottrel L, et al. A randomized trial of a parent intervention: parents can make a difference in long-term adolescent risk behaviors, perceptions and knowledge. Arch Pediatr Adolesc Med. 2004;158:947–55.

Strasburger V, Wilson BJ, Jordan AB. Children, adolescents and the media. Thousand Oaks, CA: Sage Publications; 2008.

Substance Abuse and Mental Health Services Administration, Office of Applied Studies. Results from the 2003 national survey on drug use and health: national findings. Rockville, MD: Substance Abuse and Mental Health Services Administration; 2004 (DHHS Publication No. SMA 04–3964, NSDUH Series H-25).

Tiffany J, Tobias D, Raqib A, Ziegler J. Talking with kids about AIDS: a program for parents and other adults who care (manual). New York: Cornell University; 1993a.

Tiffany J, Tobias D, Raqib A, Ziegler J. Talking with kids about AIDS: a program for parents and other adults who care (teaching guide). New York: Cornell University; 1993b.

Toulou-Shams M, Paikoff R, McKirnan DJ, Holmbeck GN. Mental health and HIV risk among African American adolescents: the role of parenting. Soc Work Ment Health. 2006;5(1/2): 27–58.

United States Census Bureau. Selected social characteristics in the United States: 2005 2007. Available via: http://factfinder.census.gov/servlet/DatasetMainPageServlet (2009). Cited 24 Jan 2009.

Vakalahi HF. Adolescent substance use and family-based risk and protective factors: a literature review. J Drug Educ. 2001;31:29–46.

Vandenhoudt H, Miller KS, Ochura J, Wyckoff SC, Otwoma N, Poulsen MN, et al. Evaluation of a US evidence based parenting intervention in rural western Kenya: from parents matter to families matter! AIDS Educ Prev. 2010;22(4):328–43.

Wang A, Peterson GW, Morphey LK. Who is more important for early adolescents' developmental choices? Peers or parents? Marriage Fam Rev. 2007;42(2):95–122.

Warren C. Parent-child communication about sex. In: Socha TJ, Stamp G, editors. Parents, children, and communication: frontiers of theory and research. Mahwah, NJ: Lawrence Erlbaum; 1995. p. 173–201.

Whitaker DJ, Miller KS. Parent-adolescent discussions about sex and condoms: impact on peer influences of sexual risk behavior. J Adolesc Res. 2000;15(2):251–73.

Whitaker DJ, Miller KS, May DC, Levin ML. Teenage partners' communication about sexual risk and condom use: the importance of parent-teenager discussions. Fam Plann Perspect. 1999;31(3):117–21.

Whitaker DJ, Miller KS, Clark LF. Reconceptualizing adolescent sexual behavior: beyond did they or didn't they? Fam Plann Perspect. 2000;32(3):111–7.

Wilder EI, Watt TT. Risky parental behavior and adolescent sexual activity at first coitus. Milbank Q. 2002;80(3):481–524.

Wingood GM, DiClemente RJ. The Willow Program: mobilizing social networks of women living with HIV to enhance coping and to reduce sexual risk behavior. In: Pequegnat W, Szapocznik J, editors. Working with children in the era of HIV/AIDS. Thousand Oaks, CA: Sage; 2000. p. 281–99.

Wu Y, Stanton B, Galbraith J, Kaljee L, Cottrell L, Li X, et al. Sustaining and broadening intervention impact: a randomized controlled trial of three adolescent risk reduction intervention approaches. Pediatrics. 2003;111(1):e32–8.

Wyckoff SC, Miller KS, Forehand R, Bau JJ, Fasula A, Long N, et al. Patterns of sexuality communication between preadolescents and their mothers and fathers. J Child Fam Stud. 2008;17:649–62.

Zimmer-Gembeck MJ, Helfand M. Ten years of longitudinal research on U.S. adolescent sexual behavior: developmental correlates of sexual intercourse, and the importance of age, gender and ethnic background. Dev Rev. 2008;28:153–224.

Chapter 5
Mothers: The Major Force in Preventing HIV/STD Risk Behaviors

Barbara Dancy and Colleen DiIorio

Abstract The focus of this chapter is on mothers serving as protective factors against high-risk sexual behaviors for their adolescents. We present information about the scope of the HIV/AIDS epidemic among adolescents in the United States, followed by a discussion of the role of mothers and the impact of mothers' influence on their adolescents' high-risk sexual behaviors. We then present several innovative HIV-risk reduction interventions designed to include mothers as key agents in the fight against HIV in the adolescent population.

5.1 Scope of the Problem

Over one million people in the United States are currently infected with the Human Immunodeficiency Virus (HIV) and some of those infected individuals having progressed to the more deadly Acquired Immunodeficiency Syndrome (AIDS) (http://www.cdc.gov/hiv/resources/reports/hiv3rddecade/chapter2.htm#serious). From the beginning of the epidemic through 2004, 40,059 adolescents and young adults have been diagnosed with AIDS accounting for 4% of all AIDS diagnoses, and 10,129 young people have died representing 2% of all AIDS-related deaths (http://www.cdc.gov/hiv/resources/factsheets/youth.htm).

Although surveillance data indicate that the number of deaths due to AIDS has decreased, the disease is not curable. People infected with HIV must live with symptoms and treatments that affect their productivity and quality of life. The most recent statistics from the Centers for Disease Control and Prevention (CDC 2009a, b) indicate that in 2004, 4,883 young people ages 13–24 years of age were diagnosed with HIV infection or AIDS, representing about 13% of all those diagnosed that year. African Americans were most likely to be diagnosed with HIV infection accounting for 55% of all HIV infections in this age group. During the same year, close to 7,800

W. Pequegnat and C.C. Bell (eds.), *Family and HIV/AIDS: Cultural and Contextual Issues in Prevention and Treatment*, DOI 10.1007/978-1-4614-0439-2_5, © Springer Science+Business Media, LLC 2012

adolescents and young people were living with AIDS, representing a 42% increase in AIDS diagnoses since 2000 in the 13–24 year old age group.

In the United States and many other parts of the world, HIV is largely transmitted among young adults through unprotected sexual intercourse and injection drug use. Data from the Youth Risk Behavioral Survey (YRBS) showed that 47% of high school students reported having had sexual intercourse, with 7.4% reporting their first sexual experience prior to age 13 years (Centers for Disease Control and Prevention (CDC) 2004). About 67.3% of African American and 51.4% of Hispanic high school students reported having had sexual intercourse, compared to 41.8% of white peers. Roughly one-third of African American males (31.8%) noted that they were 13 years of age or younger at their first sexual encounter. The number of students reporting sexual intercourse increased with year of school, so that 61.6% of all high school seniors reported sexual intercourse. Of this group, 62% of girls and 60% of boys reported having had sexual intercourse.

Sexually active adolescents can reduce their chance of contracting HIV if they use a condom every time they have sexual intercourse and only have sex with a mutually monogamous partner. Unfortunately, although many adolescents do use condoms, their rates of consistent and correct condom use are less than desired. The 2003 YRBS data showed that only 63% of sexually active high school students reported using condoms at last intercourse (Centers for Disease Control and Prevention (CDC) 2004). The rate of condom use was slightly higher for African American females at 63.6% and significantly higher for African American males at 81.2%. The lowest rates of condom use were reported among Hispanic females (52.3%) and white females (56.5%). In addition to their risk for HIV and other sexually transmitted diseases (STDs) because of inconsistent condom use, adolescents are also at risk because they tend to have more than one sexual partner. The tendency for short-term relationships means that sexually active adolescents can have several partners before reaching 20 years of age. Although adolescents may not have more than one partner during the same time period, younger age at first intercourse coupled with older age at first marriage increases the potential for multiple partners in their lifetime and thus, increases their risk of contracting HIV and other STDs (Centers for Disease Control and Prevention (CDC) 1996). Data from the 2003 NRBS revealed that 14.4% of high school students reported having sex with four or more partners. The highest rates were among African American and Hispanic males (41.7 and 20.5% respectively).

The good news is that AIDS and HIV education appear to be readily available in schools (Centers for Disease Control and Prevention (CDC) 2004). Overall, 87.9% of students reported school-based HIV/AIDS education with the highest rates among white males and females (90.3%). A slightly lower percent of African American (85.1%) and Hispanic (83.4%) students reported school-based HIV/AIDS education. Despite widespread education within the school system, the data from the Centers for Disease Control and Prevention (CDC) and the YRBS suggest that complementary educational efforts are necessary to foster protective behaviors such as abstinence and condom use. As discussed in the following sections, the family, in particular, the mother can play an important role in supporting their adolescents.

5.2   The Emerging Roles of Mothers and Fathers in Family Life

Mothers play an important and unique role in the lives of their children. By providing care, emotional support, and discipline, they contribute to the future well-being of their children (Scott et al. 2007). Much has been written about the role of the mother within the family unit and the consequences of the mother's presence or absence on children's development. Most of the research in this area has addressed consequences related to academic, psychosocial, and physical well-being of children. Less is known about the role of the mother in specific areas, such as her role in educating children about health issues, including sexual health.

Parsons and Bales (1955) first differentiated the roles of mothers and fathers. They described the traditional role of the mother as one with more expressive involvement and less instrumental involvement in the lives of their children (Finley et al. 2008; Parsons and Bales 1955). Mothers have traditionally been responsible for providing physical care for infants and young children, teaching children basic self-care skills, protecting children from harm and providing emotional support, companionship, and guidance during the school years. Fathers, on the other hand, have been more responsible for the instrumental aspects of family life, including providing protection, discipline, the economic well-being of the family, and the moral, ethical and career development of their children (Finley et al. 2008; Parsons and Bales 1955). At the time Parsons and Bales presented their ideas over 50 years ago, a two-parent family was the norm as was stay-at-home mothers who provided the primary care for their children. In the ensuing 50 years, the nature of the family has changed. Today, the percent of single-parent families has increased, and most of the single-parent households are headed by single or divorced mothers. Regardless of family structure, a greater percentage of mothers work outside the home and most of their earnings go to support the family. Thus, women are adopting some of the instrumental functions originally subscribed to men. These changes mean that mothers are assuming more of the economic burden for raising children and assuming a stronger role in disciplining their children. Fathers are more likely to share some of the care taking tasks that were once the sole responsibility of mothers.

As parental roles are merging with mothers working outside the home and contributing to the financial well-being of the family and fathers becoming more involved in expressive activities (Penn State 2008), researchers are questioning whether or not the distinction between mothers and fathers' roles first proposed by Parsons and Bales (1955) still exists. To test this idea, Finley et al. (2008) conducted a retrospective study of college students. They found that the students rated their fathers higher on instrumental functions than on expressive functions and rated their mothers higher on expressive functions than instrumental functions as would be predicted by Parsons and Bales (1955). However, when mean scores were compared, mothers were rated higher than fathers on all functions except one instrumental function that was income. These findings provide support that mothers are taking on more instrumental functions within the family. Of interest in this study is that mothers and fathers were both rated low on expressive functions related to physical development, sharing activities, and leisure activities. While this finding may not be surprising given the increased time demands in single and dual earner families, less involvement in issues related to physical development has implications for the sexual health of adolescents.

In addition to studying parental role functions, researchers have also examined the role of the family on children outcomes. Much of this research has demonstrated the advantage of children living in two-parent households. Investigators studying families uniformly agree that there are benefits to the child being raised by both the mother and father, because these children tend to consistently have a better sense of well-being than those raised in single-parent households (Amato 2005). Children raised in two-parent families are less likely to be involved in delinquent activities such as carrying weapons; engaging in theft, violence, and disorder; and running away (Carlson 2006; National Fatherhood Initiative 2008). They are also less likely to fail academically and more likely to report more favorable psychological adjustment as adults (Carlson 2006).

Interestingly, parental characteristics may be as important as family structure in predicting children outcomes. In his work, Lerner (National Fatherhood Initiative[SM] 2008) found that children raised in two-parent families demonstrated fewer delinquent behaviors than children raised in one-parent households or blended families. However, when reports of mother and father closeness were considered, the effects of family structure diminished. More specifically, those who reported greater parental closeness also reported fewer delinquent behaviors regardless of family structure. Lerner concluded that parental closeness acts as an intervening variable between family structure and delinquent behaviors. Two-parent families provide more opportunities for parental closeness, which in turn serves as a protective factor against adolescent delinquent behaviors.

Kirby and Lepore (2007) have conducted an extensive study of parent characteristics including parental closeness and its association with child health outcomes. Their work has led to the development of the parent–child connectedness (PCC) construct to capture the most influential components of the parent's role in promoting adolescent health. They define PCC as "a condition characterized by an emotional bond between a parent and a child that is both mutual and sustained over time" (Rolleri et al. 2006). The PCC construct is composed of the following components: attachment/bonding, autonomy granting, cohesion, communication, support/involvement, maternal/paternal characteristics, monitoring/control, and warmth/caring (Lezin et al. 2004). The researchers have outlined the specific parent behaviors that foster PCC and identified the determinants of these behaviors (Rolleri et al. 2006). Two of these concepts, monitoring/control and communication, have been studied extensively in regard to adolescent sexual health as discussed below.

5.2.1 Mothers' Influence

Mothers' behavior, especially their communication with their adolescents, their approval of their adolescents' behavior, and their monitoring of their adolescents' behavior, has been associated with their adolescents' participation in risky behaviors. Compared to fathers and other guardians, mothers were the main persons to discuss sexuality with their adolescents (Miller et al. 1998a, b; Romer et al. 1999). Mothers' willingness to talk openly with their adolescents about many topics, including sexuality and sexual risks, was related to the reduction of adolescents' risky sexual behavior (Dutra et al. 1999; Miller et al. 2000). This reduction included the adolescents delaying sexual initiation until a later age (Fasula and Miller 2006; Whitaker and Miller 2000), the adolescents' tendency to communicate with their sexual partners about sex (Perrino et al. 2000), and the adolescents' participation in fewer sexual activities (Hutchinson et al. 2003). Mothers' willingness to speak openly was characterized as talking and listening to their adolescents without being judgmental (Dutra et al. 1999; Miller et al. 2000).

In addition, when mothers talked to their adolescents about condom use, their adolescents tended to use condoms more consistently (Whitaker and Miller 2000). If mothers talked to their adolescents before the adolescents' sexual initiation, their adolescents were more likely to use a condom during their first and subsequent sexual intercourse (Miller et al. 1998a, b). Similarly, mothers talking to their adolescents about sexual risks was associated with the adolescents using condoms at initial sexual intercourse and more consistently (Romer et al. 1999), and with more condom use and increased condom use self-efficacy (Hutchinson et al. 2003). Lastly, mothers' communication with their adolescents about sex and condoms was associated with the adolescents not succumbing to peer pressure to engage in sex and to not use condoms (Whitaker and Miller 2000; Romer et al. 1999).

Adolescent's perception of their mother's disapproval of sex was associated with the adolescent participating in fewer sexual activities, including delaying sexual initiation (Jaccard et al. 1996, 1998; Aronowitz et al. 2005; McNeely et al. 2002). Additionally, adolescents who were monitored by their mothers tended to initiate sexual intercourse at a later age (Romer et al. 1999), especially when they perceived that their mothers were monitoring their behavior (Dancy et al. 2006a). However, maternal monitoring was not related to adolescents' condom use (Romer et al. 1999).

5.3   Innovative HIV-Risk Reduction Interventions for Adolescents

To enhance adolescents' HIV-risk reduction behaviors, several researchers have developed innovative HIV-risk reduction interventions for mothers and their adolescents. Family members, including mothers, are important in HIV-risk reduction because they can implement social control and provide adolescents HIV-risk reduction knowledge and skills on a daily basis or during "teachable moments" (Pequegnat 2005). The inclusion of parents in health interventions, including HIV/AIDS interventions, has especially been advocated for African American youths (Williams 2003).

5.3.1   A Mother–Adolescent HIV Prevention Program

DiIorio et al. (2000) developed a mother–adolescent HIV prevention program based on Bandura's social cognitive theory (SCT). In this HIV prevention program, adolescents and their mothers attended, over a 14-week period, 72-h sessions: four sessions together and three sessions separately (DiIorio et al. 2000, 2006). During the four sessions where mothers and their adolescents attended together, facilitators covered topics related to HIV transmission and protection, communication, and values. The separate sessions for adolescents focused on peer pressure, sexual decision making, and consequences of early sexual initiation. The separate sessions for mothers focused on adolescent development, reproductive health, including condom and contraceptive use, peer pressure, and communication with adolescents. The intervention consisted of role-plays, games, demonstrations, group discussions, videos, and homework assignments. This intervention was compared to a Life Skills Program (LSK) and a 1 hour intervention with a 20 minute video on HIV transmission and prevention.

A randomized cluster trial was used to explore the effectiveness of these three HIV-risk reduction interventions. Adolescents ranged in age from 11 to 14 years with a mean age of 12.2 years. These adolescents were 98% African Americans and 60% males, with 90% residing with their biological mothers, and 46% residing with their biological, step, or adoptive fathers. Their mothers had a mean age of 38 years, and 97% were African Americans, 67% were single, and 56% had completed some college. Only 11% of their mothers had less than a high school diploma (DiIorio et al. 2006).

DiIorio et al. (2006) results revealed that over the 24-month period, adolescents receiving the SCT, the LSK, and the control interventions did not differ in holding hands, touching their partners' genitals, and initiating sexual intercourse. Condom use increased for sexually active adolescents at the 6- and 12-month period for the LSK, but not for the SCT and the control groups. Knowledge increased for mothers and adolescents in the SCT at the 4-month period. Compared to mothers in the control intervention, mothers in the SCT and LSK interventions were more likely to talk to their adolescents, intended to talk to their adolescents, and were more comfortable talking to their adolescents about sexual topics.

5.3.2   Mother/Daughter HIV-Risk Reduction

Dancy (2003) and Dancy et al. (2006b) developed the Mother/Daughter HIV-Risk Reduction (MDRR) intervention. The MDRR intervention, based on the SCT and the theory of reasoned action, consisted of six weekly sessions taught by trained mothers. Each session lasted 2 hours. The content covered was sexual development, reproductive health, sexually transmitted illnesses, HIV transmission and prevention, assertiveness and decision-making, abstinence, and the correct use of the male and female condoms. Teaching strategies included didactic information, games, role-plays, group discussions, modeling, return demonstration, and constructive feedback. Over a 12-week period in a group setting, facilitators provided to mothers intensive training on the MDRR intervention. The facilitators modeled the presentation of the MDRR intervention and had mothers select portions of the intervention that they would present to their daughters in a group setting. Mothers were required to practice in-session and between-sessions to ensure that they were knowledgeable about the MDRR content and teaching strategies and were competent in their presentation. Facilitators and other mothers in the group provided mothers with constructive feedback. After the 12-week period, mothers implemented the MDRR intervention to their daughters with facilitators serving as consultants.

Using a longitudinal quasi-experimental comparison group design, Dancy et al. (2006a, b) determined the effectiveness of the MDRR intervention by comparing it to two control interventions. The first control intervention was the health expert HIV-risk reduction intervention (HERR) that consisted of the same HIV-risk reduction content and teaching strategies as the MDRR, but was taught by facilitators and not by the girls' mothers as in the MDRR intervention. The second control group was the mother/daughter health promotion (MDHP) intervention. Similar to the MDRR intervention, the MDHP intervention was taught by the girl's mothers. However, the content of the MDHP intervention focused on healthy eating and physical activity to promote health and prevent obesity-related diseases that are prevalent in the African American community, namely hypertension and diabetes.

The sample consisted of African American mother/daughter pairs. The adolescent girls ranged in age from 11 to 14 years with a mean age of 12.4 years. Their mothers ranged in age from 22 to 76 years with a mean age of 40.2 years. The majority of the mothers (45%) were single; 31% had less than a 12th grade education; 56% had completed 12th grade or received their graduation equivalency diploma (GED); and 62% had a monthly income of less than $1,100 (Dancy et al. 2006a, b).

At the 2-month posttest, compared to adolescents in MDHP interventions, the adolescents in the MDRR and HERR interventions had significantly higher scores on HIV transmission knowledge, self-efficacy to refuse sex, and intention to refuse sex. Also adolescents in the MDHP were more likely to be sexually active than the adolescents in the MDRR and HERR interventions (Dancy et al. 2006a, b).

5.3.3 Saving Sex for Later

O'Donnell et al. (2005) developed three CDs titled *Saving Sex for Later* based on the diffusion of innovation theory and the theory of planned behavior. The CDs were designed as a parent education program to increase parents' self-efficacy, attitudes, and skills to communicate with their adolescents about sexual topics and to promote their adolescents' sexual abstinence. To provide parents an opportunity to view the CDs at a convenient time in the privacy of their homes, parents received the CDs via mail one every 10 weeks over a 6-month period. Topics covered in these CDs were adolescent development, sexual attraction to the opposite sex, peer pressure, and reasons why adolescents are not ready for sex.

In a randomized experiment, parent–adolescent pairs were randomly assigned to either the CD intervention or the no treatment control intervention. The adolescents ranged in age from 10 to over 13 years. Eighty-three percent were 10 or 11 years old; 48% were males; 64% were African Americans; and 90% qualified for the public school free lunch program. Eighty-eight percent of the parents were mothers; 66% were African Americans; and 66% were 40-years-old or younger (O'Donnell et al. 2005).

At the 3-month follow-up, compared to parents in the control intervention, parents in the CD intervention had significantly higher scores on parental influence on their adolescent's behavior, communication about sexual topics, and self-efficacy to communicate about sexual topics. Adolescents in the CD intervention had significantly higher scores on perceptions of family rules and family support and reported fewer episodes of dating, kissing, and holding hands (O'Donnell et al. 2005).

5.3.4   Informed Parents and Children Together

The Informed Parents and Children Together (ImPACT) intervention was designed to reduce adolescent truancy, substance abuse, and sexual risk behaviors through promoting adolescents' parental monitoring and communication behaviors (Stanton et al. 2000, 2004). Based on the SCT, the ImPACT intervention is a one-session 20-min video. It covers parental monitoring behavior of adolescent's behavior, parental communication with adolescent about sex, factual information about HIV/AIDS and condom use, sexual risk reduction strategies, and risks related to substance use. An interventionist showed the video to the parent and the adolescent in their home. After the viewing of the video, the interventionist addressed any questions the parent and adolescent had and instructed the parent and adolescent to participate in a predetermined role-play. The interventionist reiterated the key points of the video and instructed the parent and adolescent to repeat the role-play and to incorporate the key points of the video in the role-play. The parent and adolescent then practiced putting on and removing a condom and the interventionist gave the parent the copy of the video and notes stressing the key points (Stanton et al. 2000).

Using a randomized, controlled longitudinal research design, the effectiveness of the ImPACT intervention was explored. Parent–adolescent pairs were randomly assigned to either the ImPACT intervention or the attention control intervention (Stanton et al. 2000, 2004).

All participating parents and adolescents pairs were African American. Adolescents ranged in age from 12 to 16 years (Stanton et al. 2000, 2004). Adolescents had a median age of 13.6 years (Stanton et al. 2000) and 14 years (Stanton et al. 2004) with 51% (Stanton et al. 2000) and 42% being male (Stanton et al. 2004). Approximately 96% of the parents were mothers; no other parental demographic information was provided (Stanton et al. 2000, 2004).

At 24 months, compared to the adolescents in the control interventions, the adolescents in the ImPACT intervention had significantly higher self-efficacy to practice low-risk behaviors. However, the adolescents in the control and ImPACT interventions did not differ significantly on school truancy, substance abuse, sexual risk behaviors (Stanton et al. 2000), and participation in sexual intercourse (Stanton et al. 2004). Additionally, the ImPACT intervention had no effect on increasing the use of condom and birth control (Stanton et al. 2004).

5.3.5 Chicago HIV Prevention and Mental Health Project

Paikoff et al. designed the Chicago HIV Prevention and Adolescent Mental Health Project (CHAMP) Family Program (McKay et al. 2000, 2004). CHAMP is a 12-session group intervention to promote parental communication, support, and monitoring and supervision as well as adolescents' assertiveness and problem-solving skills. Each session lasted 90 min. Topics included communication techniques, monitoring skills, the development of rules for adolescents, talking to adolescents about and preparing them for puberty and adolescents, and factual information about HIV/AIDS. Each session began with parents and their adolescents meeting together in a group where the topic for the session was presented. Then, a separate adolescent group and a separate parent group were conducted for detailed discussion of the topic. These groups were followed by the parent and adolescents meeting together again for the last 30 min to practice family activities. The 12th session was a celebration of the completion of the program.

A quasi-experimental posttest-only research design was used to compare participants in the CHAMP Family Program intervention with a comparison group of participants residing in the same community. The comparison group was assessed a year prior to the administration of the posttest to the CHAMP Family Program participants. This community was predominantly African American and 75% of the households were female-headed. Seventy-six percent of the parents in the CHAMP Family Program and 90% of the parents in the comparison group reported an annual income less than $14,000. In regards to education, 75% of the CHAMP Family Program adults and 46% of the comparison group adults had a 12th grade education. All adolescents were in the fourth and fifth grades with approximately 60% being female (McKay et al. 2004).

Posttest data were collected during the 11th weeks. Compared to the comparison group, the parents in the CHAMP Family Program made more decisions, monitored their adolescents more, had increased communication with their adolescents, and were more comfortable talking to their adolescents about HIV/AIDS and sexuality (McKay et al. 2004).

5.3.6 Parent–Adolescent Relationship Education Program

Lederman et al. developed the Parent–Adolescent Relationship Education (PARE) program for parents and their 12–14-year-old adolescents (Lederman and Mian 2003; Lederman et al. 2004). The PARE program is designed to reduce the rate of adolescent pregnancy and acquisition of STDs by increasing communication about sexuality between parents and their adolescents and by enhancing adolescents' risk reduction behaviors. Based on the social learning theory and the cognitive behavioral theory, the PARE program has four sessions that are taught over the course of 4 weeks. Each session is two and a half hours with parents and adolescents in separate classes during the first half followed by parents and adolescents together in the same class for the last half. The content focuses on adolescent development, communication between parents and adolescents with emphasis on effective and ineffective communication and communication barriers, risk reduction behavioral skills, consequences of risky behaviors, stress reduction, and the development of future goals. Teaching strategies include didactic information, behavioral rehearsal, and role-playing.

Parent–adolescent dyads were randomly assigned to either the PARE program or to the attention control group. In addition, another control group of students were included who did not receive any intervention. The adolescents ranged in age from 11 to 15 years with 46% being between 11 and 12 years and 54% between 13 and 15 years. Fifty-five percent were girls; 38% were Latino; 26% were African American; and 26% were Caucasian. No demographic characteristics were given for the parents (Lederman et al. 2004).

Lederman et al. (2004) revealed that at 3–6 months after the initiation of the intervention, compared to adolescents in the control groups, adolescents in the parent-involved social learning curriculum had higher intention to delay sex. However, there were no differences among the adolescents in the three groups on level of parent–adolescent communication. The researchers also found no relationship between parent–child communication and these three determinants of risky sexual behavior: the adolescents' intention to engage in sex, attitude about risky sexual behavior, and perception of parental disapproval of risky sexual behavior.

5.3.7 Mothers and Sexual Communication

Lefkowitz et al. (2000) designed an intervention to enhance mothers' communication skills with their adolescents (Lefkowitz et al. 2000). The intervention consisted of two communication training sessions conducted in a group setting 1 week apart. The first session focused on communication related to conflict whereas the second session focused on communication related to sexuality and dating. In both sessions, the group facilitator stressed good communication techniques, such as, using open-ended and probing questions, listening more and talking less, providing the adolescent with ample opportunity to present his/her opinion, being supportive, and making every attempt not to lecture. During the first session, the mothers listened to two two-minute audiotapes of a mother–adolescent conversation. The mothers critiqued these audiotapes for similarities and differences in communication and then role-played communication exercises. Mothers were given a communication techniques handout to use to complete the homework assignment, which was to practice the communication techniques before the second session. The second session focused on the communication techniques for discussing sexuality and dating. This session ended with a homework assignment to discuss sexuality and dating with their adolescents.

Mother–adolescent pairs were randomly assigned to the intervention or the delayed control group. The age range for the adolescents was 10.7–14.5 years with a mean age of 12.5 years for the intervention group and 12.8 years for the delayed control group. The mean age for mothers in the intervention group was 41.8 years and 44.0 years for the delayed control group mothers. Mothers in the intervention group had a mean of 15 years of education whereas those in the delayed control groups had a mean of 16.7 years of education. For both groups, the household income ranged from $10,000 to more than $100,000 with a median of $40,000 to $60,000. Half (50%) of the mothers were European–American with 18% being Latin American, 15% being African American, and 10% being Asian American (Lefkowitz et al. 2000).

The results revealed that 7 weeks after session one, compared to mothers in the delayed control group, mothers in the intervention group talked less, used more open-ended questions, were less judgmental, and communicated about sexuality and dating more. The adolescents of mothers in the intervention group, compared to those adolescents of mothers in the delayed control group, reported being more comfortable talking to their mothers and engaged in more communication with their mothers about birth control (Lefkowitz et al. 2000).

In summary, the interventions including mothers as agents to promote adolescents' sexual risk reduction behaviors have used different innovative strategies and were successful in enhancing adolescents' condom use, HIV knowledge, self-efficacy to refuse sex, intention to refuse sex, perception of family rules and support, self-efficacy to practice low-risk behaviors, comfort in talking with their mothers, and communication about birth control with their mothers. The interventions were also successful in increasing mothers' effective communication, intention to communicate, and self-efficacy to communicate with their adolescents about sexuality. Additionally, the interventions also increased maternal monitoring and influence on their adolescents' behavior. However the interventions had no long-term impact on engaging in sexual intercourse.

Innovative strategies used in some of these interventions included the enhancement of intentions, behavioral skills, and environmental constraints, three components that Fishbein et al. (1992) advocated as both necessary and sufficient to promote behavioral change (Pequegnat 2005). Intentions are plans to behave in a manner that will promote HIV-risk reduction, behavioral skills are the actions needed to implement or perform risk reduction behaviors, and environmental constraints are the external factors that promote the performance of risk reduction behaviors. For adolescents, environmental constraints can include parental monitoring and supervision, familial rules and values, parent–adolescent communication about adolescent issues and concerns, including sexuality, and peers and adults in the neighborhoods who sanction risk reduction behaviors. These components interact reciprocally to promote behavioral change. Research is needed to systematically explore the pathway by which these components interact to promote behavior for specified populations.

5.4   Translation of Research Findings into Practice

Incorporating any one or a combination of these interventions into clinical practice would require a systematic organized effort to overcome challenges. These challenges include lack of support from facility administrators and from credible clinical leaders; inconsistency between the intervention and the facility's norms, values, and goals; and inadequate plans and resources to implement and sustain the intervention (Bradley et al. 2004). In addition, the complexity of the intervention is an additional challenge (Titler 2007). To overcome these challenges, health care providers will need to secure strong support from their administrators and from key clinical leaders. Health care providers and key clinical leaders will need to thoroughly review the intervention and adapt it to their clinical practice as well as implement and evaluate the intervention. It is necessary to conduct group discussions about the role of the intervention and about the compatibility of the intervention with the facility's norms, values, and goals. Also it is imperative to develop detailed feedback mechanisms for the evaluation of the implementation of the intervention.

References

Amato PR. The impact of family formation change on the cognitive, social, and emotional well-being of the next generation. Future Child. 2005;115:75–96.

Aronowitz T, Rennells RE, Todd E. Heterosocial behaviors in early adolescent African American girls: the role of mother-daughter relationships. J Fam Nurs. 2005;11(2):122–39.

Bradley EH, Webster TR, Baker D, Schlesinger M, Inouye SK, Barth MC, et al. Translating research into practice: speeding the adoption of innovative health care programs (2004). Available via the Commonwealth Fund http://www.cmwf.org. Cited 15 July 2009.

Carlson MJ. Family structure, father involvement, and adolescent behavioral outcomes. J Marriage Fam. 2006;68:137–54.

Centers for Disease Control and Prevention (CDC). Sexually transmitted disease surveillance 1995. Atlanta, GA: CDC; 1996.

Centers for Disease Control and Prevention (CDC) (2004) Youth Risk Behavior Surveillance – United States, 2003. MMWR, 53(SS-2):1–29. Atlanta, GA: CDC.

Centers for Disease Control and Prevention (CDC) (2009) HIV/AIDS among Youth. Available via: http://www.cdc.gov/hiv/resources/factsheets/youth.htm Cited 30 January 2009.

Centers for Disease Control and Prevention (CDC) (2009) The HIV/AIDS Epidemic: what is the Magnitude? Available via: http://www.cdc.gov/hiv/resources/reports/hiv3rddecade/chapter2. htm#serious Cited January 30, 2009.

Dancy BL. Focus on solutions: a community-based mother/daughter HIV risk reduction intervention. In: Gilbert DJ, Wright EM, editors. African American women and HIV/AIDS. Westport, CT: Praeger Publisher; 2003. p. 183–9.

Dancy BL, Crittenden KS, Talashek M. Mothers' effectiveness as HIV risk reduction educators for adolescent daughters. J Health Care Poor Underserved. 2006a;17:218–39.

Dancy BL, Crittenden KS, Freels S. African-American adolescent females' predictors of having sex. J Natl Black Nurses Assoc. 2006b;17(2):30–8.

DiIorio C, Resnicow K, Denzmore P, Rogers-Tillman G, Wang DT, Dudley WN, et al. Keepin' it R.E.A.L.! A mother-adolescent HIV prevention program. In: Pequegnat W, Szapocznik J, editors. Working with families in the era of AIDS (113–132). Thousand Oaks, CA: Sage Publications; 2000.

DiIorio C, Resnicow K, McCarty F, De AK, Dudley WN, Wang DT, et al. Keepin' it R.E.A.L.! Results of a mother-adolescent HIV prevention program. Nursing Res. 2006;55(1):43–51.

Dutra R, Miller KS, Forehand R. The process and content of sexual communication with adolescents in two-parent families: association with sexual risk-taking behavior. AIDS Behav. 1999;3(1):59–66.

Fasula AM, Miller KS. African-American and Hispanic adolescents' intentions to delay first intercourse: parental communication as a buffer for sexually active peers. J Adolesc Health. 2006;38:193–200.

Finley GE, Mira SD, Schwartz SJ. Perceived paternal and maternal involvement: factor structures, mean differences, and parental roles. Fathering. 2008;6:62–82.

Fishbein M, Bandura A, Triandis HC, Kanfer FH, Becker MH, Middlestadt SE et al. (1992). Factors influencing behavior and behavior change: final report – Theorist's workshop. Rockville, M.D.: NIMH. A slightly revised version of this report was published in Baum A, Revenson T, and Singer J (eds), (2000). Handbook of health psychology. N.J: Lawrence Erlbaum and Associates.

Hutchinson MK, Jemmott III JB, Jemmott LS, Braverman P, Fong GT. The role of mother-daughter sexual risk communication in reducing sexual risk behaviors among urban adolescent females: a prospective study. J Adolesc Health. 2003;33(2):98–107.

Jaccard J, Dittus PJ, Gordon VV. Maternal correlates of adolescent sexual and contraceptive behavior. Fam Planning Perspect. 1996;28(4):159–65. 185.

Jaccard J, Dittus PJ, Gordon VV. Parent-adolescent congruency in reports of adolescent sexual behavior and in communications about sexual behavior. Child Dev. 1998;69(1):247–61.

Kirby D, Lepore G. A matrix of risk and protective factors affecting teen sexual behavior, pregnancy, childbearing and sexually transmitted disease. Santa Cruz, CA: ETR Associates; 2007.

Lederman RP, Mian TS. The parent-adolescent relationship education (PARE) program: a curriculum for prevention of STDs and pregnancy in middle school youth. Behav Med. 2003;29:33–41.

Lederman RP, Chan W, Roberts-Gray C. Sexual risk attitudes and intentions of youth aged 12–14 years: survey comparisons of parent-teen prevention and control groups. Behav Med. 2004;29(4):155–63.

Lefkowitz ES, Sigman M, Au TK. Helping mothers discuss sexuality and AIDS with adolescents. Child Dev. 2000;71(5):1383–94.

Lezin N, Rolleri LA, Bean S, Taylor J. Parent-child connectedness: implications for research, interventions, and positive impacts on adolescent health. Santa Cruz, CA: ETR Associates; 2004.

McKay MM, Baptiste D, Coleman D, Madison S, Paikoff R, Scott R. In: Pequegnat W, Szapocznik J, editors. Working with families in the era of AIDS. Thousand Oaks, CA: Sage Publications; 2000.

McKay MM, Chasse KT, Paikoff R, McKinney L, Baptiste D, Coleman D, et al. Family-level impact of the CHAMP Family program: a community collaborative effort to support urban families and reduce youth HIV risk exposure. Fam Process. 2004;43(1):79–93.

McNeely C, Shew ML, Beuhring T, Sieving R, Miller BC, Blum RW. Mothers' influence on the timing of first sex among 14- and 15- year-olds. J Adolesc Health. 2002;31:256–65.

Miller KS, Forehand R, Kotchick BA. Adolescent sexual behavior in two ethnic minority groups: a multisystem perspective. Adolescence. 2000;35(138):313–33.

Miller KS, Kotchick BA, Dorsey S, Forehand R, Ham AY. Family communication about sex: what are parents saying and are their adolescents listening? Fam Planning Perspect. 1998a;30(5):218–22.

Miller KS, Levin ML, Whitaker DJ, Xu X. Patterns of condom use among adolescents: the impact of mother-adolescent communication. Am J Public Health. 1998b;88(10):1542–4.

National Fatherhood Initiative SM. Family structure, father closeness and delinquency. Available via: http://www.fatherhood.org/download_files.asp?DownloadID=11 Cited November 13, 2008.

O'Donnell L, Stueve A, Agronick G, Wilson-Simmons R, Duran R, Jeanbaptiste V. Saving sex for later: an evaluation of a parent education intervention. Perspect Sexual Reproduct Health. 2005;37(4):166–73.

Parsons T, Bales RF. Family, socialization, and interaction process. Glencoe, IL: Free Press; 1955.

Penn State (2008, January 11). Divorce May Widen Distance Between Teens, Fathers. Science Daily. Available via: http://www.sciencedaily.com/releases/2008/01/080109094337.htm Cited 13 November 2008.

Pequegnat W. AIDS behavioral prevention: unprecedented progress and emerging challenges. In: Mayer KH, Pizer HF, editors. The AIDS pandemic: impact on science and society. Amsterdam: Elsevier; 2005. p. 236–60.

Perrino T, Gonzalez-Soldevilla A, Pantin H, Szapocznik J. The role of families in adolescent HIV prevention: a review. Clin Child Fam Psychol Rev. 2000;3(2):81–96.

Rolleri LA, Bean S, Ecker N. A logic model of parent-child connectedness: using the behavioral determinant-intervention (BDI) logic model to identify parent behaviors necessary for connectedness with teen children. Santa Cruz, CA: ETR Associates; 2006.

Romer D, Stanton B, Galbraith J, Feigelman S, Black MM, Li X. Parental influence on adolescent sexual behaviorin high-poverty settings. Arch Pediatr Adolesc Med. 1999;153:1055–62.

Scott ME, Booth A, King V, Johnson DR. Postdivorce father-adolescent closeness. J Marriage Fam. 2007;69:1194–209.

Stanton B, Cole M, Galbraith J, Li X, Pendleton S, Cottrel L, et al. Randomized trial of a parent intervention: parents can make a difference in a long-term adolescent risk behaviors, perception, and knowledge. Arch Pediatr Adolesc Med. 2004;158:947–55.

Stanton B, Li X, Galbraith J, Cornick G, Feigelman S, Kaljee L, et al. Parental underestimates of adolescent risk behavior: a randomized, controlled trial of a parental monitoring intervention. J Adolesc Health. 2000;26(1):18–26.

Titler M. Translating research into practice. Am J Nurs. 2007;107(6):26–33.

Whitaker DJ, Miller KS. Parent-adolescent discussions about sex and condoms: impact on peer influences of sexual risk behavior. J Adolesc Res. 2000;15(2):251–73.

Williams PB. HIV/AIDS case profile of African Americans: guidelines for ethnic-specific health promotion, education, and risk reduction activities for African Americans. Fam Commun Health. 2003;26(4):289–306.

Chapter 6
Fathers and HIV/AIDS: A Missing Factor in Developing Interventions But Not in the Lives of Their Children

Larry D. Icard, Colleen DiIorio, and Jay S. Fagan

Abstract This chapter provides an overview of three perspectives on fatherhood in relation to HIV prevention and treatment: an ecological approach, father identity, and father involvement. Next, four distinct subgroups are highlighted: (1) HIV-negative fathers, (2) gay and bisexual fathers, (3) incarcerated fathers, and (4) homeless fathers. An intervention study for fathers and their children, Responsible, Empowered, Aware, Living (REAL) Men is presented to illustrate the importance of fathers as effective educators on HIV prevention and sexuality for their sons. Race and culture are discussed as key factors to consider as we move forward in understanding the role of fathers in relations to HIV/AIDS. The discussion concludes with recommendations for future directions.

Public health researchers and practitioners have long recognized the importance of fathers in the promotion of optimum health and the reduction of health problems within families. Nationally and globally, little attention is given to fathers in the context of family-based HIV prevention and treatment (Desmond and Hosegood 2011; Sherr 2010). Cognizant of the staggering effect which HIV and AIDS continue to have on the lives of families, this chapter focuses on fathers affected with, and affected by, this menacing health problem. The meaning of father has traditionally referred to a male biological parent of a child. The contemporary meaning of father should be understood in the context of the dramatic shifts occurring in the socio-demographic characteristics of families, the growing diversity of fatherhood, and varying residential patterns for men in their role as primary care provider to a child. The complexities of contemporary fatherhood require thoughtful attention to the meaning of family. Worthy of consideration is the NIMH Consortium on Families and HIV definition of family as a network of mutual commitments (Pequegnat and Bray 1997; Pequegnat and Szapocznik 2000). This broad definition of the family captures populations of men who may or may not be biologically related to a child.

W. Pequegnat and C.C. Bell (eds.), *Family and HIV/AIDS: Cultural and Contextual Issues in Prevention and Treatment*, DOI 10.1007/978-1-4614-0439-2_6,
© Springer Science+Business Media, LLC 2012

6.1 Scope of the Problem

As in the early stages of the pandemic and in industrialized and developing countries, HIV infection is predominantly among men (WHO 2008). In the United States, men comprise three quarters of the HIV/AIDS diagnosed cases (Centers for Disease Control and Prevention (CDC) 2009a), and they comprise 76% of all new cases of HIV/AIDS (Centers for Disease Control and Prevention (CDC) 2009b). Although Blacks (13%) and Hispanics (12%) comprise a small portion, of the total population in the United States (Centers for Disease Control and Prevention (CDC) 2003), Black men constitute 49% of all HIV/AIDS cases. Hispanic American men make up 18% of all cases (Centers for Disease Control and Prevention (CDC) 2008). Data are currently not available on the number of men with HIV who are also fathers. Still, these statistics raise questions concerning the percentage of men living with HIV/AIDS today who might be fathers.

The survival rates of adult men and adolescent males raise additional concerns with regard to fathers with HIV/AIDS. As a result of advances in medical treatment after an AIDS diagnosis, life expectancy continues to increase. The survival rate for adult men and adolescent males is approximately 90% (Centers for Disease Control and Prevention (CDC) 2009a, b). An increased life expectancy for fathers who are now living with HIV/AIDS has enabled them to play an active role as providers and care takers for their children. There are, however, mixed blessings from advancements in HIV medical treatment. As people are living longer with the disease, new insights about fathers with HIV/AIDS are beginning to emerge.

Major concerns in being a long-time survivor of HIV/AIDS are the effects of the virus itself, coupled with treatment regiments, on the process of aging. Studies now show that HIV/AIDS patients live longer but age faster. Fathers who are long-term survivors of HIV and who adequately manage their health are able to carry out their parenting responsibilities. However, they may also find that their parenting abilities are compromised by the unanticipated negative consequences of their medical treatments.

Another issue that has implications for fathers is the decreasing age at which persons become infected with the virus. About 50% of all new HIV infections occur among young people aged 10–24 (WHO 2008). The most recent statistics from the Centers for Disease Control and Prevention (CDC) indicate that young people aged 13–24 years represent approximately 13% of the cases diagnosed with HIV infection or AIDS (Centers for Disease Control and Prevention (CDC) 2007). This age trend means that there is likely to be a growing population of adolescent fathers with HIV/AIDS. Adolescence is generally thought to be a highly stressful period of development and may be particularly challenging when the young father also has a chronic disease.

The current trend of the AIDS pandemic provides impetus for examining the role of fathers in HIV/AIDS prevention and treatment. The fact that three-fourths of people living with HIV/AIDS are men suggests that many of these men may be fathers. The shift of the epidemic from white gay men to Blacks and Hispanics raises concerns for fathers and the consequences that HIV/AIDS may have on their families. The statistics on the increasing rates of HIV among adolescents and young adults has implications for fathers in developing prevention and treatment programs.

6.2 Fathers as the Focus for Health and HIV/AIDS Research

Efforts to understand and apply knowledge about fatherhood generally follow one of three approaches. One approach focuses on fatherhood in the ecological context of the family (Bradford and Hawkins 2006; Crosby et al. 2002; Patterson et al. 1999). Other scholars approach fatherhood by focusing on father identity (Forste et al. 2009; Fox and Bruce 2001; Jordan-Zachery 2009; Olmstead et al. 2009; Palkovitz and Palm 2009; Soliz et al. 2009). A third approach concerns father involvement, particularly with regard to children's developmental outcomes (Barber and Thomas 1986; Fagan et al. 2009; Thornton and Camburn 1987; Yang et al. 2007).

6.2.1 Ecology of Fatherhood

A fundamental question being addressed by researchers exploring the ecology of fatherhood is: "What are the important contextual factors affecting fathers, and in what ways do these factors affect fathers with HIV?" Some of the important contextual variables are: (1) changing gender roles, (2) cultural shifts in what it means to be a good father, (3) economic influences, (4) changing family structures, (5) homelessness, and (6) high rates of incarceration. Bronfenbrenner and Morris (1998) suggested that ecological factors include both proximal and distal influences, with proximal influences having greater effect on parenting than distal influences. For example, the influence of relationships within the family (proximal influence) may have a greater influence on fathers' parenting than does the influence of changing gender role norms in society (distal influence).

6.2.1.1 Changing Gender Roles

Societal changes in gender roles (distal influence) include the large increase in the number of women with children in the labor market and changing norms for what it means to be a father. Several decades of research show that fathers' participation in childcare is influenced by mothers' employment. Fathers in married or cohabiting relationships with the mother are more likely to provide care for their child while the mother is at work and while both parents are at home with the children (Wang and Bianchi 2009). As mothers' work hours and responsibilities increase, fathers provide additional hours of care to the child.

A shift in what it means to be a "good" father has also taken place in the United States. Over the past several decades, good fathering has shifted from being a breadwinner and playmate to one's child to participating in the care and nurturance of one's child (Coltrane 1996). Breadwinning is still important but not at the expense of fathers' participation in direct childcare. Evidence of this shift in fathering behavior comes from national time diary studies of fathers' household activities. Data have shown that fathers engaged in approximately three times as many hours of childcare activities in 2000 as they did in the 1960s (Sayer et al. 2004).

The shifts in gender roles and definitions of fathering seem to affect many populations of fathers in the United States. For example, a recent study of nonresidential fathers showed significantly higher rates of weekly contact with children among nonresidential fathers in 2000 compared with nonresidential fathers in 1976 (Amato et al. 2009). These shifts in fathering expectations are also likely to affect fathers with HIV (and potentially receiving disability benefits) and their abilities to provide care and nurturance of one's child. A father living with HIV and receiving disability benefits may have more time to spend with his children. Similarly, a father who is HIV-negative may have to assume more responsibilities as a nurturer and provider if the mother or wife is HIV-positive.

6.2.1.2   Gender Distrust

Researchers have found high levels of generalized gender distrust in low-income populations in the United States (Edlin and Kefalas 2005). Recent findings have also suggested that gender distrust is closely linked to the decline in marriage among low-income populations (Carlson et al. 2004). Yet, gender distrust does not seem to discourage low-income women from entering other types of unions with men, including romantic and cohabiting relationships (Lincoln et al. 2008). Several researchers have suggested that gender distrust may lead couples into having many short-term cohabiting relationships (Lichter and Qian 2008). Multiple partner relationships may place low-income couples at higher risk for transmission of the HIV virus. They have possible implications also for fathers with HIV attempting to stay involved with their children because they have less legal protection. Roy and colleagues' (2008) qualitative research with low-income unmarried, nonresidential fathers showed that mothers often want their baby's father to be involved with the child, but only if the father does not have too many problems of his own and can provide for his child. The father's HIV-positive status may result in an increase in the mother's distrust of the father and, therefore, result in the mother restricting the father's access to his children.

6.2.1.3   Economic Influences

Although cultural shifts in what it means to be a good father have deemphasized fathers' breadwinning (distal influence), it is clear that fathers are still expected to be good providers to their children (Townsend 2002). Public policy continues to place primary emphasis on nonresidential fathers' financial contributions to the children rather than their childcare contributions. What has become clear, however, is that fathers contribute a smaller percentage of the total family finances than they did 30–40 years ago. These economic changes are likely to have several implications for fathers with HIV/AIDS. A father living with HIV/AIDS is challenged by the vigilant adherence to treatment regiments required to manage the chronic invasiveness of HIV throughout his body. These demands may have a negative effect on the father's employability and ability to earn a living wage. These fathers may find it difficult to keep up with child support payments if they are no longer residing with the mother and children. There is increasing evidence that regular formal child support payments are linked to fathers' visits and time spent with the child. Fathers residing with their partners and children may find that they have less influence in decisions about their children when they are unable to make significant financial contributions to the family.

6.2.1.4   Household Structure

Three major changes in household structure have occurred in the last several decades that have implications for fathers with HIV. These include the increase in the number of children living in single mother households, the increase in the number of children living with cohabiting parents, and the increase in the number of nonfamily households (Selzter 2000). According to the U.S. Census Bureau, household types are arranged into two broad groups: family households and nonfamily households (Census 2008). The Census Bureau defines a family household as one with at least two people, the householder and at minimum, one other person related to the householder by birth, marriage, or adoption. A nonfamily household is a person living alone or a householder who is not related by birth, marriage, or adoption to the other persons sharing a home (Rawlings 1994).

Over the past several years, the proportion of households containing a mother, father, and a child under 18 has declined slightly while the number of nonfamily households has increased. In terms of population growth, nonfamily households contributed about 44% of the growth of total households over the past several years (Census 2008). The number of female-headed nonfamily households has contributed largely to the growth in nonfamily households; however, male-headed nonfamily households are growing slightly faster at a rate of 1.7% annually compared to female-headed nonfamily households with an annual projected growth rate of 1.4% a year. The second trend is the increase in the number of children living in single mother households. In 1960, 89% of children lived with both biological parents. In 2005, 72% of children lived with both parents. The third trend is the growing number of parents who cohabit and either delay or never marry each other. It is well established at this time that cohabiting relationships have a much higher dissolution rate than their married counterparts (Osborne et al. 2007). Together, these trends in household type mean that fewer fathers (with or without HIV) reside in the same household with their children and may sometimes reside in households with children of their partner.

6.2.1.5 Fathering

Fathers who are HIV-positive have characteristics and experiences that can influence the well-being of their children and other family members. Until recently, having HIV meant not conceiving children. Medical advances have reduced the risk of men who are HIV-positive passing on the virus to the mother. Fathers who are HIV-positive may know their status before conceiving or learn of their status after the birth of their child.

Medical advances allow HIV-positive men to reduce the risk of HIV transmission during insemination (Klein et al. 2003). Sperm washing which involves separating the sperm from the seminal fluid provides one option (van Leeuwen et al. 2009). Even though HIV is found in seminal fluid, it is not found in sperm itself. A sample of the washed sperm is tested for HIV and if the test is negative, it can then be used for conception through insemination. The procedure for sperm washing is costly.

Another less costly option for men who have reduced their viral load with antiviral treatment entails tracking ovulation and timing unprotected intercourse to occur during the woman's most fertile period (van Leeuwen et al. 2009). Although reducing the viral load to undetectable levels reduces the amount of HIV in the semen, HIV may be present (Barreiro et al. 2007). This option consequently presents a possible risk for HIV infection to the mother. These "safer" alternatives are available for a small number of HIV-positive men desiring to father a child. Men struggling with the emotional and physical challenges of being HIV-positive and having the desire to father children, along with bearing added pressures of poverty and the struggle to meet basic needs, may view medical options as unattainable. As one HIV-positive man shared in a focus group with HIV-positive men and women: "I can't afford any of that stuff" (Icard et al. unpublished).

6.2.2 Father Identity

Another approach to understanding fatherhood focuses on father identity. Olmstead and colleagues (2009) explored men's perceptions of their role as fathers. These researchers examined how these self-perceptions are positioned in men's overall sense of self as fathers in a sample of married and divorced, nonresident fathers.

Data from 34 fathers who participated in focus group interviews revealed that men's definition of self as father is both complex and integrative. Seven fathering role identities emerged: (1) provider, (2) teacher, (3) protector, (4) disciplinarian, (5) caretaker, (6) supporter, and (7) co-parent. Similarities were found in the fathers' self-perceptions regardless of marital status. Fox and Bruce (2001) also explored the notion of father identify by focusing on role salience and satisfaction. The findings from this study underscored the importance of social psychological variables in understanding variations in men's commitment to their children. Scholars have also found that a man whose identity as a father is central to his sense of himself is highly predictive of his involvement with his children (Rane and McBride 2000).

Researchers have hypothesized that the more a father is embedded in a network of relationships that are based on his being a father the more he will be committed to his role as a father (Ihinger-Tallman et al. 1993). A father living with HIV/AIDS is challenged in managing the negative impact that HIV/AIDS can have on his family. Grodeck (2003) presents a process that newly diagnosed patients may experience in the first year of diagnosis. The first 10 months are devoted to navigating through the physical, social, and emotional hurdles in having HIV, including overcoming the emotional overload, managing stigma, physical health, nutrition, and treatment. The subject of parenting is not addressed until the final stage of the process. Although the process described by Grodeck (2003) is biographical, his description provides insights into some of the challenges of living with HIV/AIDS for newly diagnosed fathers. Fathers with HIV/AIDS may find themselves marginalized from their family at a time when they need them to cope with this life challenge. This can result in a sense of loss of self which can impede a father's responsibilities as a caregiver and provider (Icard and Nurius 1996).

6.2.3 Father Involvement

Developmental outcome studies can be especially useful in describing the involvement of fathers in the transmission of values, including that of HIV/AIDS education and prevention. A number of studies address the relationship between family structures and processes and levels of sexual activity among adolescents. These studies include investigations on the importance of parental factors such as marital status, presence of adults in the household, income, quality of parenting and communication, supervision and monitoring, parental closeness, and values in relation to children's sexual development (Jessor et al. 1992; Newcomer and Udry 1987; Udry and Billy 1987). Adolescents from single-parent families often initiate sexual intercourse at earlier ages than those from two-parent families (Santilli et al. 2000). Early initiation of sexual intercourse has also been linked to educational attainment of parents (Santilli et al. 2000; Small and Luster 1994), low SES (Lammers et al 2000), and parental divorce/separation (Devine et al. 1993).

The nature of parent–adolescent relationships, including quality and type of communication, has been associated with early initiation of sexual intercourse

(Danziger 1995; Inazu and Fox 1980). Children reporting initiation of sexual intercourse during teen years often report high levels of conflict and/or strained relationships with their parents (Longmore et al. 2009; Price and Hyde 2009). Conversely, adolescents reporting warm and supportive relationships with parents and lower levels of family conflict tended to delay initiation of intercourse (Lenciauskiene and Zaborskis 2008; Price and Hyde 2009).

Other studies that focused on father–child communication revealed interesting findings. Lehr and colleagues (2005) examined predictors of father–child communication about sexuality among a sample of 155 fathers of adolescent sons. Fathers were more likely to talk with sons who were further along in pubertal development. Fathers who had more permissive sexual values were more likely to share sexuality information with their sons. The study findings also revealed that fathers with lower education levels reported more sexuality communication with their sons. Additionally, fathers who had more communication with their own fathers about sexuality reported more sexuality communications with their sons. Likewise, fathers who had more positive outcome expectations (e.g., talking to their sons about sex would strengthen their relationship with their sons, prevent their sons from engaging in negative health behaviors) were more likely to engage in sexuality communication with their sons. Similar to other studies examining self-efficacy as a determinant of the sexuality communication between parents and children, fathers who reported greater self-efficacy for sexuality communication reported more sexuality communications with their sons (Lehr et al. 2005). Kirkman and colleagues (2002) interviewed 32 parents (including mothers and fathers) and 19 adolescents ages 12–14 with the intention of learning the difficulties fathers have in communicating about sexuality with children. Results revealed that fathers experienced difficulties in sexual communication because they felt that it was the mother's role to talk with children about sex.

6.3 Special Populations and Issues

This section focuses on subgroups that are particularly salient in discussing the role of fathers in the context of HIV and AIDS. We highlight four distinct subgroups: (1) HIV-negative fathers, (2) gay and bisexual fathers, (3) incarcerated fathers, and (4) homeless fathers. We discuss race and culture as key factors to consider as we move forward in understanding the role of fathers in relations to HIV/AIDS.

6.3.1 HIV-Negative Fathers

Fathers who are HIV-negative are distinct in their roles and responsibilities both viewed in the context of having a child with HIV/AIDS and having a wife or spouse who is HIV-positive. This relational difference (i.e., one HIV-negative and one HIV-positive person in a relationship) is also known as being in a serodiscordant relationship.

A more popular term for serodiscordant couples is magnet couples (i.e., one positive, one negative viewed synonymously as the polarities of magnets). This raises questions regarding the needs of fathers in their roles as providers and caregivers to children and adolescents with HIV/AIDS. Additional issues emerge with regard to fathers with significant others and mothers who are HIV-positive and how this impacts their roles and responsibilities as caregivers and providers as well as how their partner's status affect their own health and mental health needs.

6.3.2   Gay Fathers

The number of gay fathers is on the rise and some of these men are seropositive themselves and may be adopting seropositive children. The attention to this issue is extremely sparse. Only one report to date was located that focused on being a gay father living with HIV. In a discussion on his decision to father a child after being diagnosed with HIV, Blum (2008) wrote:

I became a father at the age of 40, after having been HIV-positive for more than 10 years. My family includes my son, his bisexual mother, and my male partner of 7 years, as well as our families and friends. Our son just celebrated his second birthday – full of laughter and in love with trucks, balls, and animals. (p. 5) Blum (2008) further discusses his father identity in relation to his gay identity. He added:

Parenthood is one of the greatest achievements of my life. There is always something new, profound, common, thrilling, and, at times, overwhelming. Although I am a gay dad, very little of my life is "gay" as I once defined it. To me, being "gay" meant pursuing cultural and political activities, engaging in an active social life with other gay people, and taking adventure-filled vacations. Now, the free time necessary to engage in these activities is a thing of the past. When I am not working, I am taking care of our son. (p. 7).

Because of the gay rights movement fatherhood is now a viable option for gay men. The role of gay fathers in the context of HIV treatment, prevention, and care is an area greatly in need of attention. As members of family systems, the potential for gay fathers to play an important role in reducing the spread of HIV among children and youth are endless. Understanding is needed regarding the role of gay fathers as caregivers for children and mothers with HIV/AIDS. Questions arise regarding the role that gay fathers play in adopting children. Focusing on the role that single and same gender coupled men can play in responding to the need for adoptive parents for children orphaned by HIV/AIDS is worthy of attention.

6.3.3   Incarcerated Fathers

Fathers who are incarcerated are vulnerable both with regard to their children's, their family members', and their own health (Robertson et al. 2004; Royal et al. 2009).

Among both state and federal prisoners who are parents with minor children, Blacks comprised the largest racial/ethnic group. In state prisons, 49% of parents were Black compared to 29% of Whites, and 19% of Hispanics (Mumola 2000). Similarly, in federal prison, Blacks (44%) are the largest racial/ethnic group among parents, followed by Hispanics (30%) and Whites (22%) (Glaze and Maruschak 2008). From 1991 to 2007, the number of parents incarcerated in state or federal correctional facilities increased by 79% while the number of children with an incarcerated parent increased by 80% (Glaze and Maruschak 2008). Black children with a parent incarcerated in a state or federal correctional facility comprise 6.7% of all minor children in the United States compared to 0.9% for White and 2.4% for Hispanics. Black children are seven times more likely to have a parent in a state or federal prison compared to Whites. Hispanic children are twice as likely to have a parent in a state or federal prison compared to Whites. Sixty-three percent of the incarcerated fathers are aged 24–34 with 58% of the incarcerated fathers in the age range of 35–44 (Glaze and Maruschak 2008). As of 2007, 1.6% of state prison inmates and 0.8% of federal inmates were known to be infected with HIV (Maruschak and Beavers 2009).

The prevalence of HIV among inmates is three times that for the general public. The effect of prisoner re-entry on Black families and communities is increasingly receiving attention among practitioners, policy makers, and researchers (Gadsen and Rethemeyer November 2001). Ex-offender fathers can influence their children's behavior, including their risk behavior (particularly their son's) (Icard et al. 2008). Specifically of concern is the role that former incarcerated fathers might play in the intergenerational transmission of attitudes and norms that may place their children at risk of exposure to HIV.

6.3.4 Homeless Fathers

The limited attention to homeless parents has focused on mothers. The marginality of homeless fathers introduces a number of issues that may have a significant effect on developing HIV treatment and prevention interventions. This includes such issues as HIV-positive fathers' relationship with their children and the implications of these relationships for the health outcomes of fathers and their children. Understanding the health consequences for foster children resulting from a deceased mother and homeless fathers is also of concern. Little is known about the mental and physical health status of HIV/AIDS homeless fathers affected by the relationship between adult children and their homeless fathers. Fathers who are homeless or experiencing unstable housing are at high risk of being exposed to HIV. Extreme poverty, the pressures of daily survival needs, substance use, and mental illness result in homeless men being highly vulnerable to HIV infection (Culhane et al. 2001). People who are homeless or experiencing unstable housing are 3–16 times more likely to be infected with HIV compared to people with similar sociodemographic characteristics (Wolitski et al. 2009). Approximately 3.5 million people may experience homelessness in a given year (National Law Center on Homelessness and Poverty 2007). Approximately 3–10% of all homeless persons are HIV-positive – 10 times the rate of infection in the general population (Culhane et al. 2004).

Homeless men who are HIV-positive are more likely to receive inadequate care and early death. Representative studies of HIV among homeless and marginally housed adults are rare. In addition, estimates of HIV infection and other health problems vary dramatically as a function of sampling strategy (Moss et al. 2004; North and Smith 1993). The limited attention to homeless parents has focused largely on mothers. Understanding is needed on homeless father–child relationships and the HIV/AIDS health status for both homeless fathers and their children.

6.4   Race, Culture, and Poverty

In his memoir, *Dreams from My Father*, President Obama relates his experience as the son of a Black African father, a white American mother, and an Indonesian step-father (Obama 2008). Obama emphasizes in his autobiographical exposition how understanding his racial heritage added to his worldview. The importance of fathers transmitting their cultural beliefs and practices to their sons cannot be underestimated in designing interventions to reduce the spread of HIV. In many cultures, fathers serve an important function in transmitting attitudes and beliefs about HIV sexual risk behavior to their sons (Khan et al 2007). Fathers also can play an important role in dissuading their sons from drinking. Using thoughtful consideration of how fatherhood is addressed culturally in the context of HIV/AIDS is crucial.

6.5   Interventions for Fathers and Their Children

Responsible, Empowered, Aware, Living (REAL) Men (Dilorio et al. 2006, 2007) was developed to promote the delay of sexual intercourse, condom use among 11- to 14-year-old adolescent boys, and communication on sexuality between fathers (or father figures) and sons. Sites were randomly assigned to the intervention and control groups. Assessments were conducted prior to the intervention and at 3-, 6-, and 12-month follow-ups. A total of 277 fathers and their sons completed baseline assessments. Eighty-seven percent ($n = 240$) completed the three follow-up assessments. Most participants were Black (97%), and most fathers lived with their sons (70%).

The REAL Men program was based on social cognitive theory, which proposes that the behaviors a person chooses to perform are based upon a complex interaction of personal, environmental, and behavioral factors (Dilorio et al. 2007). Personal factors include self-efficacy, outcome expectations, and performance goals; environmental factors include encouragement and support from others. The program was structured to include opportunities to view others performing the behavior (i.e., videotapes of fathers talking to sons about sexual topics) and to practice the behavior through role-plays. To encourage participation in the sessions, dinner was served and small nonmonetary incentives were given to both fathers and sons. All participants received 25 dollars for completing each of the four assessments (a baseline questionnaire and three follow-up interviews). The intervention, which consisted of seven 2-hour sessions for the fathers, was delivered once each week in a group format. Fathers attended the first six sessions alone, and fathers and sons attended the final session together. All sessions except the first began with a review of the previous session, a discussion of the take-home activities, and a review of personal goals set by the study participants. Session content was delivered through a combination of lectures, discussions, role plays, games, and videotapes. In the REAL Men program, fathers were taught skills to communicate with their adolescent sons, to monitor their child's relationships with peers, and to prevent high-risk sexual behavior. Participants were given a participant manual to assist with weekly take-home activities and adherence to personal goals set each week. The last session included a celebration of the end of the intervention in which fathers and sons received certificates of completion.

Significantly higher rates of sexual abstinence, condom use, and intent-to-delay initiation of sexual intercourse were observed among adolescent boys whose fathers participated in the intervention. Fathers in the intervention group reported significantly more discussions about sexuality and greater intentions to discuss sexuality than did control group fathers. Based on the results of mediation analyses, the data supported a mediation model that suggests that the effect of the intervention on father–son communication was influenced by differences in father's self-efficacy in communicating sexual information to their sons (Dilorio et al. 2006). A mediation effect for outcome expectations was weak and could not be validated using additional tests. The study demonstrated that fathers can serve as an important and effective educator on HIV prevention and sexuality for their sons.

6.6   Challenges for Fathers

The role of fathers in the context of HIV/AIDS may be considered a new frontier for researchers, practitioners, and policy makers. Although fathers have received considerable attention by health professionals and researchers, a paucity of information exists on fathers in the context of HIV/AIDS. Two broad issues emerge under the subject of fathers and HIV/AIDS. One issue is the role of fathers as agents for prevention, treatment, and care of children and youth. Another set of issues centers on the HIV prevention and treatment of fathers.

Researchers and practitioners have expanded the focus on fathers now to include stepfathers, uncles, grandfathers, and nonresidential fathers. There is limited attention to men who fulfill roles as foster parents, big brothers, and friends who perform the functions of fathers. A significant step in addressing this challenge is developing an understanding of the parental functions of fatherhood in relation to HIV/AIDS. This endeavor can be achieved by developing samples that are more reflective of the diversity of fatherhood today including stepfather, immigrant fathers, and fathers in the military.

In the U.S. mothers tend to volunteer more than fathers in health promotion research studies and particularly among racial and ethnic minorities (Icard et al. 2003). This pattern of men not volunteering to participate in studies does not appear to hold true for HIV prevention studies (Icard et al. unpublished; Jemmott 2009). Fathers marginalized by extreme poverty or other predicaments, such as returning offenders or homeless men, do volunteer to participate in HIV prevention and clinical trial studies. For some men who are struggling financially, the "compensation" received from participating in prevention studies and clinical trials may be a primary source of income (Icard et al. 2009). For other men, the knowledge and skills received through participating in HIV/AIDS prevention programs provides important life skills for better problem solving, parenting, family communication, and/or stress and anger management. In addition to developing samples reflective of the diversity of fathers, epidemiological and ethnographic studies are needed to support the design of interventions focusing on fathers.

Challenges persist in the need to better understand socio-cultural and contextual factors affecting father–child relationships (i.e., child's gender, nonresident fathers, father figures) (Sherr 2010). These challenges also apply in obtaining a deeper comprehension of the social networks of father's HIV/AIDS attitudes and behaviors and the opportunities for the transmission of these attitudes to their children and family members. AIDS prevention and treatment programs must consider the role of fathers in identifying and targeting at-risk children and youth. Numerous studies show a relation between sexual risk behavior among adults and traumatic experiences encountered during childhood. Health and social service practitioners should consider the implications for focusing on HIV prevention interventions for children subjected to abusive fathers and family violence. Similarly, for children and youth living with HIV/AIDS considerations should be given to the role of fathers as a support and as a harmful agent in the child's experiences with stigma and disclosure.

Clinicians, politicians, and researchers agree that confronting the HIV/AIDS epidemic needs to begin at home. Institutional barriers are of concern. Few HIV/AIDS service agencies and organizations focus on men and the importance of their role as fathers. Staff training is particularly needed in organizations that service fathers who are more vulnerable for HIV exposure and poor health. Lastly, a continuum of services to vulnerable fathers (including incarcerated men, homeless men, and men who are offenders and re-entering their families and communities) should be placed as a priority.

6.7 Conclusions

Reports reveal that Americans' impressions of HIV/AIDS as a national health problem have declined drastically over the past 15 years (Singh 2009). Declining public interest in HIV/AIDS would be less troublesome if the rates of infection were also declining. However, the fact is that not only are new HIV infections higher than expected, a greater number of youth are becoming infected. Additionally, HIV infection continues to occur predominantly among men. In this discussion, we have highlighted reports from several sources suggesting the importance of fathers in developing more effective responses to the HIV/AIDS epidemic. The changing demographics of families in the U.S. signal a decline in the traditional two-parent household. Single-headed male households are increasing at a faster rate than single- headed female households. There is documented evidence that fathers do play a unique role in the socialization of their children. We must examine fatherhood via the lenses of diversity in order to add understanding and bring clarity to the concept of fatherhood in the prevention, treatment, and care of HIV/AIDS today.

This shift requires focusing on race/ethnicity, class, sexual orientation, residency, and HIV status. The findings from risk-reduction interventions focusing on fathers are promising. The information presented in this discussion underscore the fact that fathers can and do play a significant role in confronting HIV/AIDS.

References

Amato P, Meyers CE, Emery RE. Changes in nonresident father-child contact from 1976 to 2002. Fam Relat. 2009;58:41–53.

Barber BK, Thomas DL. Dimensions of fathers' and mothers' supportive behavior: the case for physical affection. J Marriage Fam. 1986;48(4):11.

Barreiro P, Castilla JA, Labarga P, Soriano V. Is natural conception a valid option for HIV-serodiscordant couples? Hum Reprod. 2007;22(9):2353–8.

Blum B. How I became an HIV-positive gay dad. Focus. 2008;23:3.

Bradford K, Hawkins AJ. Learning competent fathering: a longitudinal analysis of marital intimacy and fathering. Fathering. 2006;4(3):215–34.

Bronfenbrenner U, Morris PA. The ecology of developmental processes. In: Damon W (series editor), Lerner RM (volume editor). Handbook of child psychology: vol. 1. Theoretical models of human development. 5th ed. Hoboken, NJ: Wiley; 1998. p. 993–1028.

Centers for Disease Control and Prevention (CDC). Cases of HIV infection and AIDS in the United States and dependent areas, 2007. Atlanta, GA: CDC; 2003.

Centers for Disease Control and Prevention (CDC). Cases of HIV infection and AIDS in the United States and dependent areas, 2007. Atlanta, GA: CDC; 2007.

Centers for Disease Control and Prevention (CDC). Subpopulation estimates from the HIV incidence surveillance system – United States, 2006. MMWR Morb Mortal Wkly Rep. 2008;57(36):985–9, Atlanta, GA: CDC.

Centers for Disease Control and Prevention (CDC). Cases of HIV infection and AIDS in the United States and dependent areas, 2007. HIV/AIDS Surveillance Report, 19. 2009a. Available via: http://www.cdc.gov/hiv/topics/surveillance/resources/reports/2007report/default.htm. Cited 4 Mar 2011.

Centers for Disease Control and Prevention (CDC). HIV and AIDS in the United States: a picture of today's epidemic. Atlanta, GA: CDC; 2009.

Census, U. S. Families and living arrangements. 2009b. Available via: http://www.census.gov/population/www/socdemo/hh-fam.html. Cited 7 Mar 2011.

Coltrane S. Family man: fatherhood, housework, and gender equity. New York: Oxford University Press; 1996.

Crosby RA, DiClemente RJ, Wingood GM, Harrington K, Davies S, Oh MK. Activity of African-American female teenagers in black organizations is associated with STD/HIV protective behaviors: a prospective analysis. J Epidemiol Community Health. 2002;56:549–50.

Culhane D, Gollub E, Kuhn R, Shpaner M. The co-occurrence of AIDS and homelessness: results from the integration of administrative data for AIDS surveillance and public shelter utilization in Philadelphia. J Epidemiol Community Health. 2001;55(7):5.

Culhane, J. F., Webb, D., Grim, S., Metraux, S., & Culhane, D. Prevalence of child welfare services involvement among homeless and low-income mothers: a five-year birth cohort study. Journal of Sociology and Social Welfare. 2003;30(3):79–95.

Danziger SK. Family Life and Teenager Pregnancy in the Inner City: Experiences of African-American Youth. [Reports - Research]. Children and Youth Services Review. 1995;17(1–2), 183–202.

Devine, D., Long, P., & Forehand, R. A prospective study of adolescent sexual activity: Description, correlates, and predictors. Advances in Behaviour Research & Therapy. 1993;15(3):185–209. doi: 10.1016/0146-6402(93)90016-u.

Desmond C, Hosegood V. Men, families and HIV and AIDS. New York: United Nations; 2011.

DiIorio C, McCarty F, Resnicow K, Lehr S, Denzmore P. REAL men: a group randomized trial of an HIV prevention intervention for adolescent boys. Am J Public Health. 2007;97(6): 1084–9.

DiIorio C, McCarty F, Denzmore P. An exploration of social cognitive theory mediators of father-son communication about sex. J Pediatr Psychol. 2006;31(9):917–27.

Edlin, K., & Kefalas, M. Unmarried with Children. Context. 2009;4(2):6.

Fagan J, Palkovitz R, Roy K, Farrie D. Pathways to paternal engagement: longitudinal effects of risk and resilience on nonresident fathers. Dev Psychol. 2009;45(5):16.

Forste R, Bartkowski JP, Jackson RA. "Just be there for them": perceptions of fathering among single, low-income men. Fathering. 2009;7(1):20.

Fox GL, Bruce C. Conditional fatherhood: identity theory and parental investment theory as alternative sources of explanation of fathering. J Marriage Fam. 2001;63(2):394–403.

Fox, G. L., & Inazu, J. K. Patterns and Outcomes of Mother-Daughter Communication about Sexuality. [Reports - Research]. Journal of Social Issues. 1908;36(1):7–29.

Glaze LE, Maruschak LM. Parents in prison and their minor children. Bureau of justice statistics special report. Washington, DC: Bureau of Justice Statistics; 2008.

Grodeck B. The first year-HIV: an essential guide for the newly diagnosed. New York: Marlowe; 2003.

Icard LD, Nurius PS. The loss of self in coming out: special risks for African American gays and lesbians. J Pers Interpers Loss. 1996;1:29–47.

Icard LD, Bourjolly JN, Siddiqui N. Designing theoretically based social marketing strategies to increase African Americans' access to health promotion programs. Health Social Work. 2003;28(3):169–248.

Icard LD, Rutledge SE, Eyrich-Garg K, Schmitz M, Scharff N. HIV prevention with pre-release incarcerated men and the roles of the family. Paper presented at the NIMH annual international research conference on the role of families in preventing and adapting to HIV/AIDS. Providence, Rhode Island; 2008.

Icard LD, Rutledge SE, Garg K, Schmitz M, Scharff N, Harrison M, et al. Paper presented at the 2009 National HIV prevention conference promoting synergy between science and program innovation and action to end the epidemic. Atlanta, GA; 2009.

Icard LD, Rutledge SE, Conley C, Davis N, Crawford M, Kormoff E. Positive intervention prevention: health beliefs and risk behaviors among HIV positive African American men. unpublished.

Ihinger-Tallman M, Pasley K, Buehler C. Developing a middle range theory of father involvement post divorce. J Fam Issues. 1993;14:550–71.

Jemmott J. Co-investigators meeting for being responsible for ourselves. University of Pennsylvania, Center for Health Behavior Research; October 29 2009.

Jordan-Zachery JS. Making fathers: black men's response to fatherhood initiatives. J Afr Am Stud. 2009;13(3):9.

Jessor, R. Risk Behavior In Adolescence - A Psychosocial Framework For Understanding And Action. Developmental Review. 1992;12(4):16.

Khan ME, Mishra A, Morankar S, Mishra A, Morankar S. Exploring opportunities to project a "responsible man" image: gatekeepers views of young men's sexual and reproductive health needs in Uttaranchal, India. Int Q Community Health Educ. 2007;28(1):13–31.

Kirkman M, Rosenthal DA, Feldman SS. Talking to a tiger: fathers reveal their difficulties in communicating about sexuality with adolescents. New Dir Child Adolesc Dev. 2002;2002(97):57–74.

Klein J, Peña JE, Thornton II MH, Sauer MV. Understanding the motivations, concerns, and desires of human immunodeficiency virus 1-serodiscordant couples wishing to have children through assisted reproduction. Obstet Gynecol. 2003;101(5):987.

Lammers, C., Ireland, M., Resnick, M., & Blum, R. Influences on adolescents' decision to postpone onset of sexual intercourse: A survival analysis of virginity among youths aged 13 to 18 years. Journal of Adolescent Health. 2000;26(1):42–48.

Lehr ST, Demi AS, Dilorio C, Facteau J. Predictors of father-son communication about sexuality. J Sex Res. 2005;42(2):119–29.

Lenciauskiene I, Zaborskis A. The effects of family structure, parent-child relationship and parental monitoring on early sexual behaviour among adolescents in nine European countries. Scand J Public Health. 2008;36(6):607–18.

Lichter DT, Qian Z. Serial cohabitation and the martial life course. J Fam Marriage. 2008;70:861–78.

Lincoln KD, Taylor RJ, Jackson JS. Romantic relationships among unmarried African Americans and Carribbean Blacks. Fam Relat. 2008;57:254–66.

Longmore MA, Eng AL, Giordano PC, Manning WD. Parenting and adolescents' sexual initiation. J Marriage Fam. 2009;71(4):969–82.

Maruschak LM, Beavers R. HIV in prisons, 2007–08 (No. NCJ 228307). U.S. Department of Justice; 2009.

Moss AR, Hahn JA, Perry S, Charlebois ED, Guzman D, Clark RA. Adherence to highly active antiretroviral therapy in the homeless population in San Francisco: a prospective study. Clin Infect Dis. 2004;39:1190–8.

Mumola CJ. Incarcerated parents and their children. 2000. Retrieved November 15, 2002. From http://www.ojp.usdoj.gov/bjs.

Newcomer SF, Udry JR. Parental Marital Status Effects on Adolescent Sexual Behavior. Journal of Marriage and the Family. 1987;49(2):5.

NLCHP How Many People Experience Homelessness? National Law Center on Homelessness & Poverty, 2009.

North CS, Smith EM. A comparison of homeless men and women: different populations, different needs. Community Ment Health J. 1993;29(5):423–31.

Obama B. Dreams from my father: a story of race and inheritance. Edinburgh: Canongate; 2008.

Olmstead SB, Futris TG, Pasley K. An exploration of married and divorced, nonresident men's perceptions and organization of their father role identity. Fathering. 2009;7(3):249–68.

Osborne D, Manning WD, Smock PJ. Married cohabiting parents relationships stability. J Marriage Fam. 2007;69:1345–66.

Palkovitz R, Palm G. Transitions within fathering. Fathering. 2009;7(1):19.

Patterson CJ, Chan RW, Lamb ME. Families headed by lesbian and gay parents. In: Lamb ME, editor. Nontraditional families: parenting and child development. 2nd ed. Hillsdale, NJ: Lawrence Erlbaum Associates Publishers; 1999. p. 191–219.

Pequegnat W, Bray JH. Families and HIV/AIDS: introduction to the special section. J Fam Psychol. 1997;11(1):3–10.

Pequegnat W, Szapocznik J, editors. Working with families in the era of HIV/AIDS. Thousand Oaks: Sage; 2000.

Price MN, Hyde JS. When two isn't better than one: predictors of early sexual activity in adolescence using a cumulative risk model. J Youth Adolesc. 2009;38(8):1059–71.

Rane T, McBride BA. Identity theory as a guide to understanding father's involvement with their children. J Fam Issues. 2000;21:347–66.

Rawlings SW. Households and families. Population profile of the United States. 1994. Cited from http://www.census.gov/population/www/pop-profile/hhfam.html.

Robertson M, Clark R, Charlebois E, Tulsky J, Bangsberg D, Long H, et al. HIV seroprevalence among homeless adults in San Francisco. Am J Public Health. 2004;94(7):10.

Roy KM, Buckmiller N, McDowell A. Together but not "together": trajectories of relationship suspension for low-income unmarried parents. J Fam Issues. 2008;57:198–210.

Royal SW, Kidder DP, Patrabansh S, Wolitski RJ, Holtgrave DR, Aidala A, et al. Factors associated with adherence to highly active antiretroviral therapy in homeless or unstably housed adults living with HIV. AIDS Care. 2009;21(4):7.

Santilli, F., Greene, S., & Chiarelli, F. Diabetes mellitus in the pre-school child. [Review]. Minerva pediatrica. 2000;52(12):719–729.

Sayer LC, Bianchi SM, Robinson JP. Are parents investing less in children? Trends in mothers' and fathers' time with children. Am J Sociol. 2004;110:1–43.

Selzter JA. Families formed outside of marriage. J Marriage Fam. 2000;62:1247–68.

Sherr L. Fathers and HIV: considerations for families. J Int AIDS Soc. 2010;12 Suppl 2:10.

Singh R. Less than a year after CDC announced the U.S. HIV epidemic is much larger than previously thought. 2009. Available via: http://www.kff.org/kaiserpolls/posr042809nr.cfm. Cited 2 Mar 2011.

Small, S. A., & Luster, T. Adolescent Sexual Activity: An Ecological, Risk-Factor Approach. [Reports - Research]. Journal of Marriage and the Family. 1994;56(1):181–192.

Soliz J, Thorson AR, Rittenour CE. Communicative correlates of satisfaction, family identity, and group salience in multiracial/ethnic families. J Marriage Fam. 2009;71(4):23.

Thornton A, Camburn D. The influence of the family on premarital sexual attitudes and behavior. Demography. 1987;24(3):323–40.

Townsend NW. The package deal: marriage, work, and fatherhood in men's lives. Philadelphia: Temple University Press; 2002.

Udry, J. R., & Billy, J. O. G. Initiation of Coitus in Early Adolescence. American Sociological Review. 1987;53(6):6.

van Leeuwen E, Repping S, Prins JM, Reiss P, van der Veen F. Assisted reproductive technologies to establish pregnancies in couples with an HIV-1-infected man. Neth J Med. 2009;67(8):322–7.

Wang R, Bianchi SM. ATUS fathers' involvement in childcare. Soc Indic Res. 2009;93:141–5.

WHO. HIV/AIDS data and statistics. Geneva, Switzerland: WHO; 2008.

Wolitski RJ, Pals SL, Kidder DP, Courtenay-Quirk C, Holtgrave DR. The effects of HIV stigma on health, disclosure of HIV status, and risk behavior of homeless and unstably housed persons living with HIV. AIDS Behav. 2009;13(6):1222–32.

Yang H, Stanton B, Li X, Cottrel L, Galbraith J, Kaljee L. Dynamic association between parental monitoring and communication and adolescent risk involvement among African-American adolescents. J Natl Med Assoc. 2007;99(5):517–24.

Chapter 7
Couple-Based HIV Prevention and Treatment: State of Science, Gaps, and Future Directions

Nabila El-Bassel and Robert H. Remien

Abstract This chapter focuses on three areas. First, it discusses the state of science on couple-based modalities to reduce HIV risk and STIs and improve adherence to HIV treatment. Second, it discusses the potential advantages of such a modality in both HIV prevention and treatment adherence. Third, it highlights the significant gaps and limitations of couple-based HIV prevention and treatment and makes suggestions for future directions. Fourth, it examines the status of dissemination research and transportability of effective couple-based HIV prevention and treatment to real-world settings. Although advances have been made in HIV prevention science, until a short time ago, HIV prevention approaches did not adequately focus on couples. Effective couple-based intervention strategies are needed for primary prevention for serodiscordant couples, couples who do not know their HIV status, or who are both HIV negative but vulnerable. To date, few couple-focused ART adherence interventions have been tested; even though it is well established that social support is one of the most consistent correlates of adherence across a wide range of populations and diseases. So far all couple-based studies have been efficacy trials rather than effectiveness ones. It has yet to be determined whether any of the interventions is capable of widespread effectiveness under real-world conditions.

7.1 Introduction

Accumulated research over the past 25 years demonstrates that behavioral interventions can curb individual HIV sexual risk behaviors in a variety of populations (Ehrhardt et al. 2002; Jemmott and Jemmott 2000; NIMH Multisite HIV Prevention Trial 1998; O'Leary and Wingood 2000). Studies find significant increases in self-reported condom use (Belcher et al. 1998; DiClemente and Wingood 1995;

W. Pequegnat and C.C. Bell (eds.), *Family and HIV/AIDS: Cultural and Contextual Issues in Prevention and Treatment*, DOI 10.1007/978-1-4614-0439-2_7, © Springer Science+Business Media, LLC 2012

El-Bassel and Schilling 1992; Healthy Living Project Team 2007; Jemmott et al. 1998; Kamb et al. 1998; Kelly et al. 1994, 1997; Neumann et al. 2002; NIMH Multisite HIV Prevention Trial 1998) and reductions in the self-reported frequency of unprotected sexual acts (Belcher et al. 1998; Jemmott et al. 1998, 1999; Jemmott and Jemmott 1992; Kelly et al. 1994, 1997; Neumann et al. 2002; St. Lawrence et al. 1995) among people who received HIV risk-reduction interventions, as compared to those in control groups. A number of randomized clinical trials (RCTs) have also found that HIV risk-reduction interventions lowered the incidence of biologically confirmed STIs (Jemmott and Jemmott 2000; Kamb et al. 1998; Neumann et al. 2002; NIMH Multisite HIV Prevention Trial 1998; Shain et al. 1999). The efficacy of HIV prevention models has also been supported by a number of meta-analyses. These meta-analyses have found that prevention works in reducing both HIV and drug risk behaviors, using both biological and behavioral markers (Albarracin et al. 2008; Exner et al. 1997, 1999; Johnson et al. 2003, 2006; Kalichman et al. 1996; Logan et al. 2002; Neumann et al. 2002; Noar et al. 2007; Semaan et al. 2002).

While there have been calls for developing prevention programs at the couple, family, community, and structural levels (Pequegnat and Stover 2008), a systematic review of couple-based behavioral HIV prevention interventions shows that, until recently, HIV prevention approaches did not adequately focus on couples (Burton et al. 2008), and of the few that did, most did not address relationship contexts, such as intimacy, closeness, trust, living together, and dependencies that have been found to be linked to HIV risks among women and men in committed relationships. Effective couple-based intervention strategies are needed for primary prevention for serodiscordant couples, couples who do not know their HIV status, and couples in which both are HIV negative but vulnerable to infection (El-Bassel et al. 2005; Pequegnat 2005; Pequegnat and Stover 2008).

In this chapter, we focus on heterosexual couple-based prevention and treatment, and discuss the efficacy of such a modality in reducing HIV risks and STIs and improving treatment adherence. We point out the potential advantages of this modality, as well as the gaps and limitations in the science of couple-based HIV prevention and treatment adherence. We then discuss the need for dissemination of effective couple-based prevention and treatment to real-world settings, and future directions for the advancement of HIV prevention and treatment strategies for couples.

7.2 State of Knowledge on Couple-Based HIV Prevention: What Do We Know?

7.2.1 Voluntary Counseling and Testing for Couples

The earliest evidence suggesting the efficacy of couple-based HIV prevention interventions comes from voluntary counseling and HIV testing (VCT) studies conducted mainly overseas. Deschamps et al. (1991) examined whether couple counseling reduced sexual-risk behavior among 475 serodiscordant couples participating in a retrospective study from 1988 to 1992, and followed up every 3 months. At study entry, a physician advised the HIV-infected patients about the importance of their informing their seronegative partners about their HIV status. Subsequently, a session was held with each couple about the risk of unprotected intercourse, to alleviate fears that HIV could be transmitted, and condoms were distributed at each visit. The study found that counseling and provision of condoms contributed to safer sex practices in 45% of the serodiscordant couples.

When Allen et al. (1992) conducted a study of voluntary HIV counseling and testing among 1,458 Rwandan women, some of the women asked permission to allow their husbands to come and participate in the interviews. At the 2-year follow-up, HIV-negative women whose partners had participated were 50% less likely to seroconvert than were those whose partners had not participated. Allen and her colleagues have developed a detailed counseling program for couples that have been adopted in Rwanda and Zambia.

In one of the first studies designed to evaluate a couple-based VCT in the U.S., Padian et al. (1993) examined behavioral change among 144 HIV serodiscordant heterosexual couples who received intensive couple counseling. Couple counseling focused on safer sex practices, how to purchase and use condoms, refraining from the practice of anal sex with new partners, and choosing abstinence. Sessions included role play to build self-esteem and confidence, and the discussion of social, financial, and legal issues associated with HIV infection. About half (49%) of the couples reported consistent condom use before the intervention, whereas 88% reported consistent condom use at first follow-up; but the increase in condom use was not maintained at subsequent follow-ups.

In the first multicountry RCT to test the efficacy of VCT with couples, the Voluntary HIV-1 Counseling and Testing Efficacy Study Group randomly assigned 589 couples to receive either a couple-based VCT or a basic health information intervention. Couples assigned to the VCT condition were more likely to report decreasing unprotected intercourse with each other, but reported no difference in frequency of unprotected intercourse with nonenrolled partners. The study demonstrates that bringing a couple together to discuss their serostatus in a safe environment to negotiate a risk-reduction plan is a strategy that has great potential to reduce the high risk for transmission among couples (Coates et al. 2000). In a prospective study, Farquhar et al. (2004) examined the impact of partner voluntary counseling and HIV testing involvement on prenatal uptake and condom use. The primary aim of this study was to assess the impact of partner involvement, and specifically the impact of being counseled as a couple on prenatal intervention uptake and condom use. Women attending a Nairobi prenatal clinic were encouraged to return with their partners for voluntary HIV-1 counseling and testing and offered individual or couple counseling following the test. Among 2,104 women who accepted testing, 308 (15%) had partners who participated in VCT, of whom 116 (38%) were counseled as a couple. Partner participation in VCT and couple condom use improved when couples received the intervention together.

The AIDS epidemic had been recognized for over 15 years before couple-based efficacy RCTs began to move beyond VCT. Moreover, while there has been improvement in the science of couple-based HIV prevention, the number of studies in the field remains limited. Burton et al. (2008) found that only six clinical trials had been published by the time they conducted their review. In this chapter, we review a number of these studies to highlight the scientific advances that have been made, and the challenges that have been identified in conducting these studies.

7.2.2   Relationship-Based HIV Prevention Programs

One of the first RCTs to test the efficacy of a relationship-based HIV prevention intervention was Project Connect, conducted with low-income urban couples in the U.S. (El-Bassel et al. 2003a, 2005). This study included 217 couples who reported risky sexual behavior with each other or with at least one outside partner. A woman was eligible for Project Connect if she was between 18 and 55 years of age and was involved in a relationship for at least 6 months.

The intervention emphasized relationship contexts, gender roles, communication, and intimacy, all of which contribute to HIV risk behaviors among couples. The intervention consisted of an orientation session and five relationship-based sessions. It combined content related to safer sex practices and prevention of HIV and other STIs, as well as joint HIV testing. The intervention emphasized communications, negotiation, and problem-solving skills. The goal of the intervention's relationship-based approach was to reframe safer sex not as individual "protection," but rather as a way to preserve the relationship and the community, as an act of love, commitment, and intimacy. This approach highlights how relationship dynamics may be affected by gender roles and expectations. The session content pointed out the positive contribution of each participating couple to the future health of their partnership, family, and community. Consistent with the U.S. National HIV Prevention Plan (Centers for Disease Control and Prevention (CDC) 2001), the intervention also directed prevention messages to HIV-positive individuals and serodiscordant couples. For example, the intervention emphasized reducing risk for any new STIs, including HIV, with a secondary prevention emphasis on HIV-infected individuals, and educated participants about drug-resistant strains of HIV. The intervention addressed the particular susceptibility of HIV-positive individuals to infection by other STIs, and the common, incorrect belief that individuals whose viral load is undetectable pose no transmission risk to their partners.

The intervention also emphasized responsibility for self, for each other as a couple, for family, and for the community. The intervention focused on a positive future orientation (for example, addressing change for preventive health, as opposed to past risky behaviors). It also emphasized the importance of individual contributions to enhancing the future health of ethnic communities hardest hit by AIDS by addressing the adverse effects of HIV in the African American and Latino communities; and by linking behavior change to commitment to one's community

(DiClemente and Wingood 1995; Kelly et al. 1995; Schilling et al. 1995; Van Der Straten et al. 1995). Several steps were employed in order to make the intervention in Project Connect congruent with the culture, needs, and worldviews of the community in which the study was conducted. The community and consumers had considerable opportunities to make their voices heard during the grant preparation and conceptualization, research implementation, and dissemination. In order to strengthen the cultural congruence and gender specificity of the intervention, focus groups were conducted with several couples from the target setting, and their input and voice were incorporated into the design of the intervention components. (For a more complete discussion, see Sormanti et al. 2001).

El-Bassel et al. (2003a, b, 2005) found that the HIV prevention intervention provided to the couples was efficacious in reducing unprotected sex at both the 3- and 12-month follow-up assessments. Two major factors may explain the success of the intervention. First, the content of the sessions targeted the intimate relationship as the focus of change, and defined the couple as the agent of change. The relationship context received primary emphasis even when a woman received the intervention without her partner. All exercises in each session and homework assignments were geared toward the woman who was asked to practice the communication, negotiation, and condom skills that she learned in the sessions with her partner. The intervention enabled women and their intimate partners to discuss sexual issues and to explore, together, how they could protect themselves from HIV and STIs.

Harvey et al. (2004) develop an intervention focused on young couples but delivered in a group format. The intervention was delivered in a group modality with culturally appropriate counseling. It included facilitated discussions in small groups about relationship dynamics affecting sexual risk behavior and choices about contraception, a demonstration of proper use of condoms and assistance for couples in selecting a healthy safer-sex strategy that worked for them. Strategies were designed to consider the couple's reproductive intentions and sexual expectations, including preventing an unintended pregnancy and having a healthy pregnancy, avoiding or controlling triggers leading to unsafe sex, and communicating with partners about sexual issues. At the end of each session, participants were given condoms. The findings of the study showed that no significant effects on condom use were reported at 3 and 6 months. Intervention effects were found at 3 and 6 months on self-efficacy, and effects on health protective communication skills were found at 3 months.

Finally, we would like to discuss Project Eban, a recent RCT funded by the National Institute of Mental Health (NIMH) that involved four sites across the U.S. The project was led by investigators with demonstrated leadership in culturally congruent HIV/STI prevention interventions. It showed powerful intervention effects on increasing condom use. The intervention, focusing on a single ethnic group (African Americans), was guided by an Afrocentric paradigm (Karenga 1994), and concentrated on the within-ethnic group strengths of people of African descent, as well as on the beliefs and practices that can shape an individual's understanding and worldview (Kambon 1992). The structure of the intervention promoted the individualism essential to self-protection, as well as the collectivism necessary to support relationship building and peer support for behavior change (Karenga 1988;

Triandis 1994). It was guided by the well-known paradigm of Nguzo Saba (Karenga 1994). Seven principles of Nguzo Saba (unity, self-determination, collective work and responsibility, cooperative economics, purpose, creativity, and faith) guide the Afrocentric worldview and belief systems of native groups of Africa (Karenga 1988). In the context of this study, these seven principles guided the content of the intervention, the style of delivery, and the study design. The use of these principles sanctions the ethnic matching of facilitators and participants, essential to the peer support and modeling needed in a culturally congruent intervention.

Nguzo Saba informs HIV prevention guidelines that bring couples, families, and communities together. The principles promote respect for traditions, and highlight the sociopolitical and racial realities that African-descended people affected by HIV continue to face. The intervention consisted of eight weekly 2-h sessions. It included four sessions with individual couples and four sessions with groups of three to five couples (NIMH Multiside HIV prevention trial group 2008a). Positive outcomes of the Eban study demonstrate the success of another culturally congruent adaptation of the original Connect intervention, in increasing condom use at 12 months (NIMH Multiside HIV prevention trial group 2008b).

The only couple-based HIV prevention study for injection drug users (IDUs) that has been developed outside of the USA is a HIV/STI risk-reduction intervention for IDU couples conducted in Kazakhstan (Gilbert et al. 2010). The study was conducted at a needle exchange program (NEP) site in Shu, Kazakhstan, a small city of approximately 34,000 situated along a major drug trafficking route originating in Afghanistan. The study examined the preliminary effects of a couple-based sexual risk-reduction intervention (CHSR). This pilot trial demonstrated the feasibility and preliminary effects of the CHSR in reducing sexual and drug-related HIV risks. The content of all the CHSR sessions was couple based and focused on (1) identifying HIV risks encountered by the couple and (2) introducing, modeling, and practicing couple communication and problem-solving skills, which both partners could use to reduce their transmission risks. Materials and exercises incorporated social cognitive skill-building strategies, including couple sexual communication skills, problem-solving and assertiveness skills, technical condom use, and syringe disinfection skills (Centers for Disease Control and Prevention CDC 2004). As the preferred method of reducing injection risks, participants were encouraged to obtain new needles from the NEP and not share drug use equipment. Participants were also taught problem-solving and assertiveness skills to identify and avoid triggers for unsafe sex and injection practices. Other activities included participating in games, brainstorming, role playing, and small group discussions to build group cohesion and to increase knowledge of HIV/STIs and transmission risks.

The CHSR intervention was tailored to the realities of drug-involved couples in Kazakhstan. The sessions began and ended with a ritual, such as listening to an inspirational Kazakh song, poem, or quote. At the end of each session, participants were asked to set a risk-reduction goal for the week; progress with respect to each goal was reviewed at the next session. The content for the first three single-gender groups for male and female partners was identical, except for a component that was added to sessions 2 and 3 in the female gender groups, designed to help women anticipate and manage negative partner reactions to requests to use condoms or not to share needles.

Participants were significantly more likely to increase condom use and decrease unsafe injection acts at the 3-month follow-up. This pilot trial demonstrates the preliminary benefits for a couple-based approach for reducing sexual and drug-related HIV risks. The study findings also suggest some preliminary evidence of the short-term effects of the CHSR intervention in increasing HIV/STI knowledge, condom negotiation self-efficacy, and couple's risk-reduction communication. These positive effects suggest that the modified approach of delivering the CHSR intervention using a mixed modality of single-gender group sessions and an individual couple session was effective in promoting change in the core mediators of original couple-based HIV prevention (El-Bassel et al. 2003b, 2005).

Few couple-focused Antiretroviral Therapy (ART) adherence interventions have been tested, even though it is well established that social support is one of the most consistent correlates of adherence across a wide range of populations and diseases (Kaplan et al. 1997).

7.3   State of Knowledge on Couple-Based Interventions for Adherence to HIV Care and HIV Treatment: What Do We Know?

Empirical research has identified a variety of predictors and correlates of adherence to ART. While adherence to ART is multiply determined and dynamic and its correlates differ among individuals and across time for a given individual (Remien et al. 2003), the importance of social support is particularly evident. The amount of social support received, satisfaction with that support, and extent of a person's social network are correlated with health status and clinical outcomes in patients with a wide range of chronic illnesses (Berkman 1985; Brecht et al. 1994; Cohen 1988; DiMatteo and Hays 1981). Social support can be a significant factor in enhancing adherence to treatment, leading to better health outcomes (DiMatteo 1994; Haynes 1976). Greater social support has been associated with higher levels of adherence to HIV care and treatment (Catz et al. 2000; Glass et al. 2006; Gonzalez et al. 2004; Power et al. 2003). Thus, there are many advantages to a couple-level approach, in its capacity for supporting optimal adherence to HIV care and treatment as well as for reducing transmission risk behaviors.

The Sharing Medical Adherence Responsibilities Together (SMART) Couples Study is the first and only couple-based ART adherence intervention to be tested in a RCT (Remien et al. 2006). The intervention targeted HIV serodiscordant couples to improve medication adherence among HIV-seropositive patients by fostering active support from their HIV-seronegative partner. It also addressed sexual transmission concerns within the dyad. In addition to partner support, the intervention employed other cognitive behavioral strategies based on Ewart's Social Action Theory (SAT) (Ewart 1991), which emphasizes how social context, in addition to individual cognitive and emotional factors, can influence healthcare behaviors. This trial was designed to test the efficacy of the intervention implemented in a clinical setting. The brief intervention aimed to improve patients' adherence to

HIV/AIDS medical care regimens by fostering the support of their partners. The intervention also sought to help couples address issues of sex and intimacy. To help translate SAT constructs into specific activities within the couple-focused intervention curriculum, the investigators consulted the literature on couple distress and satisfaction that describes the following critical components of an effective dyadic intervention: (1) clarify negative attributions and encourage positive ones, (2) increase expressiveness and foster effective communication, (3) create positive experiences, (4) develop strategies to protect the couple's investment in the relationship, (5) improve problem-solving skills, and (6) increase conflict management skills (Gottman 1993; Kurdek 1991; Rusbult et al. 1991). Researchers have identified two broad classes of relationship-focused coping: (1) active engagement, which involves open discussion and joint decision-making, inquiries into the partner's feelings, and problem solving, and (2) protective buffering, in which concerns are hidden, worries are denied, and accommodation is employed to avoid disagreements (Coyne and DeLongis 1986; Coyne et al. 1990; Coyne and Smith 1991). These approaches informed the development of this couple-based intervention.

The intervention was individually administered to each couple by a nurse practitioner in an outpatient treatment setting through four 45–60 minutes sessions held over 5 weeks. The session content included structured discussions and instruction, as well as specific problem-solving and couple-communication exercises. Additionally, the couple monitored and reviewed the treatment adherence of the HIV-seropositive partner over the course of the intervention through the use of the Medication Event Monitoring System (MEMS). Key intervention components included educating about HIV and its treatment, and the importance of adherence to avoid viral resistance and maintain health; teaching self-monitoring, including identifying patterns of nonadherence; identifying barriers to adherence and developing communication and problem-solving strategies to overcome them; improving adherence motivation and self-efficacy by re-framing beliefs and attitudes about treatment; optimizing partner support; and building the couple's confidence in achieving and maintaining improved adherence. Facilitators were trained to provide referrals as needed for the couple or for either individual for mental health treatment, substance abuse treatment, sexual risk-reduction counseling, and public assistance. This brief, theoretically based, dyad-focused behavioral intervention was more effective than usual clinic care in improving medication adherence. Involving a significant other in the enhancement of support for adherence to ART can benefit both the individual and public health. More couple-based treatment research is needed to affect both treatment adherence and HIV risk.

7.4 Potential Advantages of Couple-Based HIV Prevention and Treatment

A number of advantages have been identified in the literature on couple-based approaches to HIV prevention. Bringing couples together sends a message that the responsibility for HIV risk reduction is placed on both members of the dyad, and not solely on one person; underscores that both men and women can put the other at risk for HIV (El-Bassel et al. 2001); it provides a supportive environment that may enable couples to more safely disclose to each other extra-dyadic sexual relationships, STI histories, injection drug use, or past experiences in abusive relationships (El-Bassel et al. 2001); an environment in which couples can learn communication skills and discuss gender differences (how men discuss sex, the meaning of requesting and/or refusing the use of condoms, etc.) and gender power imbalances associated with sexual coercion and the inability to negotiate condom use; and gender inequalities in a couple's needle sharing practices (Basen-Engquist 1992; Ehrhardt 1994; El-Bassel et al. 2001; Fisher and Fisher 1992; Kelly 1995; Nadler and Fisher 1992; Tanner and Pollack 1988).

There are also numerous advantages to bringing couples together in terms of improved adherence to HIV care and treatment. Intervening with both members of the dyad, rather than just the patient, can produce increased (1) motivation to maintaining good health; (2) understanding of how medications work to control HIV viral load, and of the necessity for very high levels of adherence to the treatment regimen to ensure success; (3) commitment to obtain and maintain a steady supply of medications, and to provide daily reminders for medication taking; (4) ability to identify and resolve ongoing barriers to optimal adherence; (5) propensity to confront HIV-related stigma and feelings of isolation which can contribute to treatment avoidance; and (6) communications and mutual care-taking behaviors within the dyad. Furthermore, in the context of HIV infection, it is important to integrate HIV prevention into HIV care whether couples are serodiscordant or concordant-positive since, as noted earlier, there is a clear association between viral load control and transmission risk. A couple-focused approach has the benefit of significantly improving the health and well-being of the dyad, thus preventing new HIV infection and mother-to-child transmission (Remien et al. 2006, 2008).

7.5 Gaps and Limitations in HIV Couple-Based Prevention and Future Directions

7.5.1 Definition of a Couple

Existing couple-based models vary in their definition of a "couple." Most rely on the index participant to identify his or her partner. Several existing models use more stringent criteria, such as the length of the relationship and the nature of living arrangements. For example, Project Connect used the following criteria. To be considered a member of a couple, a woman had to (1) be between 18 and 55 years old; (2) have a regular, male sexual partner whom she identified as a boyfriend, spouse, or lover; (3) be in a long-term relationship, operationalized as involvement with this partner for at least the past 6 months, with the intention to stay with him for at least 1 year; (4) have had at least one episode of unprotected vaginal or anal sex with this partner within the past 30 days; (5) have not reported any severe physical or sexual abuse by this partner within the past 6 months, as defined by selected questions from the Revised Conflict Tactics Scale (Straus et al. 1996); and (6) be a patient at one of the hospital's outpatient clinics. Harvey et al. (2004), the Eban NIMH multisite study, and Project Renaissance (Gilbert et al. 2010) all use similar criteria. These criteria may limit the ability to generalize from study findings to all couples, and to men who have sex with men (MSM).

7.5.2 Methodological Challenges

Couple-based HIV interventions are still in the early stages of development. Most existing couple-based prevention studies remain limited by one or more methodological drawbacks, including relatively small sample sizes, lack of a randomized control design, and/or lack of biologically confirmed STIs as an outcome (Burton et al. 2008). Thus far, of the existing couple-based models only three studies have used biological outcomes (Coates et al. 2000; NIMH Multisite HIV/STD Prevention Trial for African American Couples Group 2008; Gilbert et al. 2010). None of the currently reported studies with couples have had sufficient power to examine any new incidence of HIV as an outcome.

7.5.3 Partner Concurrency as an Outcome

Most of the empirically tested, couple-based HIV prevention approaches reviewed have not looked at whether these approaches reduce partner concurrency. This is an important outcome to consider because partner concurrency increases the HIV risk among couples as well as within their social network (Halperin and Epstein 2004). It is also not clear whether these existing approaches have any effect on HIV risks with other partners outside of the dyad.

So far, studies of couple-based HIV prevention have been unable to determine the optimal intervention modality. Is the intervention more effective when sessions are provided individually to each couple, when sessions are provided to several couples in a group, or when they are provided to a small, single-gender group of individuals who are in coupled relationships? The HIV couple-based prevention approaches reviewed in this chapter have used one or a combination of these modalities. Research on HIV couple-based interventions should tackle these questions. Accurate answers would improve the science of couple-based HIV prevention.

7.5.4 Focusing on Couple Dynamics

Although the existing couple-based studies reviewed in this chapter are designed to address the couple dynamics, the majority of these studies did not focus on the couple's relationship and contexts – such as how gender roles, gender expectations, couple communications, and sexual dysfunction within the dyad contributes to HIV risks (Burton et al. 2008). In the context of emerging biomedical interventions for HIV prevention, such as microbicides and Pre-exposure prophylaxis (PrEP) couple-based research will be necessary to inform the most effective modes of delivery and implementation in real-world settings.

Microbicides, which are currently and likely to remain only partially effective in reducing transmission risk, need to be used vaginally or rectally prior to (and during) sexual intercourse. How they can be used effectively in the context of sexual intercourse between two people is still in need of research. While it is possible for one person, such as the woman, to use the product, early research has shown that partner acceptability and participation is necessary for successful and consistent use of such products. Thus, utilization of these produces will not be entirely under the control of one person, but will need to involve partner cooperation and participation (Abdool Karim et al. 2011; Grant et al. 2010).

PrEP thus far has also been shown to be only partially effective in reducing HIV transmission. Research is needed to identify comparative effectiveness of PrEP in the HIV-negative partner in the dyad as compared to ART in the HIV-positive partner. Also, how will the couple integrate partially effective tools such as microbicides and PrEP into their sex lives and how might the use of biomedical interventions affect the use of condoms and other barrier methods among couples (Abdool Karim et al. 2011, Grant et al. 2010).

7.5.5 Couple-Based Theories

Most couple-based HIV prevention approaches are guided by individual-based theory, such as social learning and cognitive behavioral theories (Ajzen and Fishbein 1980; Bandura 1977a, b; Bandura and Adams 1977; Beck 1975; Rosenstock et al. 1988). These theories assume that couples are motivated to take protective actions, and often overlook many relationship and dyadic factors. Moreover, it is still unclear which populations are most responsive to the interventions (moderators), and what mechanisms and mediators lead to behavioral change. To advance the science of HIV intervention with couples, the most useful theories are those that focus on fine-grained relationship structures and contexts.

7.5.6 Couple Data Analytic Approaches

Although data from existing prevention and treatment studies were collected from the couples, most of the studies reviewed employed individual-data analytical approaches. The use of couple-based data would advance HIV prevention and treatment science for this modality and answer questions on the efficacy of the intervention used in the existing studies. More attention should be given to couple-data analytical techniques.

7.5.7 Male Couples

Unfortunately, thus far, no HIV prevention intervention targeting male couples has been tested, in spite of the finding that many MSM are infected by steady partners (Sullivan et al. 2009). There are several HIV prevention interventions for MSM that have shown efficacy in reducing transmission risk behaviors among HIV-positive and HIV-negative MSM, with mixed results as to whether risk reduction took place with steady as opposed to casual partners (Johnson et al. 2005).

7.5.8 HIV Drug Risk Reduction with Couples

HIV prevention with IDU couples is also limited. Existing couple-based HIV efficacy trials have minimal content in their core components on HIV drug risk reduction behaviors, such as the proper way to clean syringes, needles, and other drug equipment, and HIV risks associated with sharing syringes and other drug paraphernalia with main sex partners (Burton et al. 2008). Moreover, couple-based HIV prevention is not an approach commonly used in drug treatment and HIV services for IDUs. Bringing IDUs and their regular sexual partners together in an HIV prevention intervention can be an effective strategy to reduce both sexual and drug risk behaviors, and to lower HIV transmission.

7.5.9 Couple-Focused Adherence to HIV Care and Treatment

There is a need for more research on couple-based approaches to improving adherence to HIV care and treatment. Since social support is an important factor in adherence to care, partners of patients with chronic illness can play an important and instrumental role in optimizing adherence, as described earlier. As with couple-based HIV prevention research, gaps remain in our knowledge of optimal intervention modalities for couple-focused interventions to improve adherence. There are gaps in research on couples' relationship dynamics and contexts, such as how gender roles, gender expectations, and a couple's communications contribute to HIV healthcare behaviors. Research is lacking on the specific forms of practical support that spouses and partners actually offer in support transactions. Research is needed on couples in which both members are HIV infected, and on how differences play out depending on the individual's stage of illness, so that interventions can be tailored for a wide range of couples.

7.6 Dissemination of HIV Couple-Based Approaches

Couple-based approaches are not broadly employed, adopted, and accepted as a standard practice in HIV community-based organizations (CBOs), primary health care settings, and drug treatment and harm reduction programs. In these settings, there is low awareness of the utility and importance of couple-based prevention interventions and couple-based adherence/treatment approaches.

Most HIV prevention approaches available in these service organizations are delivered through individual or group modalities. In many such organizations, couples are treated separately even if they present together or prefer to be treated together, many agencies and CBOs that serve HIV positive individuals, serodiscordant couples, or at-risk couples do not provide any opportunity for the presenting individuals to be treated as a couple.

Moreover, service providers have limited access to the scientific literature on couple-based approaches. Evidenced-based approaches tend to be published in scholarly articles that may not be readily accessible to service providers; and most scientific papers primarily describe the outcome of studies, with less emphasis on the core components and strategies of interventions, methods of implementation, and challenges that providers may face in delivery of the intervention. A lack of this information in published papers limits an agency's ability to successfully adopt such models. Overall, there has been little scientific focus on the significance of couple-based HIV prevention and adherence/treatment, and little movement toward the adoption of evidence-based couple approaches.

The literature on the transfer of HIV prevention interventions to community-based provider settings draws largely on the experiences of the Centers for Disease Control and Prevention (CDC) Replicating Effective Programs (REP) (Centers for Disease Control and Prevention (CDC) 2006a; Neumann and Sogolow 2000) and Diffusion of Effective Behavioral Interventions (DEBI) initiatives (Centers for Disease Control and Prevention (CDC) 2006b). Because of the urgent need for dissemination of efficacious HIV prevention interventions, the DEBI project's objective was to enhance the capacity of CBOs and state and local departments of health to implement efficacious interventions (Collins et al. 2006).

Thus far, Project Connect, described in this chapter, is the first and only couple-based study recognized by the Centers for Disease Control and Prevention (CDC) in its HIV/AIDS Prevention Research Synthesis (PRS) project (Crepaz et al. 2006; Des Jarlais and Semaan 2002; Sogolow et al. 2002 – the largest review of evidence-based HIV/STI prevention programming to date) as a best-evidence prevention intervention recommended for widespread dissemination. The Project Connect intervention has been packaged with all materials, in a format designed to replicate the manualized version for implementation in community-based settings, and is currently disseminated by a number of CBOs. However, the Eban HIV/STI Prevention Program has been submitted to Centers for Disease Control and Prevention (CDC) for consideration.

To date, there are no DEBI initiatives for behavioral interventions aimed at improving adherence to ART, although the Centers for Disease Control and

Prevention (CDC) has a process in place for selection and dissemination of evidence-based HIV treatment adherence interventions (Charania 2010). In order to scale up couple-based adherence interventions for wider applicability domestically and internationally, it will be important to apply what has been learned from couple-based interventions to a wider range of dyads. For sexually active couples in which one or both members of the dyad is HIV infected, it is important to integrate HIV prevention and treatment adherence interventions because reducing viral load is beneficial to the person living with HIV and also reduces the risk of HIV transmission should one partner be uninfected (Granich et al. 2010).

Applying available HIV prevention and treatment approaches to real-world settings – and training clinicians to use them – is an important step in making a strong public health impact on an epidemic that continues to affect many communities in the U.S., particularly the African American and Latino communities. Funding and training should look at couple-based dissemination models in real-world settings.

Two promising HIV couple-based approaches are currently underway. Two years ago, the NIMH funded a study (PI: Susan Witte) to develop the Project Connect intervention into an entirely multimedia-based, web-accessible intervention. This is the first step in a dissemination plan that includes a technology transfer study that will advance the science of HIV prevention dissemination research. This study will test whether employing multimedia and Internet-based technology for implementation of Project Connect improves adoption outcomes beyond existing technology transfer approaches that use a combination of manuals, training, and technical assistance. The Multimedia Connect study is a 5-year RCT to compare the effectiveness of disseminating the traditional, manualized package of Project Connect versus a state-of-the-art, multimedia, Internet-based version of Project Connect to clients at HIV CBOs across New York State. The design matches 80 participating HIV CBOs in New York State on selected HIV prevention services variables, and then randomly assigns, within each of 40 pairs, one agency to receive the multimedia intervention and training package (Multimedia) and the other to receive the original, manualized Project Connect intervention and training package (Traditional). The second study is funded by NIMH (PI: Robert H. Remien) to adapt and pilot test the SMART Couples intervention as a social support adherence intervention for patients and their "treatment buddies" in Cape Town, South Africa. The study goal was to adapt and enhance this effective social-support adherence intervention into a multimedia format that is applicable to a wide range of patients receiving ART in a South African clinic setting. Using a community-based participatory research methodology and Ewart's Social Action Theory (Ewart 1991), the study team is adapting the SMART described curriculum for South African adult men and women and treatment support partners (SMART + SA). Collaborators in this development process include nurses, physicians, psychologists, HIV counselors, and patients receiving HIV services in the participating clinics, as well as the local and provincial Departments of Health.

HIV prevention and treatment fields need to pay more attention to dissemination research and ensure that the efficacious couple-based interventions are adopted in real-world settings. This requires funding for dissemination research and training for service providers in couple-based approaches, as well as interventions. Dissemination of couple-based interventions in real-world settings also requires a paradigm shift in the way services, prevention, and treatments are delivered; such a shift must ensure easy access to evidence-based HIV couple models.

7.7 Summary and Conclusion

This chapter underscores the importance of couple-based approaches to HIV prevention and care. Compared to individual and group-level HIV interventions, couple-based HIV interventions are in nascent stages of development in the USA and internationally. The advantages of couple-based approaches are evident. They can reduce drug and sexual behaviors that drive transmission of HIV and improve adherence to ART that, in turn, can decrease the risks of transmission. However, there remains a need for more research on couple-based approaches, especially for drug users and MSM, as well as for seroconcordant-positive couples. Effective couple-based HIV prevention strategies are needed for primary prevention for sero-discordant couples, couples who do not know their HIV status, or who are both HIV negative; in other words, all couples in which HIV transmission is possible, especially for those whose behaviors place them at high risk for HIV (El-Bassel et al. 2005). In this chapter, we have presented a number of the advantages that accrue from using a couple-based modality as well as a number of gaps.

The science of couple-based research can be advanced by addressing the gaps and challenges discussed in this chapter, in particular biological outcomes and the impact of couple-based interventions on concurrent sexual relationships. More attention and resources must be given to the dissemination of evidence-based, couple-focused prevention and treatment research into real-world settings. All couple-based studies have been efficacy trials rather than effectiveness trials. It has yet to be determined whether any of the interventions is capable of widespread effectiveness under real-world conditions. Advancing the science of couple-based research (e.g., efficacy, effectiveness, and dissemination) has the potential to reduce HIV acquisition and transmission among vulnerable populations.

Despite their demonstrated value in reducing risk behaviors and improving adherence to HIV medication, couple-based approaches are rarely employed in HIV service settings. Reasons for the limited dissemination and scaling up of couple-based HIV interventions to date may include common ideological preferences of staff and administrators for individual or group services; agencies are not structured to provide couple services, even if partners present and want to be treated together; and there is a lack of access to evidence-based HIV interventions for couples, and lack of funding and staff training in couple-based modalities.

Expanding the scope of dissemination and scaling up couple-based HIV interventions will require government and donor commitment for funding dissemination and implementation research as well as funding for training providers in couple-based approaches.

References

Abdool Karim SS, Richardson BA, Ramjee G, Hoffman IF, Chirenje ZM, Taha T, et al. HIV Prevention Trials Network (HPTN) 035 Study Team. PMID 21330907 PMCID PMC3083640. Safety and Efectiveness of BufferGel and 0.5% PRO2000 gel for the prevention of HIV infection in women. AIDS, 2011 Apr 24;25(7):957–66.

Ajzen I, Fishbein M. Understanding attitudes and predicting social behavior. Englewood Cliffs, New Jersey: Prentice-Hall; 1980.

Albarracin J, Albarracin D, Durantini M. Effects of HIV-prevention interventions for samples with higher and lower percents of Latinos and Latin Americans: a meta-analysis of change in condom use and knowledge. AIDS Behav. 2008;12(4):521–43.

Allen S, Serufilira A, Bogaerts J, Van de Perre P, Nsengumuremyi F, Lindan C, et al. Confidential HIV testing and condom promotion in Africa: impact on HIV and gonorrhea rates. J Am Med Assoc. 1992;268(23):3338–43.

Bandura A. Cognitive processes mediating behavior change. J Pers Soc Psychol. 1977a;35:125–39.

Bandura A. Self-efficacy: toward a unifying theory of behavioral change. Psychol Rev. 1977b; 84(2):191–215.

Bandura A, Adams NE. Analysis of self-efficacy theory of behavioral change. Cogn Ther Res. 1977;1(4):287–310.

Basen-Engquist K. Psychosocial predictors of "safer sex" behaviors in young adults. AIDS Educ Prevent. 1992;4(2):120–34.

Beck TKH. An exploratory study of cognitive style based on perceptual mode, conceptual style and speech code. Atlanta, Georgia: Emory University; 1975.

Belcher L, Kalichman S, Topping M, Smith S, Emshoff J, Norris F, et al. A randomized trial of a brief HIV risk reduction counseling intervention for women. J Consult Clin Psychol. 1998; 66(5):856–61.

Berkman LF The relationship of social networks and social support to morbidity and mortality. Soc Supp Health 1985 241–262.

Brecht ML, Dracup K, Moser DK, Riegel B. The relationship of marital quality and psychosocial adjustment to heart disease. J Cardiovasc Nurs. 1994;9(1):74.

Burton J, Darbes LA, Operario D Couples-focused behavioral interventions for prevention of HIV: systematic review of the state of evidence. AIDS Behav 2008, 1–10.

Catz SL, Kelly JA, Bogart LM, Benotsch EG, McAuliffe TL. Patterns, correlates, and barriers to medication adherence among persons prescribed new treatments for HIV disease. Health Psychol. 2000;19(2):124–33.

Centers for Disease Control and Prevention (CDC). (2001) HIV/AIDS Surveillance Supplemental Report. Atlanta, GA: CDC.

Centers for Disease Control and Prevention (CDC). Epidemiology of HIV/AIDS – United States. MWWR, 2006a, 55(21), 589–592. Atlanta, GA: CDC.

Centers for Disease Control and Prevention (CDC). Twenty-five years of HIV/AIDS – United states 1981–2006, 2006b. MWWR, 55(21), 585–589. Atlanta, GA: CDC.

Centers for Disease Control and Prevention (CDC). Syringe disinfection for injection drug users. Atlanta, GA: CDC; 2004.

Charania M. CDC Review and dissemination of evidence-based HIV treatment adherence interventions. Unpublished plenary presentation at the 5th International Conference on HIV Treatment Adherence; International Association of Physicians in AIDS Care, 2010 Miami, FL.

Coates TJ, Grinstead OA, Gregorich SE, Sweat MD, Kamenga MC, Sangiwa G, et al. Efficacy of voluntary HIV-1 counselling and testing in individuals and couples in Kenya, Tanzania, and Trinidad: a randomised trial. Lancet. 2000;356(9224):103–12.

Cohen S. Psychosocial models of the role of social support in the etiology of physical disease. Health Psychol. 1988;7(3):269–97.

Collins C, Harshbarger C, Sawyer R, Hamdallah M. The diffusion of effective behavioral interventions project: development, implementation, and lessons learned. AIDS Educ Prevent. 2006;18(supp):5–20.

Coyne JC, DeLongis A. Going beyond social support: the role of social relationships in adaptation. J Consult Clin Psychol. 1986;54(4):454–60.

Coyne JC, Smith DAF. Couples coping with a myocardial infarction: a contextual perspective on wives' distress. J Pers Soc Psychol. 1991;61(3):404–12.

Coyne JC, Ellard JH, Smith DAF. Social support, interdependence, and the dilemmas of helping. In: Sarason BR, Sarason IG, Pierce GR, editors. Social support: An interactional view. Wiley series on personality processes. New York: Wiley; 1990. p. 129–49.

Crepaz N, Lyles CM, Wolitski RJ, Passin WF, Rama SM, Herbst JH, et al. Do prevention interventions reduce HIV risk behaviours among people living with HIV? A meta-analytic review of controlled trials. J Acquir Immune Def Syndr. 2006;20(2):143.

Des Jarlais DC, Semaan S. HIV prevention research: cumulative knowledge or accumulating studies?: An introduction to the HIV/AIDS Prevention Research Synthesis Project Supplement. J Acquir Immune Def Syndr. 2002;30:S1.

Deschamps MM, Pape JW, Haffner A, Hyppolite R, and Johnson WD (1991, June). Heterosexual activity in at risk couples for HIV infection. Unpublished paper presented at the International Conference on AIDS, Florence, Italy. 7: 318 (abstract no. W.C.3089).

DiClemente RJ, Wingood GM. A randomized controlled trial of an HIV sexual risk-reduction intervention for yourng African-American women. J Am Med Assoc. 1995;274:1271–6.

DiMatteo MR. Enhancing patient adherence to medical recommendations. J Am Med Assoc. 1994;271(1):79.

DiMatteo MR, Hays R. Social support and serious illness. Soc Net Soc Supp. 1981;4:117–1471.

Ehrhardt AA. "Narrow vs broad targeting of HIV/AIDS education": response. Am J Pub Health. 1994;84(3):498–9.

Ehrhardt AA, Exner TM, Hoffman S, Silberman I, Leu CS, Miller S, et al. A gender-specific HIV/STD risk reduction intervention for women in a health care setting: short-and long-term results of a randomized clinical trial. AIDS Care. 2002;14(2):147–61.

El-Bassel N, Schilling RF. 15 month follow-up of women methadone patients taught to reduce heterosexual HIV transmission. Public Health Rep. 1992;107:500–3.

El-Bassel N, Witte S, Gilbert L, Sormanti M, Moreno C, Pereira L, et al. HIV prevention for intimate couples: a relationship-based model. Fam Syst Health. 2001;19(4):379–95.

El-Bassel N, Gilbert L, Rajah V. The relationship between drug abuse and sexual performance among women on methadone: heightening the risk of sexual intimate violence and HIV. Addict Behav. 2003a;28(8):1385–403.

El-Bassel N, Witte SS, Gilbert L, Wu E, Chang M, Hill J, et al. The efficacy of a relationship-based HIV/STD prevention program for heterosexual couples. Am J Public Health. 2003b;93(6):963–9.

El-Bassel N, Witte SS, Gilbert L, Wu E, Chang M, Hill J, et al. Longterm effects of an HIV/STI sexual risk reduction intervention for heterosexual couples. AIDS Behav. 2005;9(1):1–13.

Ewart CK. Social action theory for a public health psychology. Am Psychol. 1991;46(9):931–46.

Exner TM, Seal DW, Ehrhardt AA. A review of HIV interventions for at-risk women. AIDS Behav. 1997;1(2):93–124.

Exner TM, Gardos P, Seal D, Ehrhardt A. HIV sexual risk reduction interventions with heterosexual men: the forgotten group. AIDS Behav. 1999;3:347–58.

Farquhar C, Kiarie JN, Richardson BA, Kabura MN, John FN, Nduati RW, et al. Antenatal couple counseling increases uptake of interventions to prevent HIV-1 transmission. J Acquir Immune Def Syndr. 2004;37(5):1620–6.

Fisher JD, Fisher WA. Changing AIDS-risk behavior. Psychol Bull. 1992;111(3):455–74.

Gilbert L, El-Bassel N, Terlikbayeva A, Rozental Y, Chang M, Brisson A, Wu E, Bakpayev M. Couple-based HIV prevention for injecting drug users in Kazakhstan: a pilot intervention study. Prev Interv Community, 2010 Apr;38(2):162–76 PMID:20391062.

Glass TR, De Geest S, Weber R, Vernazza PL, Rickenbach M, Furrer H, et al. Correlates of self-reported nonadherence to antiretroviral therapy in HIV-infected patients: the Swiss HIV Cohort Study. J Acquir Immune Def Syndr. 2006;41(3):385.

Gonzalez JS, Penedo FJ, Antoni MH, Duran RE, McPherson-Baker S, Ironson G, et al. Social support, positive states of mind, and HIV treatment adherence in men and women living with HIV/AIDS. Health Psychol. 2004;23:413–8.

Gottman JM. The roles of conflict engagement, escalation, and avoidance in marital interaction: a longitudinal view of five types of couples. J Consult Clin Psychol. 1993;61:6–15.

Granich R, Crowley S, Vitoria M, Lo YR, Souteyrand Y, Dye C, et al. Highly active antiretroviral treatment for the prevention of HIV transmission. J Acquir Immune Def Syndr. 2010;13:1.

Grant RM, Lama JR, Anderson PL, McMahan V, Liu AY, Vargas L, et al. Preexposure chemoprophylaxis for HIV prevention in men who have sex with men. New Engl J Med. 2010;363(27):2587–99.

Halperin DT, Epstein H. Concurrent sexual partnerships help to explain Africa's high HIV prevalence: implications for prevention. Lancet. 2004;364(9428):4–6.

Harvey SM, Bird ST, Henderson JT, Beckman LJ, Huszti HC. He said, she said: concordance between sexual partners. Sex Transmit Dis. 2004;31(3):185.

Haynes RB. Strategies for improving compliance: a methodological analysis And review. In: Sackett DL, Haynes RB, editors. Compliance with therapeutic regimens. Baltimore, MD: Johns Hopkins University Press; 1976. p. 69–82.

Healthy Living Project Team. Effects of a behavioral intervention to reduce risk of transmission among people living with HIV: the Healthy Living Project randomized controlled study. J Acquir Immune Def Syndr. 2007;44(2):213–21.

Jemmott LS, Jemmott III JB. Increasing condom-use intentions among sexually active inner-city black adolescent women: effects of an AIDS prevention program. Nurs Res. 1992;41:273–9.

Jemmott JB, Jemmott LS. HIV behavioral interventions for adolescents in community settings. In: Peterson J, DiClementi R, editors. Handbook of HIV prevention. AIDS prevention and mental health. New York: Kluwer Academic/Plenum Publishers; 2000. p. 103–27.

Jemmott JB, Jemmott LS, Fong GT. Abstinence and safer sex HIV risk-reduction interventions for African American adolescents: a randomized controlled trial. J Am Med Assoc. 1998;279(19): 1529–36.

Jemmott III JB, Jemmott LS, Fong GT, McCaffree K. Reducing HIV risk-associated sexual behavior among African American adolescents: testing the generality of intervention effects. Am J Commun Psychol. 1999;27:161–87.

Johnson BT, Carey MP, Marsh KL, Levin KD, Scott-Sheldon LAJ. Interventions to reduce sexual risk for the human immunodeficiency virus in adolescents, 1985–2000: a research synthesis. Arch Pediatr Adol Med. 2003;157(4):381.

Johnson WD, Holtgrave DR, McClellan WM, Flanders WD, Hill AN, Goodman M. HIV intervention research for men who have sex with men: a 7 year update. AIDS Educ Prevent. 2005; 17(6):568–89.

Johnson BT, Carey MP, Chaudoir S, Reid AE. Sexual risk reduction for persons living with HIV: research synthesis of randomized controlled trials, 1993–2004. J Acquir Immune Def Syndr. 2006;41:642–50.

Kalichman SC, Carey MP, Johnson BT. Prevention of sexually transmitted HIV infection: a meta-analytic review of teh behavioral outcome literature. Ann Behav Med. 1996;18(1):6–15.

Kamb ML, Fishbein M, Douglas JMJ, Rhodes F, Rogers J, Bolan G, et al. Efficacy of risk-reduction counseling to prevent human immunodeficiency virus and sexually transmitted diseases: a randomized controlled trial. J Am Med Assoc. 1998;280(13):1161–7.

Kambon K. The African personality in America: An African-centered framework. Tallahasee: NUBIAN Nation Publications; 1992.

Kaplan MS, Marks G, Mertens SB. Distress and coping among women with HIV infection: preliminary findings from a multiethnic sample. Am J Orthopsychiatr. 1997;67(1):80–91.

Karenga M. Black studies and the problematic paradigm. J Black Stud. 1988;18:395–414.

Karenga M. Maat, the moral ideal in ancient Egypt: A study in classical African ethics. Los Angeles: University of Southern California; 1994.

Kelly JA. Advances in HIV/AIDS education and prevention. Fam Relat. 1995;44:345–52.

Kelly JA, Murphy DA, Washington CD, Wilson TS, Koob JJ, Davis DR, et al. The effects of HIV/AIDS intervention groups for high-risk women in urban clinics. Am J Public Health. 1994;84(12):1918–22.

Kelly JA, Murphy DA, Washington C, Wilson T, Koob J, Davis D, et al. The effects of HIV/AIDS intervention groups for high-risk women in urban primary health care clinics. Am J Public Health. 1995;84:1918–22.

Kelly JA, Murphy DA, Sikkema KJ, McAuliffe TL, Roffman RA, Soloman LJ, et al. Randomised, controlled, community-level HIV prevention intervention for sexual-risk behavior among homosexual men in U.S. cities. Lancet. 1997;350(9090):1500–5.

Kurdek LA. Correlates of relationship satisfaction in cohabiting gay and lesbian couples: integration of contextual, investment, and problem-solving models. J Pers Soc Psychol. 1991;61(6):910–22.

Logan TK, Cole J, Leukefeld C. Women, sex, and HIV: social and contextual factors, meta-analysis of published interventions, and implications for practice and research. Psychol Bull. 2002; 128(6):851–85.

Nadler A, Fisher JD. Volitional personal change in an interpersonal perspective. In: Klar Y, Fisher JD, Chinsky J, Nadler A, editors. Initiating Self Change: Social Psychological and Clinical Perspectives. New York: Springer; 1992. p. 213–30.

Neumann MS, Sogolow ED. Replicating effective programs: HIV/AIDS prevention technology transfer. AIDS Educ Prevent. 2000;12(5):35–48.

Neumann MS, Johnson WD, Semaan S, Flores SA, Peersman G, Hedges LV, et al. Review and meta-analysis of HIV prevention intervention research for heterosexual adult populations in the United States. J Acquir Immune Def Syndr. 2002;30:S106–17.

NIMH Multiside HIV prevention trial group. Eban HIV/STD risk reduction intervention: conceptual basis and procedures. J Acquir Immune Def Syndr. 2008a;49:S15.

NIMH Multiside HIV prevention trial group. Formative study to develop the Eban treatment and comparison interventions for couples. J Acquir Immune Def Syndr. 2008b;49:S42.

NIMH Multisite HIV Prevention Trial. The NIMH Multi-site HIV prevention Trial: Reducing HIV sexual risk behavior. Science. 1998;280:1889–94.

NIMH Multisite HIV/STD Prevention Trial for African American Couples Group. Measure of HIV/STD risk-reduction: strategies for enhancing the utility of behavioral and biological outcome measures for African American couples. J Acquir Immune Def Syndr. 2008;49(1): S35–41.

Noar SM, Benac CN, Harris MS. Does tailoring matter? Meta-analytic review of tailored print health behavior change interventions. Psychol Bull. 2007;133(4):673.

O'Leary A, Wingood GM. Interventions for sexually active heterosexual women. In: Peterson JL, DiClemente RJ, editors. Handbook of HIV prevention. New York: Plenum Publishing Corporation; 2000. p. 179–97.

Padian NS, O'Brien TR, Chang YC, Glass S, Francis D. Prevention of heterosexual transmission of human immunodeficiency virus through couple counseling. J Acquir Immune Def Syndr. 1993;6:1043–8.

Pedraza MA, del Romero J, Roldán F, García S, Ayerbe MC, Noriega AR, et al. Heterosexual transmission of HIV-1 is associated with high plasma viral load levels and a positive viral isolation in the infected partner. J Acquir Immune Def Syndr. 1999;21(2):120.

Pequegnat, W. AIDS behavioral prevention: unprecedented progress and emerging challenges. In: Mayer KH and Pizer HF, editors. The AIDS pandemic: impact on Science and society. New York: Elsevier Academic Press; 2005. p. 236–260.

Pequegnat W and Stover E. Payoff from AIDS behavioral prevention research. Mayer KH and Pizer HF, editors. HIV prevention: a comprehensive approach. New York: Elsevier Academic Press; 2005. p. 169–202.

Power R, Koopman C, Volk J, Israelski DM, Stone L, Chesney MA, et al. Social support, substance use, and denial in relationship to antiretroviral treatment adherence among HIV-infected persons. AIDS Patient Care STDs. 2003;17(5):245–52.

Remien RH, Hirky AE, Johnson M, Weinhardt LS, Whittier D, Le GM. Adherence to medication treatment: a qualitative study of facilitators and barriers among a diverse sample of HIV positive men and women in four US cities. AIDS Behav. 2003;7(1):61–71.

Remien RH, Stirratt MJ, Dognin J, Day E, El-Bassel N, Warne P. Moving from theory to research to practice: implementing an effective dyadic intervention to improve antiretroviral adherence for clinic patients. J Acquir Immune Def Syndr. 2006;43:S69.

Remien RH, Berkman A, Myer L, Bastos FI, Kagee A, El-Sadr WM. Integrating HIV care and HIV prevention: legal, policy and programmatic recommendations. J Acquir Immune Def Syndr. 2008;22:S57.

Rosenstock IM, Strecher VJ, Becker MH. Social learning theory and the health belief model. Health Educ Behav. 1988;15(2):175.

Rusbult CE, Verette J, Whitney GA, Slovik LF, Lipkus I. Accommodation processes in close relationships: theory and preliminary empirical evidence. J Pers Soc Psychol. 1991;60(1):53–78.

Schilling RF, El-Bassel N, Hadden B, Gilbert L. Skills-training groups to reduce HIV transmission and drug use among methadone patients. Soc Work. 1995;40:91–101.

Semaan S, Des Jarlais DC, Sogolow E, Johnson WD, Hedges LV, Ramirez G, et al. A meta-analysis of the effect of HIV prevention interventions on the sex behaviors of drug users in the United States. J Acquir Immune Def Syndr. 2002;30:S73.

Shain RN, Piper JM, Newton ER, Perdue ST, Ramos R, Champion JD, et al. A randomized, controlled trial of a behavioral intervention to prevent sexually transmitted disease among minority women. New Eng J Med. 1999;340(2):93–100.

Sogolow E, Peersman G, Semaan S, Strouse D, Lyles CM. The HIV/AIDS Prevention Research Synthesis Project: scope, methods, and study classification results. J Acquir Immune Def Syndr. 2002;30:S15.

Sormanti M, Pereira L, El-Bassel N, Witte S, Gilbert L. The role of community consultants in designing an HIV prevention intervention. AIDS Educ Prevent. 2001;13(4):311–28.

St. Lawrence JS, Jefferson KW, Alleyne E, Brasfield TL. Comparison of education versus behavioral skills training interventions in lowering sexual HIV-risk behavior of substance-dependent adolescents. J Consult Clin Psychol. 1995;63(1):154–7.

Straus MA, Hamby SL, Boney-McCoy S, Sugarman DB. The revised conflict tactics scales (CTS2): development and preliminary psychometric data. J Fam Issues. 1996;17:283–316.

Sullivan PS, Salazar L, Buchbinder S, Sanchez TH. Estimating the proportion of HIV transmissions from main sex partners among men who have sex with men in five US cities. J Acquir Immune Def Syndr. 2009;23(9):1153.

Tanner WM, Pollack RH. The effect of condom use and erotic instructions on attitudes toward condoms. J Sex Res. 1988;25:537–41.

Triandis HC. Culture and social behavior. New York: McGraw-Hill; 1994.

Van Der Straten A, King R, Grinstead O, Serufilira A, Allen S. Couple communication, sexual coercion and HIV risk reduction in Kigali, Rwanda. J Acquir Immune Def Syndr. 1995;9:935–44.

Chapter 8
The Role of Families Among Orphans and Vulnerable Children in Confronting HIV/AIDS in Sub-Saharan Africa

Susannah Allison

Abstract This chapter provides an overview of the impact of the HIV/AIDS epidemic on vulnerable children and families in sub-Saharan Africa. There is a discussion of the terms used to describe HIV-affected vulnerable children. As a result of the generalized epidemic and widespread poverty, many children and families are in need of services. This chapter covers the research on the impact of HIV/AIDS on children and their families in four key areas: (1) care arrangements, (2) educational opportunities, (3) mental health, and (4) HIV risk behaviors. This is followed by a review of the emerging literature on services and programs. The chapter concludes with a discussion of the shortcomings of the research and what has been learned from the studies and programs to date.

8.1 Introduction

This chapter provides an overview of the impact of the HIVAIDS epidemic on vulnerable children and families in sub-Saharan Africa. There is a discussion of the terms used to describe HIV-affected vulnerable children. The impact of HIV/AIDS on children and their parents and caregivers is described followed by a review of the emerging literature on services and programs. The chapter concludes with a discussion of the limitations in the current research and the status of the research field.

8.2 Epidemiological HIV/AIDS Data for Children and Their Families

In 2007, 1.9 million individuals were newly infected with HIV in sub-Saharan Africa, bringing the total to 22 million people living with HIV in this region (UNAIDS 2008). This represents over two-thirds of the individuals living with

W. Pequegnat and C.C. Bell (eds.), *Family and HIV/AIDS: Cultural and Contextual Issues in Prevention and Treatment*, DOI 10.1007/978-1-4614-0439-2_8,
© Springer Science+Business Media, LLC 2012

HIV in the world. The epidemic has exacted a devastating toll on the health and well-being of millions resulting in increased morbidity and mortality rates (Andrews et al. 2006). Fifteen million people have died from HIV/AIDS since the beginning of the pandemic (UNAIDS 2008), resulting in diminished levels of productivity and declining national revenues (Barnett et al. 2001; Zuniga et al. 2008).

Adolescents and young adults represent the most vulnerable group of individuals for HIV infection. In 2007, 45% of all new infections were among those between the ages of 15 and 24 years old (UNAIDS 2008). In sub-Saharan Africa, 3.3 million youth are currently living with HIV, 76% of who are women. Unlike other areas of the world, young women are 2–4.5 times more likely to be HIV seropositive than young men in sub-Saharan Africa (UNAIDS 2008). Additionally, HIV/AIDS is the leading cause of death among adolescents and young adults (15–29 years old) and life expectancy gains have been reversed (Newell et al. 2004; Nicoll and Gill 1999).

The epidemic has subsequently had a tremendous impact on children and families. Deaths of parents have resulted in millions of orphans and there has been an increase in the number of children seeking health care services (Dowdney 2000;Walraven et al. 1996). The rate of orphans appears to be on the rise, especially in Eastern and Southern Africa (Bicego et al. 2003; Watts et al. 2005). In this region alone, 43 million children have lost one or both of their parents, with over 12 million children having lost a parent due to HIV/AIDS (UNAIDS 2006). This translates to one out of every nine children having lost a parent in this region (Monasch and Boerma 2004). In some countries, there are higher numbers of orphans in rural areas (Botswana: Arnab and Serumanga-Zake 2006), while in other countries, the difference is not that striking (South Africa: UNICEF 2003).

Because of the lag time between infection and illness, the number of orphans is expected to increase (Levine et al. 2005). The percentage of children who have been orphaned increases with age (Monasch and Boerma 2004; Watts et al. 2005). In a study across sub-Saharan countries, which only included children orphaned under the age of 15, approximately 15% of the orphans were between birth and 4 years of age, 35% were between 5 and 9 years, and 50% fell in the 10–14-year-old age range (Monasch and Boerma 2004). Paternal orphans have been more prevalent than maternal orphans or double orphans (Bicego et al. 2003; Watts et al. 2005; Monasch and Boerma 2004).

In sub-Saharan Africa, five million children are living with a HIV-infected, chronically ill family member (UNICEF 2006) which places children at risk because they assume the caretaker role and, later, they become orphans. Millions of children have experienced the death of an adult family member or live in communities that have been hard hit by the epidemic resulting in fewer economic and social opportunities (Greener 2004; Mishra and Assche 2008). For adolescents and young adults, the high HIV prevalence rates and lack of parental role models provide a daunting backdrop to their emerging sexual lives.

8.3   Definition of Terms Used to Describe Children

8.3.1   Terms Associated with HIV/AIDS and Poverty

There is controversy about the terms and definitions used to describe vulnerable children affected by HIV/AIDS and achieving consensus on definitions has been difficult. The most common definition for an orphan is a child under the age of 18 whose mother or father has died (UNAIDS 2004). This is a change from a prior UNAIDS definition (UNAIDS and UNICEF 2002) because it increases the upper age limit to 18 years of age (UNAIDS 2004). More specific terms have been identified, whereby a single orphan is a child who has lost one parent (a maternal orphan has lost their mother and a paternal orphan lost their father) and a double orphan has lost both parents. When these terms are used to identify children for services, unintended adverse consequences occur, such as the stigmatization of orphans and exclusion of other vulnerable children.

Because of the generalized epidemic and widespread poverty, many other children need services. This has led to the adoption of the term "children affected by HIV/AIDS." This term encompasses children who are infected with HIV, have lost a parent to HIV/AIDS, have parents or caregivers infected with HIV, live in a household that fosters children affected by HIV/AIDS, or live away from their family as a result of HIV/AIDS (UNICEF 2006). While this term broadened the potential pool of children that were identified as being vulnerable due to HIV/AIDS and needing services, it failed to account for other factors that can contribute to vulnerability among children. As a result, the term "highly vulnerable children" has been adopted by the U.S. Agency for International Development (USAID) to cover all children who are vulnerable and therefore in need have services (USAID 2008).

8.3.2   Terms Associated with Biological and Social Orphans

Some people who work with children have advocated for terms that differentiate between biological and social orphans (Evans 2005; Richter and Desmond 2008). Biological orphans are children who have lost both parents, while social orphans are children whose family is unable to provide for them. However, these definitions have not yet gained wide acceptance.

8.3.3   Terms Associated with Requirements for Services

Others have argued that children requiring services should be characterized in terms of their needs (Earls et al. 2007). The Joint Learning Initiative on Children and

HIV/AIDS (Irwin et al. 2009) has supported this approach and advocates targeting children based on need and not simply on whether children have lost a parent due to HIV/AIDS. This represents a paradigm shift from individual orphans to highly vulnerable children within highly vulnerable families in the context of widespread, chronic poverty (Irwin et al. 2009).

Because of the lack of consensus and the complexity, when discussing a specific study in this chapter, I have used the term used by the authors.

8.4 Impact of HIV/AIDS on Children

While awareness about the number of children affected by HIV/AIDS is growing, there is still a paucity of data focused on these vulnerable children and their families. The HIV epidemic not only affects children's health but has had an impact on four other important domains: (1) care arrangements, (2) educational opportunities, (3) mental health, and (4) HIV risk behaviors. The macro effects on the socioeconomic and health of families is not addressed, but for more information on this topic, see McNally et al. (2006). While the majority of the literature focuses on children who have been orphaned, where possible, information on vulnerable children has been included.

8.4.1 Care Arrangements

The majority of children who have been orphaned by HIV/AIDS are being cared for by a family member, such as siblings or extended family members (Ankrah 1993; Foster et al. 1995; Freeman and Nkomo 2006a, b; Jacobs et al. 2005; Monasch and Boerma 2004). The majority of children remain with their mother if the child's father is deceased, while extended family members step in if the mother dies (Richter and Desmond 2008). Orphans frequently live in households headed by a woman (Monasch and Boerma 2004; Yamano et al. 2006), an elderly person (Foster et al. 1995; Howard et al. 2006), and in households where more people are dependent on fewer income earners (Ansell and van Blerk 2004; Ansell and Young 2004; Bicego et al. 2003; Howard et al. 2006; Masmas et al. 2004; Monasch and Boerma 2004; Oleke et al. 2005). Child-headed households have generated a lot of concern; while children assume adult roles when the parents are ill, the prevalence of child-headed households after the parents die is low (Boris et al. 2006; Donald and Clacherty 2005; Foster et al. 1995; Germann 2006; Howard et al. 2006; Jones 2006; Monasch and Boerma 2004; Thurman et al. 2006a).

Little is known about how the decision is made to place children in different care arrangements when they are orphaned. Cultural norms in some places dictate that children should be placed with paternal or maternal kin; however, these norms appear to be changing in areas with high rates of orphans because extended families may not be able to absorb any more children (Oleke et al. 2005; Jones 2006). When possible, family members are preferred over other caregivers (Rotheram-Borus et al. 2002; Heymann et al. 2007; Beard 2005).

Among mothers living with HIV in South Africa, 12% could not identify a caregiver for their child and described their child's future as bleak (Freeman and Nkomo 2006a, b). Factors that have been proposed as playing a role in a child's placement include: (1) the child's HIV status (Freeman and Nkomo 2006a, b; Townsend and Dawes 2004, 2007); (2) age (male caregivers were less willing to accept younger children; Freeman and Nkomo 2006a, b); orphan girls younger than six were more likely to be offered foster care (Townsend and Dawes 2004, 2007); (3) gender [caregivers reported more willingness to take in female orphans (Townsend and Dawes 2004, 2007)]; (4) additional costs [e.g., school fees (Townsend and Dawes 2004; Matshalaga and Powell 2002)]; and (5) poverty (Howard et al. 2006). These factors may also be changing due to the increasing number of orphans and potentially limited number of family caregivers (Nyambedha et al. 2003).

8.4.2   Education

Children's schooling is affected by the HIV/AIDS epidemic in a number of ways, but the data on schooling is mixed. The differing results may be partially explained by the various indicators used to assess educational outcomes. Some studies focus on enrollment in primary or secondary school and on whether the children are at the age-appropriate grade level. Even when focusing on enrollment in primary school, the results of studies examining the impact of parental illness and death on schooling are mixed. While some studies have documented lower school enroll-ment among orphans, foster children, or children of HIV-infected parents (Mishra et al. 2007; Urassa et al. 1997), other studies have failed to find significant differ-ences (Ainsworth et al. 2005; Floyd et al. 2007; Timaeus and Boler 2007). In a large multicountry study, orphans were approximately 13% less likely to attend school than nonorphans (Monasch and Boerma 2004). Makame et al. (2002) also found higher rates of children who were out of school among those orphaned by HIV/AIDS compared to nonorphans from the same poor community. Among chil-dren in Tanzania, maternal orphans and children in households that had recently experienced an adult death were likely to delay beginning primary school; but there was no evidence that they were dropping out of primary school due to their orphan status or adult death (Ainsworth et al. 2005). While having a parent who was HIV positive did not have an impact on primary school enrollment in Malawi, children of HIV-positive parents were less likely to attend secondary school (Floyd et al. 2007).

The impact of HIV could reduce a family's ability to pay for school fees or an orphaned child could be left with a caregiver who is less willing to support education than their parents would have been (Ainsworth et al. 2005). In a sample of 200 orphaned girls, Kang et al. (2008) found that paternal orphans were more likely to be out of school than maternal orphans because of lack of funds. Additionally, the gender of the parent or caretaker with whom the child is living may impact educational outcomes. Better educational outcomes have been found for orphans living in a female-headed household (Nyamukapa and Gregson 2005), an elderly headed household (Oleke et al. 2007), and in households with greater access to external resources (Nyamukapa and Gregson et al. 2005; Oleke et al. 2007). While school enrollment data are mixed, school attendance frequently drops immediately prior to and following a parent's death (Ainsworth et al. 2005; Evans and Miguel 2007). These results are particularly true for children who lost a mother and those with low baseline academic performance (Evans and Miguel 2007). Girls sharply reduced their school hours immediately following the death of a parent due to the increased household responsibility (Ainsworth et al. 2005). Maternal orphans and young women with an infected parent appear to be at increased risk for poor educational outcomes when compared to paternal orphans, double orphans, or nonorphans (Beegle et al. 2006, 2009; Case and Ardington 2006; Nyamukapa and Gregson 2005). Maternal orphans had 1 year less of schooling (Beegle et al. 2009), were less likely to be enrolled in school, had completed significantly fewer years of schooling (Case and Ardington 2006), and had lower primary school completion rates (Nyamukapa et al. 2003; Nyamukapa and Gregson 2005).

There appear to be several reasons for low levels of primary school completion among maternal orphans. If the father is alive, others view him as being responsible for his children's needs but surviving fathers are less committed than surviving mothers to securing their children's education and are more committed to the needs of children from subsequent marriages. Means testing procedures applied by government, donor agencies, and NGOs disproportionately exclude children from receiving resources if their fathers are still alive (Nyamukapa and Gregson 2005;Rosenberg et al. 2008).

Given the mixed findings on educational outcomes and the fact that the differences in enrollment rates are small, researchers have begun to explore other factors that may be driving differences in school enrollment. Ainsworth and Filmer (2006) presented data indicating that the gap between the enrollment rate of poor and rich is greater than the gap between orphans and nonorphans. Lloyd and Blanc (1996) found that the household resources available to children were associated with school enrollment while children with living parents had slightly higher rates of school enrollment. Although there are some exceptions, Ainsworth and Filmer (2006, p. 1114) conclude that "orphan status in most countries may not be a good targeting criterion for 'traditional' programs aimed at raising enrollment rates." However, there is consensus that keeping orphans in school is a part of HIV control (Gregson et al. 2001).

8.4.3 Mental Health and Well-Being

There has been increasing focus and concern regarding the psychological well-being of children who are affected by HIV/AIDS (Foster 2002a; Omigbodun 2008). Children living in areas where there is a high prevalence of HIV/AIDS are likely to have experienced multiple stressors and losses as a result of the disease. When a child's parent is ill, a child frequently watches as their parent's health deteriorates. During this time, children can experience a range of emotions, including heightened levels of anxiety and depression (Bauman et al. 2006; Sengendo and Nambi 1997). A staggering two-thirds of children with an ill mother had depression scores in the clinically significant range (Bauman et al. 2006). Anxiety is expressed by children who are concerned about the family's source of income and concerns about being separated from siblings (Sengendo and Nambi 1997). The loss of a parent is typically the focus in research; however, losses of other family members, teachers, and other adults in their community can have an adverse mental health effect on children.

8.4.3.1 Internalizing Disorders

Following the death of a parent, children have higher rates of internalizing behavior problems, such as depression and anxiety (Atwine et al. 2005; Cluver et al. 2007; Makame et al. 2002; Sengendo and Nambi 1997). In a large study of 1,200 youth, Cluver and colleagues assessed three groups: (1) children orphaned by HIV/AIDS, (2) children orphaned by other causes, and (3) and children who are not orphans in South Africa (Cluver et al. 2007, 2008; Cluver and Gardner 2006). They found high levels of psychopathology across all three groups, with the highest rates for posttraumatic stress disorder (PTSD) (50%) and depression (17%), but these rates could not be explained by differences in exposure to community and household violence (Cluver et al. 2007). Social support, however, was found to moderate this relationship, whereby children orphaned by HIV/AIDS with higher levels of social support reported lower levels of PTSD symptoms compared to those that perceived their social support as low (Cluver et al. 2009). They also compared rates of depression among these three groups and found that children who were orphaned due to HIV/AIDS reported the highest rates of depression and peer problems when compared to both nonorphaned children and children orphaned as a result of other causes. While poverty, stigma, and caregiver's illness are risk factors, receipt of social support and school attendance were protective factors (Cluver et al. 2007, 2009; Hamra et al. 2006).

Makaya et al. (2002) conducted clinical interviews with 354 Congolese orphans and found that 20% were experiencing psychological difficulties, including depression, anxiety, irritability (34%), and PTSD (39%). Suicide is a major concern because 12% of orphans that were interviewed reported wishing they were dead compared to 3% of the nonorphan children (Atwine et al. 2005); while in another study, 34% of children had contemplated suicide compared to 12% of nonorphans (Makame et al. 2002).

Stigma and discrimination may compound the emotional distress that many children experience (Foster et al. 1997). Stigma can contribute to social isolation, bullying, shame, and a lack of opportunity to discuss their loss and access social support (Cluver and Gardner 2007; Cluver et al. 2009). These findings across multiple studies on psychological distress reflect a significant cause for concern when addressing the needs of orphans affected by HIV/AIDS.

8.4.3.2   Externalizing Disorders

Externalizing reactions have also been documented among orphans, such as stealing, truancy, aggression, and running away, but these are not as common as internalizing behavior problems (Forsyth et al. 1996). Rates of conduct problems and delinquency were higher among the children orphaned due to HIV/AIDS when compared to those orphaned for other reasons and a group of nonorphans (Cluver et al. 2008).

8.4.4   HIV Risk Behaviors

Despite increasing access to HIV prevention education and programs in the region, levels of HIV knowledge remain low. Only 28% of 10–14 year olds were able to identify how to prevent the transmission of HIV (Arnab and Serumanga-Zake 2006). Similar to findings from developed countries, parental presence is associated with sexual health among adolescents in sub-Saharan Africa. When adolescents are living with both parents, they are less likely to have had sex (Ngom et al. 2003; Magnani et al. 2002; Karim et al. 2003), but some studies have found that parental presence has a stronger effect on adolescent females (Karim et al. 2003). For this population, HIV disease is inextricably associated with having discussions of risky sexual behavior with adults. When adolescent orphans were asked about their preference for communication within the family about HIV, youth reported wanting to have candid discussions with adults about parental illness and death. Adults, however, reported not feeling prepared to be able to have these discussions (Wood et al. 2006).

Orphans have therefore been identified as a population at high risk for HIV infection (Birdthistle et al. 2008; Kang et al. 2008; Thurman et al. 2006b). Orphans are more likely to report sexual debut at a younger age (Thurman et al. 2006b), to be sexually active (Kang et al. 2008), and to have had multiple partners. Higher rates of HIV and other STIs as well as pregnancies are also higher among orphans (Birdthistle et al. 2008; Kang et al. 2008; Operario et al. 2007).

When the results have been evaluated by orphan type, maternal and double orphans appear to be at highest risk for HIV infection (Gregson et al. 2005). Maternal orphans have been found to have the highest rates of HIV when compared to other adolescent girls (Kang et al. 2008) as they are more likely to initiate sex early and to have had multiple partners. Paternal loss has not been found to be related to HIV infection or behavioral risk factors (Gregson et al. 2005).

Marital status has also been shown to modify the relationship between orphan status and HIV risk. Girls who were or had been married were more likely to test positive for HIV and HSV-2, but married orphans were not at higher risk for HIV or HSV-2 than married nonorphans (Birdthistle et al. 2008). Heightened risk is related to reduced educational opportunities and living with an HIV seropositive parent that is associated with poorer household circumstances which could result in earlier initiation of sex and marriage to a man who is much older (Gregson et al. 2005).

8.5 Impact on Caregivers

The impact of HIV/AIDS issues on caregivers is important to understand because they can have a direct impact on the family by the way they cope with the situation. The care of orphans is associated with both benefits and challenges for the caregivers. Elder HIV seropositive caregivers have economic, emotional, physical, and stresses that unduly impact their well-being (Sssengonzi 2007; de Wagt and Connolly 2005). In a study of grandparents providing foster care or assisting in the care of their grandchildren in Kenya, there were higher rates of stress among older, full-time grandparents (Oburu and Palmerus 2003). Many adults are caring for additional children from multiple families which can involve a significant amount of physical, mental, and emotional stress (Howard et al. 2006).

Ankrah (1993) and Sarker et al. (2005) failed to find any significant difficulties among families caring for orphans. Other studies, however, have documented challenges of caring for additional children: financial burden (Howard et al. 2006; Heymann et al. 2007) and problems meeting their own children's needs (Heymann et al. 2007). However, Kuo and Operario (2009) report that there were many intergenerational families living together to manage the children when the parents worked as migrants in other communities. The major impact from parental death on these households was the significant reduction in income to support an extended family.

A number of studies have documented the financial challenges associated with providing care to additional children (Miller et al. 2006; Freeman and Nkomo 2006a, b; Jones 2006). Caregivers have also raised concerns about the educational needs of the children in their care (Freeman and Nkomo 2006a, b); food security (Schroeder and Nichola 2005); difficulties managing conflicts between work and home responsibilities (Heymann et al. 2007); and less time caring for their own children (Heymann et al. 2007).

More research is needed to understand how caregivers cope effectively with the challenges of caring for orphans and other vulnerable children and enlist community support, especially around the issue of food insecurity. Zachariah et al. (2006) examined how caregivers utilized sources of community support in Malawi to train 1,694 orphans in vocational skills and help 900 orphans organize 12 vegetable gardens and three maize farms. This met a twofold need of integrating the orphans into the community and providing food to sustain them. A multiple country, community-based study of 2,205 orphans and vulnerable children (7–17 years old) corroborated the benefits of agricultural training and home and community gardens in providing sufficient food for these families (Senefeld et al. 2008). Communities have not always provided positive support to families affected by HIV/AIDS; stigma has been found to weaken social ties between families and their communities, leading to marginalization at the exact time when more support is needed (International HIV/AIDS Alliance and HelpAge International 2003).

8.6 Strategies for Intervening to Support Vulnerable Children and Families

8.6.1 Targeting the Most Vulnerable Children and Their Families

Policy makers and service providers struggle with which children and families will receive scarce services. Targeting effective prevention and treatment programs will result in beneficial effects on children and families. In one study, access to antiretroviral therapy among adults led to an 81% reduction in mortality in their under 10-year-old uninfected children and orphanhood was estimated to be reduced by 93% (Mermin et al. 2008).

While orphans and their families are faced with multiple challenges, they are not the only children who are at risk for poor developmental outcomes. Programs that only target children that have been orphaned are missing large numbers of children who are vulnerable, either due to their parent's illness or other social or economic reasons. Resources may then be distributed inappropriately and inequitably (Foster 2006).

Targeting vulnerability based on need reflects a paradigm shift from individual orphans to highly vulnerable children within highly vulnerable families in the context of widespread, chronic poverty (Irwin et al. 2009). This is based on findings that vulnerability is inextricably tied to poverty. Local community input can help to develop context-specific criteria for resource distribution (Schenk et al. 2008). Characteristics which are associated with children most in need of external support are (1) children living with someone chronically ill, (2) children taken in from another household, (3) children living with other children who have been taken in from another household, and (4) children living in a household headed by someone who is female, elderly, or widowed.

Having identified the children and families most in need of support, the report entitled *Children on the Brink* (UNICEF 2006) proposes five core strategies to guide the response to those children and families most in need of external support: (1) strengthen and support the capacity of families and communities to cope and care for their children; (2) mobilize and strengthen community-based responses; (3) strengthen the economic capacity of children and adolescents to realize their rights and fulfill their basic needs; (4) build on the ability of government to protect the most vulnerable children and provide essential services; and (5) raise awareness within societies to create a supportive environment for affected children and families. Additional reports issued by UNICEF since the Children on the Brink report have continued to lay out concrete goals for those working to help children and families affected by HIV/AIDS (UNICEF 2010).

8.6.2   Economic Strengthening

Considerable attention has been focused on strategies to improve the economic circumstances of families. Economic strengthening has been defined as "approaches to strengthen the capacity of caregivers and communities to address the financial issues to ensure vulnerable children are able to access essential services, including safety, healthcare, education, and other basic needs" (USAID 2008 p.11). A range of programs have been developed: (1) cash transfer programs, (2) child support grants, and (3) youth savings accounts.

8.6.2.1   Cash Transfer Programs

Cash transfer programs or income transfers provide support to poor families for a range of needs, including food, transportation, education, and health care (Adato and Bassett 2008). Transfers can be tied to requirements that the recipients must follow such as attending health care appointments and attending school (conditional cash transfers, CCT) or they can be provided without any requirements (unconditional cash transfers, UCT). CCT programs have proven to be effective in reducing poverty in the short term and health outcomes by increasing household incomes among poor families (Lagarde et al. 2009). They have also increased school enrollment and attendance, especially in middle school. Substantial improvements in health and nutrition have been observed in the children enrolled in these programs. While most cash transfer programs have been developed in Latin America, there is increasing interest in adopting this strategy in sub-Saharan Africa. Because the economy in South Africa is the most similar to Latin America, an experiment called Scaling Up is currently underway. There are also pilot programs in Malawi (Baird et al. 2009; Schubert et al. 2007) and Zambia (Schubert et al. 2007) which are both areas with high HIV prevalence. Most of these cash transfer programs have focused on health outcomes and the use of health services (Adato and Bassett 2008; Lagarde et al. 2009), and school enrollment and attendance (de Janvry and Sadoulet 2004; Schultz 2004). A cash transfer study by The World Bank (Baird et al. 2009) found that there were strong effects on schooling after 1 year among students who had already dropped out of school at baseline as well as for those who were still in school. The baseline dropouts tended to be older, more sexually active, and from poorer households that are more likely to be female headed. Researchers are beginning to document more distal outcomes such as sexual behavior (Baird et al. 2009), whereby youth receiving cash transfers reported less sexual activity.

A report on children, AIDS, and poverty reviewed over 50 studies and suggested that "income transfers as 'a leading edge' intervention to rapidly improve outcomes for extremely vulnerable children and families" (Irwin et al. 2009). This report suggests that cash transfers to women in households improve children's outcomes. A review of cash transfer programs found that even though families were targeted on the basis of poverty, 70% of cash transfer programs ended up targeting HIV/AIDS affected families (Adato and Bassett 2008).

8.6.2.2 Child Support Grants

In order to address the needs of children living in poverty, a number of sub-Saharan countries provide child support grants to families in need. One of the largest programs is in South Africa which is a nonconditional means-tested cash transfer targeted at poor children. The program initially targeted children under 7 years old, but this has been periodically raised and now includes all children under the age of 18 years old (Kibel et al., 2010). Child support grant systems identify a child's primary caregiver as the person who has the primary responsibility for the child on a daily basis and that person receives the support. In an evaluation of the program, 36% of all children under the age of seven have had some contact with the child support grant system, with no difference in the contact for girls and boys (Case et al. 2005). Children for whom the grant is being obtained have parents who are less well educated and who are less likely to be employed. Children whose fathers have died are significantly more likely to be receiving a grant. While there has not been a controlled study, an evaluation did find that school enrollment among 6 and 7 years old children was higher for those who had received a grant. An added benefit of these programs is the likelihood that more adults are willing to take in an orphan if there is assistance to the family and nondirect financial assistance, such as paying for the child's education and providing for a trained person to assist in care, were included (Freeman and Nkomo 2006a, b). However, 28% of best friends, 29% of strangers, 15% of fathers, and 17% of grandparents said they would decline to take children if they were HIV positive.

8.6.2.3 Children Savings Accounts

Asset theory predicts that an orphaned adolescent who does not believe that there will be family funds to support postprimary education is more likely to experience high levels of depression, academic difficulties, drop out of school, and experience negative health consequences (Zhan and Sherraden 2003; Sherraden 1990). If families and children can be provided with the economic means, children's expectations for the future and their well-being lead to continued schooling, and positive health behaviors. Ssewamala et al. (2008a, b) implemented a family centered child savings program in rural Uganda for children orphaned by HIV/AIDS. A study of 268 adolescent orphans who were on average 13.7 years old; were paternal (41%), maternal (19%), and double orphans (40%) (Ssewamala et al. 2009); and were in their last year of primary school in Uganda. The intervention consisted of three components: (1) workshops that focused on asset building and future planning, (2) a mentor that the child met with monthly who provide guidance on life choices and avoiding risk situations, and (3) a child savings account to pay for postprimary schooling or a small family business (Ssewamala and Ismayilova 2009). Children saved an average of $8.85 per month and when compared to a matched control group, the children with the savings account had higher rates of educational plans and improved HIV prevention attitudes.

Adolescents who had participated in the economic empowerment program had significantly better self-esteem and health measures than the control group. Girls reported greater increases in self-esteem than boys and self-esteem was positively related to better health functioning. Of note is the fact that adolescents with increased self-esteem were more likely to report that they intended to practice safer sexual behaviors.

Benefits from savings programs generalize to other areas of family well-being. A study conducted in Kenya (Taoka et al. 2008) of 228 orphans and vulnerable children demonstrated that those with a head of household (95% of whom were women) involved in saving and loans associations (SLAs) had more diverse diets, ate more regularly, and had better nutritional status than those from a household with a head not involved in SLAs. These households had significantly higher agricultural productivity and income generating activities after 2 years.

8.6.3 Mental Health Services/Psychosocial Support Services

Access to mental health services was found to benefit orphans (Atwine et al. 2005). A study conducted in Benin (Odjo et al. 2008) from 2005 to 2007 with 91 children (51% female, aged 5 months to 15 years) found that psychological disorders were successfully treated after 2 months of ongoing psychological care provided to the children and their parents or caregivers. Children with diagnosed psychological problems were treated weekly until the child was stable. This psychological care was integrated into an overall program for HIV exposed or infected children that provided clinical, social, nutritional, education, and pediatric community-based care.

However, there are not enough trained individuals to deliver mental health services to all the vulnerable families that could benefit from them. Other strategies for delivering mental health services need to be explored. Some health care providers have argued that a good strategy would be to integrate mental health care into the primary care structure and this might enhance the delivery of mental health services (Pillay and Lockhat 1997). Kayombo et al. (2005) have suggested another way is to collaborate with traditional healers in Tanzania, many of whom they found were already providing psychosocial support to orphans in their communities.

Another potential strategy is to provide psychosocial support through support groups (Kumakech et al. 2009). A study of 6,127 children ages 8–14 in four orphan and vulnerable children programs in Kenya and Tanzania found that kids' clubs had mixed results in improving children's psychosocial outcomes (Nyangara et al. 2009). One successful kids' club, which met once a month and had a standardized curriculum and a supervisor on staff, was associated with the children's feeling that they had adult support, improved pro-social behavior, and experiencing fewer emotional problems. Another study of a school-based peer-group support intervention was conducted with 326 AIDS orphans (aged 10–15 years old, 42.6% of whom were double orphans) in Uganda (Kumakech et al. 2009). The investigators found that when peer-group interventions were supported by teachers and by healthcare checkups. The intervention provided twice-weekly peer-group support meetings conducted by a trained teacher over the course of 10 weeks and supplemented these sessions with monthly healthcare examinations and treatment. At the end of the study period, the children in the intervention group had lower scores for anxiety, depression, and anger when compared to the control group.

8.6.4   Community-Based Interventions

Community-based interventions offer broad programs that can impact multiple outcomes (Foster 2002b). A community development project that incorporated income-generating activities for women's cooperatives in Côte d'Ivoire identified 409 orphans and vulnerable children and their families (Bossou et al. 2008). They received school kits and fees, medical care, psychosocial support, and monthly food supplements. HIV testing was offered to members of the community. Because members of the community perceived this effort as community development rather than an HIV/AIDS program, it served to reduce the stigma for HIV-affected families. Linking HIV prevention, testing and care with income generation for women may increase care and support for orphans and vulnerable children.

Another community-oriented program conducted in Kenya (Thurman et al. 2008) with 2,472 orphans and vulnerable children and their caretakers (92% female) showed that caretakers who attended antistigma community meetings had more positive attitudes towards orphans and vulnerable children than caretakers who did not. The caretakers who participated in the community meetings were twice as likely (51%) as nonattendees (27%) to have ever been tested for HIV.

Unfortunately, a study of 6,127 children ages 8–14 and 4,591 caregivers in four programs in Kenya and Tanzania found that services targeting orphans and vulnerable children and families affected by HIV/AIDS may also elicit stigma (Nyangara 2009). Between 22 and 57% of the children experienced jealousy from others in the community because of all the services they received, while 27–67% of the caregivers experienced even higher stigma. This suggests that involving the community in making decisions about allocation of health and welfare services and broadening eligibility based on need might alleviate this negative backlash.

The Young citizens' Program was initiated in 2003 to evaluate the effectiveness of training children and adolescents ages 10–14 to strengthen community approaches toward reducing the risks and stigma of HIV/AIDS (Earls et al. 2007). The goal of the Young Citizens Program is to promote a range of HIV community mobilizing skills and behaviors in adolescents, their families, and their community. In the context of the HIV/AIDS epidemic, children and adolescents have the most to gain in achieving HIV-competent communities by taking action to prevent their own orphanhood because of AIDS and to promote their own sexual health.

A program that trains youth to provide care and support to people living with HIV/AIDS in rural Zambia was conducted but no outcome data are available (Esu-Williams et al. 2006). Youth were trained to provide help with household chores and personal care tasks as well as spend time with the individuals' children to decrease their sense of isolation, encourage them to stay in school, and access other needed services when necessary. Both the youth and people living with HIV/AIDS expressed frustration at not being able to meet the material needs of the families coping with HIV/AIDS.

8.6.5 Institutions and Orphanages

Long-term institutionalization is associated with high costs and separates children from their families and communities. Many believe that institutionalized care for children is not economically, psychologically, or socially desirable (Drew et al. 1998; MacLean 2003). However, there have been concerns raised that care provided by extended families or in-home foster care will not be sufficient to care for all of the children who are orphaned or are made vulnerable by HIV/AIDS (Foster 2002a, b; Miller et al. 2006). These concerns have led to the development of other forms of care for orphans, such as residential community centers (Jackson and Kerkhoven 1995) and orphanages (Matshalaga and Powell 2002). In a recent report on residential care settings, Meintjes et al. (2007) found that the majority of children living in an orphanage had at least one living parent (53%) and over 30% of the children were in the orphanage because of parental abuse and neglect. Of the children whose status was known, 34% were HIV seropositive. While more data exists on orphanages in other parts of the world (Sheridan et al. 2010), there are only a few studies reporting on institutional care in sub-Saharan Africa.

In an evaluation of the Godfrey's Children's Center in Tanzania which is a community run orphanage, Center orphans were compared with orphans in the community and village children living with both parents (Wallis et al. 2010). Orphans at the center reported lower rates of depression when compared to orphans in the community and children living with both parents. There were no differences between the three groups on other measures of emotional or behavioral functioning. Orphans at the center also reported as many social supports as the village children and did not report feeling stigmatized or isolated. School attendance was higher among the children at the orphanage than orphans in the community. In qualitative interviews, center orphans expressed greater optimism and hopefulness. Unfortunately, because of a disagreement between the funding NGO and the local NGO, the center was closed.

Another example is an orphan day care center in Botswana which provides centralized care to over 355 orphans of ages 2–18 in a safe, supervised environment during the workday, relieving the caregiving burden and facilitating their ability to work or care for relatives with HIV (Kidman et al. 2007). Older children come to the center after school to receive meals, participate in activities, and receive counseling. The family outreach program delivers counseling to children's caretakers during home visits.

8.7 Conclusions

A number of methodological weaknesses exist in the studies reviewed within this chapter. Only a subset of studies used an appropriate comparison or control group. Without an appropriate comparison group, it is not prudent to draw conclusions about how the risks of highly vulnerable children and their families compare to other children within their community. Many of the studies are based on small, convenience samples and therefore are not as likely to be representative of the larger population of interest. Additionally, there are concerns about generalizing from one area within sub-Saharan Africa to another due to the variations in social, cultural, and economic circumstances. Lastly, the majority of studies are cross-sectional which does not take into account the dynamic nature of development as well as the changing impact of the epidemic.

Despite the shortcomings in the design and conduct of studies of children and their families confronting HIV and the mixed results, there is some convergence of the findings in the studies that suggest positive directions. Programs that offer microenterprise programs or other economic assistance can be effective in raising the goals of orphans and vulnerable children and improving their health and economic situation. Providing good medical treatment and therapy for adults can reduce the number of orphans and improve the health and education outcomes for orphans and vulnerable children. Program that strengthen the fabric of the family and support family centered economic, mental and physical health, and social support programs contribute to improved outcomes for these families and their children. Community-based programs can improve the status of orphans and vulnerable children and their families confronting AIDS and reduce stigma. Given the great need, it is vital that efficacious programs for vulnerable children, some of which were discussed in this chapter, be scaled up as quickly as possible.

References

Adato M, Bassett L. What is the potential of cash transfers to strengthen families affected by HIV and AIDS? A review of the evidence on impacts and key policy debates. Washington, DC: Joint Learning Initiative on Children and HIV/AIDS; 2008.

Ainsworth M, Filmer D. Children's Schooling: AIDS, Orphanhood, Poverty, and Gender. World Dev. 2006;34(6):1099–128.

Ainsworth M, Beegle K, Koda G. The impact of adult mortality and parental deaths on primary schooling in North-western Tanzania. J Dev Stud. 2005;41:412–39.

Andrews G, Skinner D, Zuma K. Epidemiology of health and vulnerability among children orphaned and made vulnerable by HIV/AIDS in sub-Saharan Africa. AIDS Care. 2006;18(3):269–76.

Ankrah M. The impact of HIV/AIDS on the family and other significant relationships: the African clan revisited. AIDS Care. 1993;5(1):5–22.

Ansell N, van Blerk L. Children's migration as a household/family strategy: coping with AIDS in Lesotho and Malawi. J South Afr Stud. 2004;30(3):673–90.

Ansell N, Young L. Enabling household to support successful migration of AIDS orphans in southern Africa. AIDS Care. 2004;16(1):3–10.

Arnab R, Serumanga-Zake A. Orphans and vulnerable children in Botswana: the impact of HIV/AIDS. Vulnerable Children Youth Stud. 2006;1:221–9.

Atwine B, Cantor-Graae E, Bajunirwe F. Psychological distress among AIDS orphans in rural Uganda. Soc Sci Med. 2005;61(3):555–64.

Baird S, Chirwa E, McIntosh C, and Ozler B. The short-term impacts of a schooling conditional cash transfer program on the sexual behavior of young women. Health Econ. 2009 published on-line 2009

Barnett T, Whiteside A, Desmond C. The social and economic impact of HIV/AIDS in poor countries: a review of studies and lessons. Prog Dev Stud. 2001;1(2):151–70.

Bauman LJ, Foster G, Silver EJ, Berman R, Gamble I, Muchaneta L. Children caring for their ill parents with HIV/AIDS. Vulnerable Children Youth Stud. 2006;1(1):56–70.

Beard B. Orphan care in Malawi: current practices. J Commun Health Nurs. 2005;22(2):105–15.

Beegle K, De Weerdt J, Dercon S. Orphanhood and the long-term impact on children. Am J Agricult Econ. 2006;88(5):1266–77.

Beegle K, De Weerdt J, and Dercon S (2009) The Intergenerational Impact of the African orphans crisis: a cohort study from an HIV/AIDS affected area. Forthcoming: Int J Epidemiol (doi:10.1093/ije/dyn197).

Bicego G, Rutstein S, Johnson K. Dimensions of the emerging orphan crisis in sub-Saharan Africa. Soc Sci Med. 2003;56:1235–47.

Birdthistle IJ, Floyd S, Machingura A, Mudziwapasi N, Gregson S, Glynn JR. From affected to infected? Orphanhood and HIV risk among female adolescents in urban Zimbabwe. J Acquir Immune Def Syndr. 2008;22:759–66.

Boris NW, Thurman TR, Snider L, Spencer E, Brown L. Infants and young children living in youth-headed households in Rwanda: implications of emerging data. Infant Ment Health J. 2006;27(6):584–602.

Bossou S, Gbaguidi A, Djahan Y, Kousassi H, N'zin L, and Irie B. Income-generating activities to overcome stigma and discriminization. Abstract-TUPDE102, XVII International AIDS Conference. 2008 Mexico City, Mexico.

Case A, Ardington C. The impact of a parental death on school outcomes: longitudinal evidence from South Africa. Demography. 2006;43(3):401–20.

Case A, Hosegood V, Lund F. The reach *and impact of Child Support Grants: evidence from KwaZulu-Natal*. Development Southern Africa. 2005;22:467–82.

Cluver L, Gardner F. The psychological well-being of children orphaned by AIDS in Cape Town, South Africa. Ann Gen Psychiatr. 2006;5:8.

Cluver L, Gardner F. Risk and protective factors for psychological well-being of children orphaned by AIDS in Cape Town: a qualitative study of children and caregivers' perspectives. AIDS Care. 2007;19(3):318–25.

Cluver L, Orkin M. Cumulative risk and AIDS-orphanhood: interactions of stigma, bullying, and poverty on child mental health in South Africa. Soc Sci Med. 2009;69(8):1186–93.

Cluver L, Gardner F, Operario D. Psychological distress amongst AIDS-orphaned children in urban South Africa. J Child Psychol Psychiatr. 2007;48:755–63.

Cluver L, Gardner F, Operario D. Effects of stigma and other community factors on the mental health of AIDS-orphaned children. Journal of Adolescent Health. 2008;42:410–7.

Cluver L, Fincham DS, Seedat S. Posttraumatic stress in AIDS-orphaned children exposed to high levels of trauma: the protective role of perceived social support. J Trauma Stress. 2009;22(2):106–12.

de Janvry A, Sadoulet E. Conditional cash transfer programs: are they really magic bullets? ARE Update. 2004;7(6):10.

de Wagt A, Connolly M. Orphans and the impact of HIV/AIDS in sub-Saharan Africa. Food, Nutrition and Agriculture. 2005;34:1–9.

Donald D, Clacherty G. Developmental vulnerabilities and strengths of children living in child-headed households: a comparison with children in adult-headed households in equivalent impoverished communities. Afr J AIDS Res. 2005;4(1):21–8.

Dowdney L. Childhood bereavement following parental death. J Child Psychol Psychiatr. 2000;41:819–30.

Drew RS, Makufa C, Foster G. Strategies for providing care and support to children orphaned by AIDS. AIDS Care. 1998;10 Suppl 1:S9–15.

Earls F, Raviola GJ, Carlson M. Promoting child and adolescent mental health in the context of the HIV/AIDS pandemic with a focus on sub-Saharan Africa. J Child Psychol Psychiatr. 2007;49(3):295–312.

Esu-Williams E, Schenk KD, Geibel S, Motsepe J, Zulu A, Bweupe P, et al. We are no longer called club members but caregivers: involving youth in HIV and AIDS caregiving in rural Zambia. AIDS Care. 2006;18(8):888–94.

Evans D. The Spillover Impacts of Africa's Orphans. Rand Corporation Working Paper. (pp. 10–11). 2005 Santa Monica, CA: The Rand Corporation.

Evans DK, Miguel E. Orphans and schooling in Africa: a longitudinal analysis. Demography. 2007;44(1):35–57.

Floyd S, Crampin AC, Glynn JR, Madise N, Mwenebabu M, Mnkhondia S, et al. The social and economic impact of parental HIV on children in northern Malawi: retrospective population-based cohort study. AIDS Care. 2007;19(6):781–90.

Forsyth BWC, Damour L, Nagler S, Adnopoz J. The psychological effects of parental human immunodeficiency virus infection on uninfected children. Arch Pediatr Adolesc Med. 1996;150:1015–20.

Foster G. Beyond education and food: psychological well-being of orphans in Africa. Acta Paediatr. 2002a;91:502–4.

Foster G. Supporting community efforts to assist orphans in Africa. N Eng J Med. 2002b;36:1907–10.

Foster G. Children who live in communities affected by AIDS. Lancet. 2006;367:700–1.

Foster, G, Makufa, C, Drew, R et al., Perceptions of children and community members concerning the circumstances of orphans in rural Zimbabwe. AIDS Care. 1997;9:391–405.

Foster, G, Shakespeare, R, Chinemana, F, et al., Orphan prevalence and extended family care in a peri-urban community in Zimbabwe. AIDS Care. 1995;7:3–17.

Freeman M, Nkomo N. Guardianship of orphans and vulnerable children. A survey of current and prospective South African caregivers. AIDS Care. 2006a;18(4):302–10.

Freeman M, Nkomo N. Assistance needed for the integration of orphaned and vulnerable children: view of South African family and community members. Sahara J. 2006b;3(3):503–9.

Germann SE. An exploratory study of quality of life and coping strategies of orphans living in child headed households in an urban high HIV-prevalent community in Zimbabwe, Southern Africa. Vulnerable Children Youth Stud. 2006;1(2):149–58.

Greener R. The Impact of HIV/AIDS on poverty and inequality. In: Haacker M, editor. The macroeconomics of HIV/AIDS. Washington, D.C: International Monetary Fund; 2004.

Gregson S, Waddell H, Chandiwana SK. School education and HIV control in sub-Saharan Africa: from discord to harmony? J Int Dev. 2001;13:467.

Gregson S, Nyamukapa CA, Garnett GP, Wambe M, Lewis JJ. HIV infection and reproductive health in teenage women orphaned and made vulnerable by AIDS in Zimbabwe. AIDS Care. 2005;17(7):785–94.

Hamra M, Ross MW, Orrs M, D'Agostino A. Relationship between expressed HIV/AIDS-related stigma and HIV-beliefs/knowledge and behaviour in families of HIV infected children in Kenya. Trop Med Int Health. 2006;11(4):513–27.

Heymann J, Earle A, Rajaraman D, Miller C, Bogen K. Extended family caring for children orphaned by AIDS: balancing essential work and caregiving in a high HIV prevalence nation. AIDS Care. 2007;19(3):337–45.

Howard BH, Phillips CV, Matinhure N, Goodman KJ, McCurdy SA, Johnson CA. Barriers and incentives to orphan care in a time of AIDS and economic crisis: a cross-sectional survey of caregivers in rural Zimbabwe. BMC Public Health. 2006;6(12):1–11.

International HIV/AIDS Alliance and HelpAge International, (2003). Forgotten families: older people as caregivers of AIDS orphans and vulnerable children. Available via: http://www.helpage.org. Cited on 21 February 2011.

Irwin, A., A. Adams, and A. Winter. 2009. Home Truths: Facing the Facts on Children, AIDS, and Poverty – Final Report of the Joint Learning Initiative on Children and HIV/AIDS. Boston, MA: Joint Learning Initiative on Children and HIV/AIDS (JLICA).

Jackson H, Kerkhoven R. Developing AIDS care in Zimbabwe: a case for residential community centres? AIDS Care. 1995;7:663–73.

Jacobs M, Shung-King M, Smith C, editors. South African child gauge, 2005. Cape Town, South Africa: Children's Institute, University of Capetown; 2005.

Joint United Nations Programme on HIV/AIDS (UNAIDS) and World Health Organization (WHO). AIDS epidemic update. Geneva, Switzerland: UNAIDS and WHO; 2006.

Joint United Nations Programme on HIV/AIDS (UNAIDS), United Nations Children's Fund (UNICEF). (2004). Children on the Brink 2004. A joint report of new orphan estimates and a framework for action. Geneva, Switzerland; New York, NY, USA; Washington, DC: UNAIDS, UNICEF, USAID.

Jones L. Childcare in poor urban settlements in Swaziland in an era of HIV/AIDS. Afr J AIDS Res. 2006;4:161–71.

Kang M, Dunbar M, Laver S, Padian N. Maternal versus paternal orphans and HIV/STI risk among adolescent girls in Zimbabwe. AIDS Care. 2008;20(2):221–4.

Karim AM, Magnani RJ, Morgan GT, Bond KC. Reproductive health risk and protective factors among unmarried youth in Ghana. Int Fam Plann Perspect. 2003;29:14–24.

Kayombo EJ, Mbwambo ZH, Massila M. Role of traditional healers in psychosocial support in caring for the orphans: a case of Dar-es Salaam City, Tanzania. J Ethnobiol Ethnomed. 2005;1:3.

Kibel M, Lake L, Pendlebury S & Smith C (eds) (2010) South African Child Gauge 2009/2010 Cape Town: Children's Institute, University of Cape Town.

Kidman R, Petrow SE, Heymann SJ. Africa's orphan crisis: two community-based models of care. AIDS Care. 2007;19(3):326–9.

Kumakech E, Cantor-Graae E, Maling S, Bajunirwe F. Peer-group support intervention improves the psychosocial well-being of AIDS orphans: cluster randomized trial. Soc Sci Med. 2009;68(6):1038–43.

Kuo C, Operario D. Caring for AIDS-Orphaned children: a systematic review of studies on caregivers. Vulnerable Children Youth Stud. 2009;4(1):1–12.

Lagarde M, Haines A, Palmer N. The impact of conditional cash transfers on health outcomes and use of health services in low and middle income countries. Cochrane Database Syst Rev. 2009;7(4):CD008137.

Levine C, Foster G, Williamson J, Levine C, Foster G, Williamson J. HIV/AIDS and its long-term impact on children. In: Foster G, Levine C, Willamson J, editors. A generation at risk: the global impact of HIV/AIDS on orphans and vulnerable children. New York: Cambridge University Press; 2005. p. 6.

Lloyd CB, Blanc AK. Children's schooling in sub-Saharan Africa: the role of fathers, mothers, and others. Popul Dev Rev. 1996;22(2):265–98.

Maclean K. The impact of institutionalization on child development. Dev Psychopathol. 2003;15:853–84.

Magnani RJ, Karim AM, Weiss LA, Bond KC, Lemba M, Morgan GT. Reproductive health risk and protective factors among youth in Lusaka, Zambia. J Adolesc Health. 2002;30:76–86.

Makame V, Ani C, Grantham-McGregor S. Psychological well-being of orphans in Dar es Salaam, Tanzania. Acta Pediatr. 2002;91:459–65.

Makaya J, Mboussou F, Bansimba T, Ndinga H, Latifou S, Ambendet A, et al. (2002). Assessment of Psychological Repercussions of AIDS next to 354 AIDS Orphans in Brazzaville, 2001. Paper presented at the XIV International AIDS Conference, Barcelona, Spain.

Masmas TN, Jensen H, da Silva D, Hoj L, Sandstrom A, Aaby P. The social situation of motherless children in rural and urban areas of Guinea-Bissau. Soc Sci Med. 2004;59(6):1231–9.

Matshalaga NR, Powell G. Mass orphanhood in the era of HIV/AIDS. Br Med J. 2002;324:185–6.

McNally LM, Hadingham J, Archary D, Moodley R, Coovadia HM. HIV-exposed but uninfected children: why are they vulnerable? Vulnerable Children Youth Stud. 2006;1(2):139–48.

Meintjes H, Moses S, Berry L, and Mampane R. (2007). Home truths: the phenomenon of residential care for children in a time of AIDS. Cape Town, South Africa: Children's Institute, University of Cape Town and Centre for the Study of AIDS, University of Pretoria.

Mermin J, Were W, Edwaru JP, Moore D, Downing R, Behumbiize P, et al. Mortality in HIV-infected Ugandan adults receiving antiretroviral treatment and survival of their HIV-uninfected children: a prospective cohort study. Lancet. 2008;371:752–9.

Miller CM, Gruskin S, Subramanian SV, Rajaraman D, Heymann J. Orphan care in Botswana's working households: growing responsibilities in the absence of adequate support. Am J Public Health. 2006;96:1429–35.

Mishra V, Assche B-V. Orphans and vulnerable children in High HIV-prevalence countries in Sub-Saharan Africa, DHS analytical studies 15. Washington, DC: USAID; 2008.

Mishra V, Arnold F, Otieno F, Cross A, Hong R. Education and nutritional status of orphans and children of HIV-infected parents in Kenya. AIDS Educ Prev. 2007;19(5):383–95.

Monasch R, Boerma JT. Orphanhood and childcare patterns in sub-Saharan Africa: an analysis of national surveys from 40 countries. J Acquir Immune Def Syndr. 2004;18 Suppl 2:55–65.

Newell ML, Brahmbhatt H, Ghys PD. Child mortality and HIV infection in Africa: a review. J Acqiur Immune Def Syndr. 2004;18 Suppl 2:S27–34.

Ngom P, Magadi MA, Owuor T. Parental presence and adolescent reproductive health among the Nairobi urban poor. J Adolesc Health. 2003;33:369–77.

Nicoll A, Gill ON. The global impact of HIV infection and disease. Comm Dis Public Health. 1999;2:85–95.

Nyambedha E. O. "Change and Continuity in Kin-based Support Systems for Widows and Orphans Among the Luo in Western Kenya", African Sociological Review. 2004;Vol. 8 (1): 139–154.

Nyamukapa C, Gregson S. Extended family's and women's roles in safeguarding orphans' education in AIDS-afflicted rural Zimbabwe. Soc Sci Med. 2005;60(10):2155–67.

Nyangara F, Obiero W, Kalungwa Z, Thurman TR. Community-based psychosocial intervention for HIV-affected children and their caregivers: evaluation of the Salvation Army's Mam Mkubwa Program in Tanzania. 2009. Available at http://www.cpc.unc.edu/measure/publications/pdf/sr-09-50.pdf.

Nyamukapa C, Foster G, Gregson S. Orphans' household circumstances and access to education in a maturing HIV epidemic in eastern Zimbabwe. J Soc Dev Africa. 2003;18:7–32.

Oburu PO, Palmerus K. Parenting stress and self-reported discipline strategies of Kenyan caregiving grandmothers. Int J Behav Dev. 2003;27:505–12.

Odjo F, Azondekon A, Adeyandju I, Monzorgui A, Ketichion A, Sagui A, et al. (2008). Management of HIV children psychological conditions in resource constrained settings: what can be gained? Abstract WEAD0104, XVII, International AIDS Conference, Mexico City, Mexico.

Oleke C, Blystad A, Rekdal OB. When obvious brother is not there: political and cultural contexts of the orphan challenge in Northern Uganda. Soc Sci Med. 2005;61:2628–38.

Oleke C, Blystand A, Fylkesnes K, Turnwine JK. Constraints to educational opportunities of orphans: a community-based study from northern Uganda. AIDS Care. 2007;19(3):361–8.

Omigbodun O. Developing child mental health services in resource-poor countries. Int Rev Psychiatr. 2008;20(3):225–35.

Operario D, Pettifor A, Cluver L, MacPhail C, Rees H. Prevalence of parental death among young people in South Africa and risk for HIV infection. J Acquir Immine Def Syndr. 2007;44(1):93–8.

Pillay AL, Lockhat MR. Developing community mental health services for children in South Africa. Soc Sci Med. 1997;45(10):1493–501.

Richter LM, Desmond C. Targeting AIDS orphans and child-headed households? A perspective from national surveys in South Africa, 1995–2005. AIDS Care. 2008;18:1–10.

Rosenberg A, Hartwig K, Merson M. Government-NGO collaboration and sustainability of orphans and vulnerable children projects in southern Africa. Evaluat Prog Plann. 2008;31:51–60.

Rotheram-Borus MJ, Leonard NR, Lightfoot M, Franzke LH, Tottenham N, Lee SJ. Picking up the pieces: caregivers of adolescents bereaved by parental AIDS. Clin Child Psychol Psychiatr. 2002;1:115–24.

Sarker M, Neckermann C, Muller O. Assessing the health status of young AIDS and other orphans in Kampala, Uganda. Trop Med Int Health. 2005;10(3):210–5.

Schenk KD, Ndhlovu L, Tembo S, Nsune A, Nkhata C, Walusidku B, et al. Supporting orphans and vulnerable children affected by AIDS: using community-generated definitions to explore patters of children's vulnerability in Zambia. AIDS Care. 2008;20(8):894–903.

Schroeder EA, Nichola T. The adoption of HIV/AIDS orphans and food security in rural Ingwavuma, South Africa. Int J Technol Sustain Dev. 2005;5(2):173–87.

Schubert B, Webb D, Temin M, and Masabane P (2007). The impact of social cash transfers on children affected by HIV and AIDS: evidence from Zambia, Malawi, and South. UNICEF/ESARO.

Schultz TP. School subsidies for the poor: evaluating the Mexican Progresa Poverty Program. J Dev Econ. 2004;7(Suppl):105–24.

Senefeld S, Farmer M, Ahmed S, and Lee C (2008) Food and nutrition security of orphans and vulnerable children: programatic implications resulting from a five-country evaluation. Abstract WEPE0624, XVII International AIDS Conference, Mexico City, Mexico.

Sengendo J, Nambi J. The psychological effect of orphanhood: a study of orphans in Rakai district. Health Transit Rev. 1997;7 Suppl 1:105–24.

Sheridan M, Drury S, McLaughlin K, Almas A. Early institutionalization: neurobiological consequences and genetic modifiers. Neuropsychol Rev. 2010;20(4):414–29.

Sherraden M. Stakeholding: notes in a theory of welfare based on assets. Soc Ser Rev. 1990;64(4):580–601.

Ssewamala FM, Ismayilova L. Integrating children's savings accounts in the care and support of orphaned adolescents in rural Uganda. Soc Ser Rev. 2009;83(3):453–72.

Ssewamala FM, Alicea S, Bannon WM, Ismayilova L. A novel economic intervention to reduce HIV risks among school-going AIDS orphans in rural Uganda. J Adolesc Health. 2008a;42:102–4.

Ssewamala FM, Han C-K, Neilands TB, Ismayilova L, Sperber E. Effect of economic assets on sexual risk-taking intentions among orphaned adolescents in Uganda. Am J Public Health. 2008b;100:483–8.

Ssewamala F, Han CH, Neilands T. Asset-ownership and health and mental health functioning among AIDS-orphaned adolescents: findings from a randomized clinical trial in rural Uganda. Soc Sci Med. 2009;69:191–8.

Sssengonzi R. The plight of older persons as caregivers to people infected/affected by HIV/AIDS: evidence from Uganda. J Cross Cult Gerontol. 2007;22(4):339–53.

Taoka S, Baggaley R, Hughes K, Ndondoo E, Masila N, Wambua N (2008) Do Savings and Loans Associations (SLAs) improve diets and nutritional status of orphans and vulnerable children (OVC)? Abstract TUPE0661, XVII International AIDS Conference, Mexico City, Mexico.

Thurman TR, Snider L, Boris N, Kalisa E, Murguria E, Ntaginira J, et al. Psychosocial support and marginalization of youth-headed households in Rwanda. AIDS Care. 2006a;18(3):220–9.

Thurman TR, Brown L, Richter LM, Maharaj P, Magnani R. Sexual risk behavior among adolescents in South Africa: is orphan status a factor? AIDS Behav. 2006b;10(6):627–35.

Thurman TR, Snider LA, Boris NW, Kalisa E, Nyirazinyoye L, Brown L. Barriers to the community support of orphans and vulnerable youth in Rwanda. Soc Sci Med. 2008;66(7):1557–67.

Timaeus IM, Boler T. Father figures: the progress of orphans in South Africa. J Acquir Immune Def Syndr. 2007;7 Suppl 7:S83–93.

Townsend L, Dawes A. Willingness to care for children orphaned by HIV/AIDS: a study of foster and adoptive parents. Afr J AIDS Res. 2004;3:69–80.

Townsend L, Dawes A. Intentions to care for children orphaned by HIV/AIDS: a test of the theory of planned behavior. J Appl Soc Psychol. 2007;37(4):822–43.

UNAIDS. (2004). AIDS Epidemic Update 2004. Geneva, Switzerland: Joint United Nations Programme on HIV/AIDS (UNAIDS) and World Health Organization (WHO). Available via: http://whqlibdoc.who.int/unaids/2004/9291733903.pdf. Cited 14 March 2011.

UNAIDS. (2006). AIDS Epidemic Update 2006. Geneva, Switzerland: Joint United Nations Programme on HIV/AIDS (UNAIDS). Available via: http://data.unaids.org/pub/epireport/2006/2006_epiupdate_en.pdf. Cited 18 March 2011.

UNAIDS. (2008). AIDS Epidemic Update 2008: Executive Summary. Geneva, Switzerland: Joint United Nations Programme on HIV/AIDS (UNAIDS) http://data.unaids.org/pub/GlobalReport/2008/jc1511_gr08_executivesummary_en.pdf. Cited 18 March 2011.

UNICEF. Africa's orphaned and vulnerable generations. Children affected by AIDS. New York: UNICEF; 2006.

UNICEF & UNAIDS (2010). Children and AIDS: Fifth Stocktaking Report, 2010 (UNICEF). Available via: http://www.unicef.org/aids/files/ChildrenAndAIDS_Fifth_Stocktaking_Report_2010_EN.pdf Cited 18 March 2011.

Urassa M, Walraven G, and Boerma T (1997). Consequences of the AIDS epidemic for children. In HIV Prevention and AIDS Care in Africa. A District Level Approach, (337–349). In: Ng'weshemi J, Boerma T, Bennett J, and Schapink D, (eds.). Amsterdam, The Netherlands: Royal Tropical Institute.

USAID. (2008). Third Annual Report on Orphans and Vulnerable Children in Developing Countries. Washington, D.C.: USAID. Available via: http://pdf.usaid.gov/pdf_docs/PDACM265.pdf. Cited 16 March 2011.

Wallis A, Dukay V, Mellins C. Power and empowerment: fostering effective collaboration in meeting the needs of orphans and vulnerable children. Glob Public Health. 2010;5(5):509–22.

Walraven G, Nicoll A, Njau M, Timaeus I. The impact of HIV-1 infection on child health in sub-Saharan Africa: the burden on the health services. Trop Med Int Health. 1996;1(1):3–14.

Watts H, Lopman B, Nyamukapa C, Gregson S. Rising incidence and prevalence of orphanhood in Manicaland, Zimbabwe, 1998 to 2003. J Acquir Immune Def Syndr. 2005;19(7):717–25.

Wood K, Chase E, Aggleton P. Telling the truth is the best thing: teenage orphans' experiences of parental AIDS-related illness and bereavement in Zimbabwe. Soc Sci Med. 2006;63(7):1923–33.

Yamano T, Shimamura Y, Sserunkuuma D. Living arrangements and school of orphaned children and adolescents in Uganda. Econ Dev Cult Change. 2006;54(4):833–56.

Zachariah R, Teck R, et al. How can the community contribute in the fight against HIV/AIDS and tuberculosis? An example from a rural district in Malawi. R Soc Trop Med Hyg. 2006;100:167–75.

Zhan M, Sherraden M. Assets, expectations, and children's educational achievement in female-headed households. Soc Ser Rev. 2003;72(2):191–211.

Zuniga JM, Whiteside A, Ghaziani A, Bartlett JG, editors. A decade of HAART: the development and global impact of highly active antiretroviral therapy. Oxford, UK: Oxford University Press; 2008.

Chapter 9
Collaborating with Families and Communities to Prevent Youth HIV Risk Taking and Exposure

Mary M. McKay, Clair A. Blake, Mari Umpierre, Hadiza Osuji, and Carl C. Bell

Abstract Decades into the HIV epidemic, those impacted by this stigmatizing disease disproportionately reside in urban communities of color. Early HIV prevention efforts experienced a myriad of challenges reaching large numbers of African American and Latino youth residing in the most deeply affected communities. Over time, it has become increasingly clear that in order to decrease barriers to implementation and increase access and service use, preventative efforts must shift focus to include collaboration with families, social networks and communities. There have been calls to maximize collaboration between prevention scientists and key HIV prevention stakeholders, particularly parents and family members, in order to design relevant risk reduction programs for youth living within high risk urban contexts. This chapter describes models of collaboration with families in connection with their communities which can create sustainable HIV prevention and overall health promotion platforms within inner-city community contexts.

9.1 Introduction

Decades into the HIV epidemic, those impacted by this still life threatening, stigmatizing disease disproportionately reside in urban communities of color. HIV is affecting vulnerable inner-city populations, particularly those impacted by high rates of poverty, substance abuse, exposure to community and familial violence and stressors associated with urban living (Annunziata et al. 2006; Beautrais 2001; Kotchick et al. 2006; Samuolis et al. 2005; Wild et al. 2004). The African American and Latino communities have been disproportionately impacted by these health risks and stressors. For example, although African Americans account for approximately 12% of the total US population, they are likely to live in poverty-impacted communities within large urban centers, such as New York City, Chicago, Los Angeles, and Miami, all with high rates of HIV infection. Thus, it is not surprising that African Americans comprise nearly 50% of all newly reported HIV infections (Centers for Disease Control and Prevention (CDC) 2009). An additional 18% of new infections

W. Pequegnat and C.C. Bell (eds.), *Family and HIV/AIDS: Cultural and Contextual Issues in Prevention and Treatment*, DOI 10.1007/978-1-4614-0439-2_9, © Springer Science+Business Media, LLC 2012

are accounted for by Latinos (Centers for Disease Control and Prevention (CDC) 2009). Almost one-half of the over 40,000 yearly new HIV infections in the United States are among people aged 25 years and younger. Thus, African American and Latino youth appear to be most at risk for HIV infection (Centers for Disease Control and Prevention (CDC) 2009).

Early HIV prevention efforts consisted of largely individual-level interventions. Beginning in the late 1990s, the Centers for Disease Control and Prevention (CDC) created a compendium of the "first generation" of empirically supported interventions, referred to as "Programs that Work" (Centers for Disease Control and Prevention (CDC) 2008). Several of these interventions focused on reducing minority youth risk taking behaviors. However, even programs with empirical support experienced difficulty reaching large numbers of youth within urban communities or sustaining HIV prevention efforts after research or demonstration funding ended. Barriers to implementation of evidence-informed HIV prevention programming focused on sexual and drug risk behaviors of youth included the perception by family and community members that these programs were created by "outsiders" (Dalton 1989; Stevenson and White 1994). Further, there were insufficient community-level supports and resources (Galbraith et al. in press; Kirby et al. 1991) necessary for widespread dissemination of the program or ongoing sustainability.

Thus, it became clear that if youth risks were to be diminished, then preventative efforts needed to shift focus away from targeting the individual youth at risk and towards their families and social networks, nested within surrounding neighborhoods and communities (Baptiste et al. 2005; DeVoe et al. 2005; Madison et al. 2000). Marshaling family, social network and community-level resources around vulnerable urban youth was thought to be a critical, HIV prevention and health promotion strategy as the epidemic progressed into the second decade. Therefore, this chapter focuses on models of collaboration with families in connection with their communities which can create sustainable HIV prevention and overall health promotion platforms within inner-city community contexts.

9.2 Collaborative Approaches to Family-Based HIV Prevention Research

Increasingly, there have been calls to maximize collaboration between prevention scientists and key HIV prevention stakeholders, in this case parents and family members, in order to design relevant risk reduction programs for youth living within high risk urban contexts (Trickett 1998; McKay and Paikoff 2007). A range of descriptions and definitions of participatory or collaborative research have been offered (Altman 1995; Arnstein 1969; Chavis et al. 1983; Singer 1993). There is agreement on some central themes and core foundational principles of such collaborative efforts. For example, on the most basic level, collaborative research has been described as "providing direct benefit to participants either through direct intervention or by using the results to inform action for change" (Israel et al. 1998; p. 175).

Further, what distinguishes collaborative research efforts is the emphasis on the intensive and ongoing participation and influence of key stakeholders, in this case family members, in creating knowledge (Israel et al. 1998).

Collaborative research activities are defined by: (1) a recognition that investment and development of individuals set within their contexts are important foci of research activities; (2) a commitment to build upon existing strengths and resources; (3) ongoing attention to involvement of collaborators across all phases of a research study; (4) an integration of knowledge and action for mutual benefit of all; (5) a process that actively addresses social inequalities; (6) opportunities for feedback; (7) addressing health from both strength and ecological perspectives; and (8) disseminating findings and knowledge gained to a range of audiences, including partners, service providers, community-based organizations, as well as to academic audiences (Israel et al. 1998; pp. 178–179).

Although one of the core tenants of collaborative research is the involvement of key stakeholders in every aspect of the research process, there have been few systematic attempts to operationalize the choices available to family-centered partnerships throughout a given research study. McKay and colleagues (2007) have identified a range of concrete opportunities to collaborate and conceptualized possible levels of intensity during each research phase of co-creating, co-implementing and co-examining family-based HIV prevention approaches based upon prior work of Hatch and colleagues (1993).

For example, collaborative partnerships meant to increase recruitment and retention in family-focused prevention research projects might develop strategies, such as incorporating parents as paid staff or as interviewers or recruiters. Parent HIV educators drawn from the target community can fulfill liaison roles between youth and families in need and prevention programs (Elliott et al. 1998; Koroloff et al. 1994; McCormick et al. 2000). In some cases, community parents can be the first contact that a youth or adult caregiver has with a specific family-based prevention project. The involvement of parent collaborators in these roles has been associated with significant increases in involvement by potential families in prior research efforts (McCormick et al. 2000; 2010; Elliott et al. 1998; Koroloff et al. 1994). Collaborative partnerships can also focus on facilitating the implementation of family-based prevention approaches. For example, preventative interventions can be delivered by "naturally existing community resources," specifically parents (Alicea et al. in press; McKay et al. 2000, 2010).

In relation to collaborative intensity, Hatch and colleagues (1993) indicate that although additional input is sought as collaborative efforts intensify, key decisions regarding who has ultimate control over research questions and decisions regarding research methods, procedures and interpretation of study results are critical. At the highest level of collaboration, the research partners, representing university and families in the community, work together to develop the focus of the research and an action agenda. Then, both university and family partners are responsible for pursuing these shared goals. At the most intense level of collaboration, there is true partnership between parent collaborators and researchers in shared decision-making and recognition of the *specific talents of both researchers and parents.*

9.3   Vehicles to Achieve High Levels of Collaboration with Families

One model of achieving high levels of partnership with families around urban youth HIV prevention efforts has been the formation of a Collaborative Board (CB), consisting of key stakeholders within a specific neighborhood or community. McKay and colleagues have previously described the workings of a CB in overseeing a number of youth-focused, family-based HIV prevention programs and related research activities (see McKay and Paikoff 2007 for complete description). A CB is a formalized partnership between key stakeholders in urban communities and child/ family focused researchers. Beginning with initial funding by the National Institute of Mental Health (NIMH) in 1995 as part of the CHAMP (Chicago HIV prevention and Adolescent Mental health Project) Family Program study (McKay and Paikoff 2007), CBs have expanded and been replicated to oversee a number of federally and locally funded family-based HIV prevention research studies across the US and internationally (Mckay and Paikoff 2007). Typically, a CB consists of 30 members, including urban youth, adult caregivers, school staff, representatives from youth-serving agencies, and researchers.

Board members are involved in every aspect of the research study from development to dissemination. Specific issues are addressed by the full board and within its' subcommittees, which can include Implementation, Finance, Grant Writing and Curriculum committees. For example, the Curriculum committee oversees the development of the intervention protocol and is largely comprised of parents and youth, the potential consumers of any family-based HIV prevention program. Thus, academic and family partners work together to develop the focus of the research, an action agenda, and are responsible for designing, delivering and testing preventative interventions based upon both stakeholder input and existing evidence (McKay et al. 2010).

9.4   Influence of the CB on the Design, Delivery and Testing of Family-Based HIV Prevention Programs

The collaborative development and implementation of multiple family-based HIV prevention programs has been facilitated by CB curriculum committees, the working groups of urban parents, school staff members, and research staff for more than a decade (see McKay et al. 2010 for additional details). More specifically, this group reviews: (1) existing knowledge regarding the prevention needs of families in the target urban communities; (2) expressed perspectives of families and staff regarding priorities and preferences related to focus and process of implementation; and (3) existing evidence-based, family-focused approaches and related articles summarizing associated evidence for each. Following intensive study and discussion, choices are made regarding specific focus of intervention sessions, as well as related content for presentation, discussion questions and in-session activities for any new family-based preventative intervention being introduced to the community. As members of the curriculum committee, research staffs are charged with noting all decisions made in committee meetings and drafting portions of intervention protocol for review at subsequent meetings until consensus is reached regarding final intervention guide for each of the study conditions.

9.5   CB Review of Existing Knowledge: Parent and Family-Level Influences on Youth HIV Risk

As mentioned above, CB members review findings from prior studies regarding how parents and family members can reduce youth HIV risk taking and thus, decrease probability of HIV exposure. HIV risk taking and substance use among vulnerable youth appear to be explained by a range of contextual factors, importantly family influences. Parental support and family connectedness have been associated with lower risk taking among adolescents generally. For youth with any additional vulnerability, such as mental health needs, high levels of family conflict and low levels of protective family processes can lead to early sexual debut and heightened HIV risk and substance use.

The effects of poverty on parenting skills and qualities of family life have been linked with poor outcomes for youth. Stressors associated with subsistence living can disrupt all aspects of family life. For example, experiences of housing transition, displacement and homelessness have been found to disrupt parenting practices and are often compounded by adult caregivers attempt to cope with high levels of stress and the fact that they are not completely in control of their child's environment (e.g., sharing space with other adult caregivers with conflicting expectations when living in a homeless shelter).

9.6   Family-Strengthening Approaches to Youth HIV Prevention Efforts

HIV prevention programs for adolescents have led to greater AIDS knowledge, more realistic beliefs about susceptibility and self-efficacy and positive perceptions concerning the benefits of risk reduction (Centers for Disease Control and Prevention (CDC) 2008). In addition, several programs have been associated with significant reductions in adolescent sexual risk taking. However, these outcomes have proven difficult to achieve and sustain, thus, there is now widespread recognition that multi-level, contextually oriented HIV prevention approaches, particularly family-based interventions are needed (McKay et al. 2000; McKay and Paikoff 2007).

The use of family-based interventions for youth exhibiting behavioral risk taking behaviors and their families has also gained substantial empirical support McKay et al. 2000; McKay and Paikoff 2007). Many evidence-based family interventions focus on parent management training or parenting skills, as well as on goal setting, family communication, action plans and building on family strengths.

9.7 Underpinnings of the Collaborative Process

The work of the CB curriculum committee is guided by a set of collaborative principles: (1) agreement on shared research goals; (2) equitable distribution of power, including opportunities for all to modify the research process; (3) recognition of skills and expertise associated with both university training and consumer experience; (4) ongoing opportunities for communication based upon commitment to honest exchanges and willingness to raise concerns without blame; and (5) continual development of trust.

9.7.1 Shared Goals

First, the development of shared goals that are acceptable to both researchers and family members is necessary to ensure productive collaborative efforts (Israel et al. 1998). Clearly, a goal shared by researchers and consumers, families, and providers is to support the health and mental health of youth. However, specifying the goals that will guide specific partnerships and focus research efforts can require a melding of perspectives and priorities that often appear divergent initially.

9.7.2 Distribution of Power

Many authors have voiced concern that unless power is shared among partners, rather than being largely held by university-based researchers, then the collaboration is essentially a facade (Hatch et al. 1993). We expect researchers and parent collaborators to exercise their power in unique ways. The power of researchers takes the form of specialized expertise (e.g., research and proposal writing skills) and access to research funding. Family members in communities, on the other hand, exercise their power by both supporting research efforts and opening access to participants or by blocking opportunities to conduct research within their settings or communities. Collaborative partnerships bring their collective power to bear in order to achieve the agreed upon goals.

9.7.3   Recognition of Skills and Competencies

An important activity early in the partnership is to concretely identify what skills and competencies each partner brings to the collaboration (McKay and Paikoff 2007). For example, in collaborations with family members, there could be recognition that they have knowledge regarding acceptable recruitment strategies or cultural practices that could be incorporated into innovative service delivery approaches.

9.7.4   Communication

All the processes described above require ongoing communication between members of the partnership and a willingness to engage in productive conflict resolution. A "researcher needs skills and competencies in addition to those required in research design and methods, for example, listening, communication (e.g., use of language that is understandable and respectful), group process, team development, negotiation, conflict resolution, understanding and competency to operate in multicultural contexts, ability to be self-reflective and admit mistakes, capacity to operate within different power structures, and humility" (Israel et al. 1998, p. 187).

9.7.5   Trust

Unfortunately, many families, and communities can recount prior negative experiences with university-based research projects (Stevenson and White 1994). There is often substantial concern regarding researchers' motivation to conduct children's research projects and questions regarding whether the researchers are committed to the setting or *community once research funding is expended* (McKay and Paikoff 2007).

9.7.6   Theoretical Models Guiding Collaborative Partnership with Families

Creating, nurturing, and sustaining such collaborative HIV prevention focused partnerships requires a theoretical approach to organize the influences necessary to support enhanced family-level involvement in HIV prevention efforts, and to maximize supports necessary for individual adult caregivers to play more active roles than are typical. McKay and colleagues relied on the Unified Theory of Behavior (Jaccard et al. 1999) to form the basis for understanding processes critical to galvanizing parents in the community to become HIV educators for youth. The Unified Theory of Behavior also guided collaborative training and mentoring programs meant to prepare parents to become involved in the design, delivery and testing of youth-focused HIV prevention programs within their neighborhoods.

As part of a NIMH sponsored study, CHAMPions (CHAMP In Our Neighborhoods collaborative training and mentoring intervention for parents in the community was developed. CHAMPions focused on maximizing a potential parents' attitude toward learning about sexual risk reduction strategies and the content of the evidence-based programs. Further, the training attempted to increase a parents' perception about the importance or salience of becoming involved in community-based STD and HIV prevention activities. Parents also received the training within a supportive context intended to increase the normative pressure to provide leadership within their community. Further, the training and ongoing mentorship was meant to bolster parents' self-efficacy and alter self-concept so that members of the community would view themselves as being able to contribute to helping youth reduce their sexual health risk. Further, the training was meant to enhance parents' knowledge regarding STD and HIV prevention, while ongoing mentoring from more experienced community HIV prevention experts helped to create problem solving skills necessary to address environmental obstacles to program delivery.

Prior publications support the impact of this collaborative training and mentoring approach (e.g., Alicea et al. in press; Chowdhury et al. in press). Briefly, community parent HIV educators who received collaborative training and mentoring evidenced significant increases in HIV knowledge following the training. They also reported significantly fewer environmental constraints, higher endorsement of habitual behaviors related to participation in HIV prevention activities, enhancements in social network support for HIV prevention leadership in the community and an enhanced self-concept relative to those community members who received standard exposure to evidence-based HIV prevention program materials. Further, when community parent HIV educators attempted to deliver the program to youth in their communities, collaboratively trained adults were able to help three times as many youth complete an HIV prevention program relative to those adults trained in more standard ways.

9.7.7 Maintaining HIV Prevention Collaborative Partnerships

Recently, a number of factors have been identified as influential to maintaining family-level HIV prevention momentum. For example, concepts such as self-efficacy, egalitarianism, and personal empowerment have been identified as prime motivators to remaining actively engaged in a Community CB or as a community HIV educator over time (Savard et al. in press).

More specifically, self-efficacy was described in these ways by parent collaborators:

"I have also learned how to validate myself as a person,"

"I can do this without having letter, I say letter like, you know Ph.D., all of those letters behind my name."

Further, parent partners described a strong appreciation for the ability to express their views and opinions within a forum, where they would be respected. This sense of egalitarianism was described in the following ways:

"It was when we all sat down and now the whole board has a voice in saying something about what we do, how we do it, and when we do it, whether we approve of it or disapprove, and majority rules."

"It felt good to be heard. Freedom of speech to say how you feel, about any area, and have someone actually listen without being judgmental," and,

"We're all working together making decisions and we have equal power and say-so on the Board. That's how the program is run."

Parents also identified a sense of personal empowerment as a reason for their continued involvement with community HIV prevention efforts. For instance, community members noted:

"I am a human being and I need to get things done for myself," and

"I think everyone feels empowered and that's basically what it is. I saw a lot of people talking about college and empowering their children."

"And now I'm more independent, I do things on my own and it's like if you don't like it that's fine! It's been very good."

Another main theme that emerged regarding why parent partners remained actively involved in community HIV prevention efforts over time related to the process of giving back to their community, as reflected in the following comments:

"I was straight into it because of the condition of the community. And I did want to help,"

"I believe in giving back to your community. Because if you don't help your community, who is going to help?" "I see a lot of people there involved and they care about the community and so they're excited, and it's something I can give back,"

"I live in this community and I'm planting here. I'm not going to move from here, so I want the community to change. I want this community to grow in the right way."

9.8   Future of Collaborative Family-Focused HIV Prevention Research

In the last decade, HIV prevention efforts have been intensified (Dworkin et al. 2008) with the Centers for Disease Control and Prevention (CDC) taking a leadership role in this process. Diffusion of Effective Behavioral Interventions (DEBI) is the largest centralized effort to diffuse evidence-based behavioral interventions to prevent HIV in the U.S. As with other centralized health prevention efforts, empirically supported HIV prevention programs are meant to be replicated, disseminated and implemented in communities across the U.S.

Dworkin and colleagues (2008) reviewed these efforts with the aim of identifying, whether collaborative principles were integrated into this effort. The authors highlighted important missed opportunities where collaborative processes could facilitate DEBI efforts. Particularly noteworthy in this review is the lack of emphasis on the use of family-based approaches and the possibility of family collaboration as being key to implementation efforts for youth. For example, family and community choice regarding, which evidence-based intervention to implement appears to be limited. In contrast, Dworkin and colleagues recommend that implementation and adaptation should honor and be guided by local knowledge, as it is essential to bolstering evidence-based interventions and to adapting them to real world settings. Not paying attention to local preferences and expertise, particularly those of parents and family members in relation to their children, may result in a missed opportunity to galvanize community-level support. Further, relying on local knowledge may serve to erode existing prevention efforts that may already be working.

The continued threat of HIV to young people calls for new models of HIV prevention research that can increase health protective behaviors and reduce risk taking. Collaborative models hold promise for addressing these serious issues as they bring together researchers who have substantial expertise, knowledge of the literature, and access to resources with family stakeholders who bring strong commitment to the health of youth and expertise related the needs of youth and their families, and an understanding of the practical realities of agency settings and communities.

There are multiple ways to consider collaboration within the field of HIV prevention. In this chapter, there has been a focus on core collaborative principles that could serve to guide family-based HIV prevention researchers. In addition, opportunities for increasing collaboration across the research process at varying degrees of depth are presented for those invested in HIV prevention to consider.

Although, opportunities to collaborate more intensely are available to researchers, these collaborative efforts are not without a specific set of challenges. Collaborative research efforts are labor intensive for both the researcher and family members. Further, they require a level of communication and sharing of power that has not necessarily been a part of the majority of research projects previously. However, there is a great need to develop new ways to serve our nation's youth given that innovative prevention services are likely to fail in community-based settings, if they attempt to integrate new services and involve service providers in a non-collaborative manner (Aponte et al. 1991; Boyd-Franklin 1993; Fullilove and Fullilove 1993).

We know from prior research that the potential effectiveness of HIV prevention services are limited, when those services have been designed and implemented in ways that do not appreciate stressors, scarce contextual resources, target groups' core values, or the skills and capabilities of "real world" providers (Boyd-Franklin 1993; Jensen et al. 1999a, b; McLoyd 1990). Prevention researchers encounter significant obstacles, such as poor participation or tensions and suspicions between community residents and outside researchers. Therefore, the establishment of strong partnerships with families is critical to ensuring that effective HIV prevention programs are well received within community-based settings and that innovative programs can be sustained once research funding has ended (Gustafson et al. 1992; Galbraith et al. in press). Ongoing research attention to the impact of collaborative partnerships on family-based HIV prevention outcomes is clearly needed to further refine the science of collaborative research efforts, and might be considered one of the major agenda items for the field of HIV prevention research for at least the next decade.

Acknowledgements Funding from the National Institute of Mental Health (R01 MH069934; R01 MH 63662; R01 MH069934) is gratefully acknowledged. In addition, members of the Community Collaborative Boards in Chicago and New York greatly expanded our understanding of key processes needed to create and sustain urban collaborations, as well as the substantial benefits of collaborative research efforts.

References

Alicea S, Bannon W, Cavaleri M, McKay M. Understanding urban parents' motivation to collaborate with a behavioral and preventive health program for youth: the utility of contact theory. In press.

Altman DG. Sustaining interventions in community systems: on the relationship between researchers and communities. Health Psychol. 1995;14(6):526–36.

Annunziata D, Hogue A, Faw L, Liddle HA. Family functioning and school success in at-risk, inner-city adolescents. J Youth Adolesc. 2006;35(1):105–13.

Aponte HJ, Zarskl J, Bixenstene C, Cibik P. Home/community based services: a two-tier approach. Am J Orthopsychiatry. 1991;61(3):403–8.

Arnstein S. The ladder of citizen participation. J Am Inst Plann. 1969;35(4):216–24.

Baptiste D, Paikoff R, McKay M, Madison-Boyd S, Coleman D, Bell C. Collaborating with an urban community to develop an HIV/AIDS prevention program for Black youth. Behav Modif. 2005;27:1–10.

Beautrais AL. Suicides and serious suicide attempts: two populations or one? Psychol Med. 2001;31(5):837–45.

Boyd-Franklin N. Black families. In: Walsh F, editor. Normal family process. New York: Guilford Press; 1993.

Centers for Disease Control and Prevention. Replicating effective programs plus. Available via: http://www.cdc.gov/hiv/topics/prev_prog/rep/index.htm (2008). Cited 6 February 2011.

Centers for Disease Control and Prevention. HIV/AIDS. Available via: http://cdc.gov/hiv/ (2009). Cited 5 Feb 2011.

Chavis DM, Stucky P, Wandersman A. Returning basic research to the community: a relationship between scientist and citizen. Am Psychol. 1983;38:424–34.

Chowdhury J, Alicea S, Elwyn L, Rivera-Rodriguez A, Miranda A, Watson J, et al. Collaboration with urban parents to deliver a community-based youth HIV prevention program. In press.

Dalton HL. AIDS in blackface. Daedalus. 1989;118(3):205–27.

DeVoe E, Dean K, McKay M. The SURVIVE community project: a family based intervention to reduce the impact of violence exposures in urban youth. J Aggress Maltreat Trauma. 2005;11:95–116.

Dworkin SL, Pinto RM, Hunter J, Rapkin B, Remien RH. Keeping the spirit of community partnerships alive in the scale up of HIV/AIDS prevention: critical reflections on the roll out of DEBI (diffusion of effective behavioral interventions). Am J Community Psychol. 2008;42(1–2):51–9.

Elliott D, Koroloff N, Koren P, Friesen B. Improving access to children's mental health services: the family associate approach. In: Epstein M, Kutash K, editors. Outcomes for children and youth with emotional and behavioral disorders and their families: programs and evaluation best practices. Austin, TX: PRO-ED; 1998. p. 581–609.

Fullilove MT, Fullilove RE. Understanding sexual behaviors and drug use among African-Americans: a case study of issues for survey research. In: Ostrow DG, Kessler RC, editors. Methodological in AIDS behavioral research. New York: Plenum Press; 1993. p. 117–32.

Galbraith J, Ricardo I, Stanton B, Black M, Feigelman S, Kaljee L. Evolution of risk behaviors over 2 years among a cohort of urban African American adolescents. Health Educ Q. 1996;23(3):383–94.

Gustafson KE, McNamara JR, Jensen JA. Informed consent: risk benefit disclosure practices of child clinicians. Psychother Private Pract. 1992;10:91–102.

Hatch J, Moss N, Saran A, Presley-Cantrell L. Community research: partnership in Black communities. Am J Prev Med. 1993;9(6 Suppl):27–31.

Israel BA, Schulz AJ, Parker EA, Becker AB. Review of community-based research: assessing partnership approaches to improve public health. Annu Rev Public Health. 1998;19:173–202.

Jaccard J, Litardo H, Wan C. Subjective culture: social psychological models of behavior. In: Adamopolis J, Kashima Y, editors. Social psychology and cultural context. Newbury Park, CA: Sage; 1999. p. 95–106.

Jensen PS, Hoagwood K, Trickett EJ. Ivory towers or earthen trenches? Community collaborations to foster real-world research. Appl Dev Sci. 1999a;3(4):206–12.

Jensen PS, Bhatara VS, Vitiello B, Hoagwood K, Keil M, Burke LB. Psychoactive medication prescribing practices for U. S. children: gaps between research and clinical practice. J Am Acad Child Adolesc Psychiatry. 1999b;38:557–65.

Kirby D, Barth RP, LeLand N, Fetro JV. Reducing the risk: impact of a new curriculum on sexual risk-taking. Fam Plann Perspect. 1991;23(6):253–63.

Koroloff NM, Elliott DJ, Koren PE, Friesen BJ. Connecting low-income families to mental health services: the role of the family associate. J Emot Behav Disord. 1994;2(4):240–6.

Kotchick BA, Armistead L, Forehand RL. Sexual risk behavior. In: Wolfe DA, Mash EJ, editors. Behavioral and emotional disorders in adolescents: nature, assessment, and treatment. New York, NY: Guilford Publications; 2006. p. 563–88.

Madison S, McKay M, Paikoff RL, Bell C. Community collaboration and basic research: necessary ingredients for the development of a family-based HIV prevention program. AIDS Educ Prev. 2000;12:281–98.

McCormick A, McKay M, Gilling G, Paikoff R. Involving families in an urban HIV preventive intervention: how community collaboration addresses barriers to participation. AIDS Educ Prev. 2000;12:299–307.

McKay M, Paikoff R, editors. Community collaborative partnerships: the foundation for HIV prevention research efforts in the United States and internationally. West Hazleton, PA: Haworth Press; 2007.

McKay M, Baptiste D, Coleman D, Madison S, Paikoff R, Scott R. Preventing HIV risk exposure in urban communities: the CHAMP Family Program. In: Pequegnat W, Szapocznik J, editors. Working with families in the era of HIV/AIDS. Thousand Oaks, CA: Sage; 2000.

McKay M, Jensen PS, The CHAMP, Board C. Collaborating with consumers, providers, systems and communities to enhance child mental health services research. In: Hoagwood K, Jensen PS, McKay M, Olin S, editors. Redefining the boundaries: creating partnerships for research to improve children's mental health. New York, NY: Oxford University Press; 2010. p. 14–39.

McLoyd VC. The impact of economic hardship on Black families and children: psychological distress, parenting, and socioemotional development. Child Dev. 1990;61:311–45.

Samuolis J, Hogue A, Dauber S, Liddle HA. Autonomy and relatedness in inner-city families of substance abusing adolescents. J Child Adolesc Subst Abuse. 2005;15(2):53–86.

Savard MC, McKay MM, Cavaleri MA, Udell W, Shvayetsky T, CHAMP Collaborative Board – New York, et al. Community involvement: key ingredients to university/community research partnerships that last over time. In press.

Singer M. Knowledge for use: anthropology and community-centered substance abuse research. Soc Sci Med. 1993;37(1):15–25.

Stevenson HC, White JJ. AIDS prevention struggles in ethnocultural neighborhoods: why research partnerships with community-based organizations can't wait. AIDS Educ Prev. 1994;6(2):126–39.

Trickett EJ. Toward a framework for redefining and resolving ethical issues in the protection of communities involved in primary prevention projects. Ethics Behav. 1998;8(4):321–37.

Wild LG, Flisher AJ, Bhana A, Lombard C. Associations among adolescent risk behaviors and self-esteem in six domains. J Child Psychol Psychiatry. 2004;45(8):1454–67.

Chapter 10
Families and HIV Medication Adherence

Jane M. Simoni, Joyce P. Yang, and Maura Porricolo

Abstract The arrival of highly active antiretroviral therapy (ART) has heralded an era in which AIDS, once a specter of imminent death, has become a serious but survivable illness to those with access to ART. However, optimal adherence to ART regimes is critical to their efficacy. Growing literature on interventions to promote adherence points to numerous effective strategies, yet few have capitalized on the potentially powerful role of family members and the influence of family context on adherence. In this chapter, we consider the literature on ART adherence among children and then adults from a family-based perspective. We examine the factors implicated in a successful adherence to treatment and the research on interventions to promote adherence. We consider the importance of including culturally relevant factors in family-based treatment and conclude with a case example exemplifying the potency of clinical care that embraces patients within their family context.

10.1 Introduction

The arrival of highly active antiretroviral therapy (ART) has heralded an era in which AIDS, once a specter of imminent death, has become a serious but survivable illness to those with access to ART (Hogg et al. 1997; Palella et al. 1998; Gallant 2000). There are currently 28 federally approved antiretroviral medications, with new ones continuing to appear on the market; pediatric formulations are available for about half (FDA 2010).

Unlike earlier medication regimens, many of which were complex, required dietary restrictions, led to severe and sometimes disfiguring side effects, and were unforgiving of less-than-perfect adherence (Paterson et al. 2000), the new medications are more tolerable and less prone to resistance (Weiser et al. 2004). For instance, Bangsberg and colleagues (2001) reported that the viral

W. Pequegnat and C.C. Bell (eds.), *Family and HIV/AIDS: Cultural and Contextual Issues in Prevention and Treatment*, DOI 10.1007/978-1-4614-0439-2_10, © Springer Science+Business Media, LLC 2012

suppression was common with a 54–100% mean adherence level to nonnucleoside reverse-transcriptase-inhibitor regimens, suggesting that with potent regimens even moderate adherence can lead to good clinical outcomes (Weiser et al. 2004). Nevertheless, adherence remains the primary driver of medication efficacy (Bangsberg et al. 2001) and has been called the Achilles' heel of these otherwise potent drugs.

The promise of renewed health on ART given optimal adherence, coupled with the dire consequences for less than optimal adherence, led to an explosion of research on medication adherence fueled with funding from the National Institutes of Health (Simoni et al. 2003). A review of the literature on "compliance" interventions across diseases in 1996 revealed only 13 that were methodologically sound, none of which led to substantial improvements in adherence (Haynes et al. 1996). By 2007, there were 19 published reports of sophisticated randomized controlled trials evaluating adherence interventions in the field of HIV alone (Simoni et al. 2006). A meta-analysis demonstrated that overall they led to improvements in adherence and viral load outcomes. Successful behavioral strategies include peer support and pager text messaging (Simoni et al. 2009); modified directly observed therapy (Pearson et al. 2007); and cognitive-behavioral, problem-solving, and motivational interviewing techniques (Safren et al. 2001).

One glaring shortcoming in the adherence literature is the dearth of interventions that capitalize on or even consider the powerful family context of the individual living with HIV. This is a major omission, as families may be integral to the success of HIV treatment, especially in the developing world, where the majority of new AIDS cases are occurring and non-familial caregivers and healthcare professionals are scarce.

Family factors may be particularly influential in pediatric HIV, as children are largely dependent and infants completely dependent upon their families for care and support. Although the role of family involvement is gaining increasing attention in the field of medical family therapy (McDaniel et al. 2004) and in preventing high-risk behavior in their children (Pequegnat and Szapocznik 2000), researchers in the area of adherence, especially among adults with HIV, have only recently begun to acknowledge the potential of familial support and to investigate ways to target, enhance, and evaluate it (Davey et al. 2009; Peterson et al. 2003; Lyon et al. 2010).

In this chapter, we consider the literature on ART adherence among children and then adults from a family-based perspective. We examine factors implicated in successful adherence to treatment and the research on interventions to promote adherence. We conclude with a discussion of a case example that exemplifies the potency of interventions that truly consider the individual living with HIV within the family context.

10.2 Framework for Understanding Family Role in Adherence

The Adherence Pyramid, which is analogous to Maslow's Hierarchy of Needs (Maslow 1943), provides a framework to address the complexity of adherence and the need for long-term sustainability (Fig. 10.1). According to the Pyramid, the

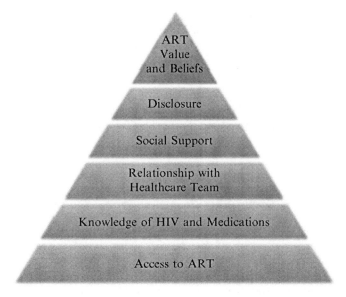

Fig. 10.1 Adherence pyramid

clinician must assure the basic foundation for adherence before addressing issues higher on up that will increase the likelihood of sustainable adherence. The family is influential at every stage.

10.3 Antiretroviral Treatment Among Children

Across the globe, from 2 to 2.5 million children are living with HIV (UNAIDS 2006, 2008). Of the 2.7 million new HIV infections worldwide in 2007, youth from the ages of 15 to 24 years accounted for half the cases (UNAIDS 2008). Also in that year, 1,000 children were born with HIV every day because of the limited access to prevention of mother-to-child transmission programs (WHO 2009). Less than half of the children born with HIV in Africa are expected to survive until their second birthday (Newell et al. 2004).

With early diagnosis and access to ART, however, chances for survival improve significantly (Leeper et al. 2010). For example, one program demonstrated a 76% reduction in mortality for children born with HIV when ART was initiated within the first 3 months of birth (Violari et al. 2008). In sub-Saharan Africa, ART has been shown to decrease hospital admissions, pneumonia, and diarrhea as well as increase probability of 1-year survival to 84–97% (Akileswaran et al. 2005).

Adherence to life-saving ART is critical in these cases. In a review of pediatric adherence in high-income countries, Simoni, Montgomery et al. (2007) reported adherence estimates of 20–100%, with 56% of studies reporting ART adherence greater than 75%. Vreeman and colleagues (2008) found that estimates of ART adherence levels in low- and middle-income countries ranged from 49 to 100%, with 76% of articles reporting greater than 75% adherence. Although initial reports of high levels of pediatric adherence in developing countries are promising, experience in the West suggests that long-term adherence may be difficult (Haberer and Mellins 2009).

10.4 Factors Associated with Adherence Among Children Living with HIV

Successful adherence among children living with HIV is determined by a constellation of inter-related factors. Initial reviews focused on factors related to the medications, the child, and the family or caregiver (Pontali 2005; Simoni, Montgomery et al. 2007). Steele and colleagues (2007) proposed a more comprehensive social ecological framework for understanding the individual, family, and societal factors contributing to adherence in children, which Haberer and Mellins (2009) extended by including cultural factors such as stigma and preferences for traditional versus Western medicine. As summarized in these comprehensive reviews, the literature on pediatric HIV adherence has identified salient factors within each of these categories.

10.4.1 Medication Regimen-Related Factors

Medication regimen-related factors that influence adherence have been addressed with new medications, although low palatability, large-volume doses, side effects, liquid formulations, as well as limited availability (i.e., stock outs), and changing doses as the children age are barriers to optimal adherence.

10.4.2 Child-Related Factors in Adherence

Child-related factors that affect adherence include psychosocial functioning and mental health, cognitive deficits, treatment fatigue, and expectations about treatment efficacy. However, much of the work in pediatric HIV adherence has been done with young children, and factors vary by the developmental stage of the child (Davey et al. 2009). Adolescence, in particular, is a developmental period characterized by marked physical, emotional, and social changes. As children age, they assume greater responsibility for making decisions about their medication regimen and adhering to it, which often leads to worse adherence (Marhefka et al. 2008). Older children are more aware of their HIV disease, which is encouraged, although awareness can lead to behavioral problems and denial. Davey and colleagues (2009) have pointed out that, in contrast to the research on individual and interpersonal factors affecting ART adherence in young children and adults, only a few studies have examined factors associated with adherence among youth with HIV – particularly the role of family support (Hosek et al. 2005; Lyon et al. 2003; Rotheram-Borus et al. 2001). One study of 231 older adolescents (aged 15–22 years) who had been infected as teens primarily through sexual behavior indicated that decreased adherence to ART regimens was related to more alcohol use, dropping out of high school, and worse outcomes (i.e., later HIV disease stage and lower CD4 count) (Murphy et al. 2005). Most of the research on pediatric HIV adherence has involved smaller sample sizes and restricted age ranges. One exception involved a US study of 2,088 perinatally infected children aged 3–18 years, conducted by the Pediatric AIDS Clinical Trials Group (Williams et al. 2006). Factors found to be associated with nonadherence in a multivariate model included older age, female gender, diagnosis of depression or anxiety, occurrence of recent stressful life events, and repeating a grade in school. Having a primary caregiver other than a biological parent, higher caregiver education, and using a buddy system for dose reminding were each associated with improved adherence. In analyses accounting for these factors, race and awareness of HIV status, medication burden, and current therapy were not related to adherence.

10.4.3 Factors Related to the Caregiver

Factors related to the caregiver are critical to pediatric adherence, especially among infants and younger children who must depend on caregivers for their medications. Their adherence to treatment, therefore, is determined by their caregiver's social, psychological, and material resources; treatment knowledge and beliefs; and efficacy. Factors associated with worse adherence in children include having caregivers who come and go, are biologically related to the child, are HIV-positive themselves, use drugs and alcohol, have a poor relationship with the child, or limit disclosure of the child's diagnosis to others.

10.5 Familial Context and ART Adherence in Children

The specific ways in which families are involved in their children's adherence to HIV medication and how they affect adherence levels have received limited attention (Williams et al. 2006). Marhefka and colleagues (2008) argued that the studies on individual characteristics of the child or caregiver, which constitute the bulk of the literature in this area, are deficient because they fail to investigate the more important influences of family processes and family member roles. They underscored the need to understand who in the family is responsible for regimen-related tasks and what are the barriers and facilitators of performing those tasks.

Relationships in organized and structured families are linked to good health outcomes in persons living with HIV, perhaps due to the routines that maintain order in families, which would otherwise be disrupted by the introduction of HIV (Rotheram-Borus et al. 2010). These factors are important across cultures. Among 409 persons living with HIV in Thailand, ART adherence was related to better family functioning, defined as cohesion, expressiveness of conflictual feelings, problem solving, and daily routines (Rotheram-Borus et al. 2010). In a domestic study of 43 caregivers, family functioning (assessed with similar subscales from a different measure than used in the aforementioned study) was not associated with adherence, although the small sample size and low reliability of the measures may have reduced the statistical power to demonstrate an effect (Naar-King et al. 2006).

10.6 Adults Living with HIV on Antiretroviral Treatment

There are approximately 30.8 million adults living with HIV worldwide; in 2009, 2.2 million adults were newly infected with HIV and 1.6 million died of AIDS (WHO 2009). Although ART is readily accessible in high-income countries (Marks et al. 2010), in low- and middle-income countries, only 5.3 million people are receiving ART of the estimated 14.6 million who need it; the gap is largest in sub-Saharan Africa and South-East Asia (WHO 2010). The benefits of ART have been astounding in the developing world, as illustrated by García de Olalla et al. (2002) with reports of the "Lazarus effect" of persons brought into clinics in wheelbarrows who were soon living lives with renewed hope and vigor.

As in the case of pediatric HIV infection, adherence to ART has been crucial to achieving optimal outcomes in adults (Bangsberg et al. 2000). One meta-analysis of data from almost 30,000 adults on ART based on self-report indicated that 77% of persons in Africa and 55% of persons in North America are achieving adequate levels of adherence (Mills et al. 2006). Maintenance of these levels in the developing world, which may be difficult to achieve (Bangsberg et al. 2006), will be crucial to continued successful treatment and prevention of new infection.

10.7 Factors Associated with ART Adherence Among Adults

Although most adults with HIV are not dependent on their caregivers to the extent that children and adolescents are, they often lead lives embedded in a family context, particularly those living in rural areas and most of the developing world.

Unfortunately, most of the early research on adults living with HIV has been based on Western samples of adults isolated from their families.

Ickovics and Meisler (1997) categorized factors associated with adherence to prescribed medication regimens across illnesses into five groups: (1) patient variables, (2) treatment regimen, (3) disease characteristics, (4) patient–provider relationship, and (5) clinical setting.

10.7.1   Patient Variables

Patient variables include socio-demographic factors (which are generally not strongly related to nonadherence) and psychosocial factors such as active alcohol or other drug use, depression or psychiatric illness, degree of social support, concerns regarding body image, and self-efficacy, which are more strongly associated with adherence.

10.7.2   Variables Related to the Treatment Regimen

Variables related to the treatment regimen include the regimen's complexity (i.e., large number of medications, frequent doses, dietary restrictions, long-term duration, and various forms of administration) as well as the number and severity of side effects. Also included in treatment regimen are patients' own perceptions of the efficacy of treatment, which may have important influences on adherence.

10.7.3   Disease Characteristics

Disease characteristics include severity of symptomatology, illness chronicity, asymptomatic periods, and lack of immediate effects of treatment on health.

10.7.4   Patient–Provider Relationship

Aspects of the patient–provider relationship include the patient's beliefs in the provider's competence; the provider's ability, knowledge, and time to implement interventions to help his or her patients; and the extent to which the patient–provider relationship is characterized by consistency, openness, friendliness, genuine interest, empathy, mutual trust, and respect.

10.7.5   Aspects of the Clinical Setting

Aspects of the clinical setting that may influence adherence include access to ongoing primary care, involvement in a dedicated adherence program, availability of transportation and child care, appeal of the clinical environment, convenience in scheduling appointments, perceived confidentiality, and satisfaction with past experiences in the health care system.

Later research has indicated that factors often associated with nonadherence to ART include the presence of adverse drug effects, neuropsychological dysfunction, psychological distress, substance use, lack of social support, low patient self-efficacy, inconvenience of treatment, and low literacy (Ammassari et al. 2002).The majority of studies examining family or social support demonstrated an association with adherence, even in multivariate analyses controlling for other factors. Although the authors were not referring specifically to family support, they reasoned that tangible and emotional support likely reduces barriers to adherence and enhances motivation.

In a review of 84 studies across the globe and almost 2,000 adults living with HIV, Mills and colleagues (2006) identified barriers and facilitators related to ART adherence grouped (according to findings in the qualitative studies they reviewed) as patient-related factors, beliefs about medication, daily schedules, and interpersonal factors/relationships. They found that in both developed and developing countries, the common barriers were fears around disclosure, substance abuse, forgetting, negative beliefs about treatment, complex regimens with high pill burden, decreased quality of life, occupational and family responsibilities, fatigue, and access to medication. In resource-poor countries, the most frequently cited barriers included restricted access to medication, often due to limited finances; interestingly, no facilitators of adherence were discussed in any study conducted in a developing country. Important facilitators noted in studies from developed countries included high self-worth, accepting one's HIV-positive status, seeing the beneficial effects of treatment, understanding the need for strict adherence, making use of reminder tools, and having a simple regimen.

10.8   Familial Context and ART Adherence in Adults

Although the studies on correlates of adherence are ignored in the literature, the specific situation and familial context of the individual adult living with HIV bear on the ability to adhere to medications. Specifically, those who are parents have unique challenges (Chaps. 4–6). Parents often have caregiving responsibilities that trump their own when it comes to taking their medication (Ickovics et al. 2002). In one study of 97 inner-city women with HIV, psychiatric problems, substance abuse, stressful life events, more household members, and parenting stress were significantly associated with both missed pills and missed medical appointments at follow-ups (Mellins et al. 2003). Disclosure, which often facilitates adherence, can involve wrenching decisions for a parent living with HIV (Müller et al. 2011). In one study of 188 HIV-positive mothers and their 267 children of minor age in New York City, only half the mothers had disclosed their HIV diagnosis to at least one of their children (Simoni et al. 2000), with usually older children being more informed than younger children. In this study, maternal disclosure was not related to ethnicity, advanced illness, improved psychological well-being, or greater or more satisfying social support resources. Moreover, when parents have children who were perinatally infected with HIV, treatment can become a reminder of the parents' guilt about their role in their child's acquisition of infection, which is another challenge to both their own and their child's adherence (Wrubel et al. 2005).

The relationship context of adults living with HIV is also critical to consider when addressing adherence (see also Chap. 7). Many individuals are living with long-term life partners who are also infected, meaning their attention may be shared between their own and their partner's treatment needs. Many adults living with HIV are in caregiving dyads, either as the recipient of or provider of care. Unfortunately, much of the caregiving research had focused on the caregiver, and most of the adherence research has focused on the experiences of the person living with HIV, ignoring the dyadic and reciprocal natures of the caregiving relationship.

In one exception, Beals et al. (2006) examined the role that middle-life and older wives and mothers play in promoting medication adherence among their husbands or adult sons living with HIV. Their conceptual model posits that caregiver characteristics can influence medication adherence, either directly or indirectly through behaviors and attitudes. Caregiver behaviors such as refilling prescription and providing reminders at dosing times may influence adherence, as well as their attitudes about adherence (concerns about treatment failure and perceptions of daily hassles). Data from their survey of 112 care-giving dyads in the U.S. indicated that the female caregivers reported strong attitudes about medication hassles as well as concerns over treatment failure and adherence. Although they often reminded the person living with HIV to take medications, these behaviors were not significantly associated with adherence. As evidence of the shared influence within the caregiving dyad, the authors report that caregivers' perceptions of adherence hassles were associated with poor adherence. Similarly, in a qualitative study of 144 adults with advanced HIV disease and their informal/familial caregivers in the Bronx, concordance of patient and caregiver perceptions of treatment was related to positive feelings about the patient's healthcare experience, supporting the importance of providers including both patients and their caregivers in treatment discussions about HAART (Sacajiu et al. 2009).

10.9 Interventions to Promote ART Adherence: Where is the Family?

The observational research on ART adherence has identified multiple potential targets for intervention, and there is a growing literature of studies that systematically evaluate intervention programs in this area. However, few consider the need to address adherence within the family context. Mary Jane Rotheram-Borus has duly noted that, "As the epidemic has unfolded, the early focus on individuals has become inadequate: families live with HIV, not just individuals…yet intervention models consistently focus on medical and psychosocial interventions for individuals" (p. 978; Rotheram-Borus et al. 2005 as cited in Davey et al. 2009). This is particularly apt with respect to field of adherence intervention research.

Several reviews of intervention research in HIV have been published, yet none has specifically examined family-focused interventions to promote ART in either pediatric or adult HIV infection. Rather, they have reviewed ART adherence interventions of any type for any target (Simoni et al. 2006; Amico et al. 2006; Sandelowski et al. 2009); home-based care interventions for individuals, adults, or children living with HIV (Young and Busgeeth 2010); family-centered HIV care programs for children living with HIV (Leeper et al. 2010); and interventions of any type to promote adherence in pediatric HIV infection (Simoni, Montgomery et al. 2007). Although the methodological rigor of the individual studies varies, with many of the pediatric studies in particular suffering from small sample sizes and lack of comparison groups, overall they indicate that a variety of intervention modalities can have a beneficial impact on ART adherence, biomarkers such as HIV-1 RNA viral load and CD4 count, and well-being among persons living with HIV.

Earlier adherence-promotion strategies targeting adults involved the provision of didactic information on HAART; discussions addressing cognitions, motivations, and expectations about taking HAART (e.g., motivational interviewing, group therapy); behavioral strategies such as cue dosing and cognitive-behavior therapy; and reminder systems such as diaries and electronic pagers (Simoni et al. 2006; Chadoir et al. 2011). Increasingly, attention has focused on directly observed therapy, contingency management, and computer-supported technologies to support individually tailored education and support (Simoni et al. 2008a, b). Although HIV-positive peers have been introduced to patients as a way of promoting adherence (Simoni, Pantalone et al. 2007; Simoni et al. 2009), only one of the studies in the recent meta-analysis involved a family component. Specifically, in an intervention study targeting serodiscordant couples, Remien et al. (2005) reported that treatment focused on improving communication, enhancing problem solving, and educating participants about the importance of adherence led to improvements in medication adherence and reductions in VL.

A more recent ART adherence study targeting adults with HIV did attempt to capitalize on family and caregiver support. Feaster and colleagues (2010) evaluated the effect of a systemic family therapy intervention called Structural Ecosystems Therapy (SET) on HIV medication adherence relative to a person-centered condition and a community control condition. Adherence data for this secondary analysis from 156 women in Miami indicated SET was significantly more likely to move women to high levels of adherence (defined as at least 95% adherence) than a person-centered therapy. Although SET also reduced family hassles, the effect of SET on adherence did not appear related to diminished family hassles.

One review examined the extent to which 88 studies evaluating antiretroviral promotion interventions incorporated targets shown in the observational literature to be linked to adherence (Sandelowski et al. 2009). The authors reported consistency between the frequent identification of family and provider support as a facilitator of adherence in the descriptive studies and social support as an intervention component or outcome variable in the trials. They noted social support was an explicit intervention component in 12 of the intervention studies and an outcome variable in 13; however, they used a very broad definition of social support, at one point suggesting that social support was an implicit component in all interventions using cognitive-behavioral or psycho-educational strategies. In fact, an examination of the components of the intervention studies they cite reveals none involved a family member.

Interventions to promote ART adherence among children are more likely to prioritize family involvement. Simoni, Montgomery et al. (2007) identified nine ART adherence interventions in pediatric populations, although most were small feasibility or pilot investigations. Four interventions involved comprehensive family components: Lyon et al. (2003), Ellis et al. (2006), Berrien et al. (2004), and New et al. (2005). Specifically, Lyon et al. (2003) had 23 HIV-positive black youths aged 15–23 years and 23 family members or other "treatment buddies" participate in a 12-week educational program. Six meetings included family members, and six meetings were with the youths only; all meetings were 2 h and included a meal. Devices such as watches, pill boxes, and calendars were introduced. Three months post-intervention, 91% self-reported improved adherence and four demonstrated immune improvement, but none showed improvements in VL. Ellis and colleagues (2006) evaluated a clinical program that used home-based multi-systemic family therapy delivered by mental health specialists, averaging 46 therapy sessions over 7 months. Among the 19 children, aged 1–16 years, who participated, caregiver-reported adherence did not change (possible due to very high reports of adherence at baseline), but chart-abstracted VLs were found to decrease significantly from referral to the end of treatment and persisted through the 3-month follow-up. In the only study employing a randomized controlled trial, Berrien and colleagues (2004) evaluated home nursing visits as a means of increasing adherence with 67 families. The home visits were designed to identify and resolve barriers to medication adherence, but the specific barrier addressed by the intervention that was reported in the paper was difficulty with pill swallowing. In the treatment group, knowledge scores significantly improved, and self-reported adherence marginally improved. Finally, Pediatric Impact was a large multisite randomized, controlled trial of an intervention to improve adherence to ART. It involved children aged 5–13 years and their primary caregivers in New York City and Washington, DC (New et al. 2005). The intervention included a dedicated adherence coordinator, an initial needs assessment, and tailored modular interventions, including home-based services. Enrolled children and their caregivers were randomly assigned to either a "minimal" or "enhanced" arm and offered an individualized combination of the following six modules: HIV education, HIV diagnosis-disclosure education to children, behavior modification, medication swallowing, medication management, and referrals to social and mental health services. Results of the intervention have not yet been published.

In a systematic review of explicitly family-centered models of care for the treatment of children living with HIV (not specifically focused on ART adherence), Leeper and colleagues (2010) identified 22 cohorts of between 43 and 657 children. Limited outcome data were available, yet excellent adherence and retention and low mortality were reported. They cited the need to target difficult-to-reach populations, identify high-risk patients at treatment initiation, and use evidence-based intervention that promote individualized care. In a Cochrane review of home-based care for children and adults living with HIV (also not specifically focusing on ART adherence), Young and Busgeeth (2010) identified 13 studies that evaluated home-based care provided by family, lay persons, or professionals and that included all forms of care as long as it was offered in the home. The home-based care evaluated included nursing, comprehensive case management by trans-professional teams, total parenteral nutrition, exercise programs, and safe water systems, with varying results. Sample sizes were small, with few studies conducted in developing countries.

10.10 Incorporating Culture into Family-Based ART Adherence Interventions

The worldwide impact of HIV suggests ART adherence interventions targeting families may need to attend to a vast array of diverse cultural influences. Specifically, within the U.S., the majority of persons living with HIV (about 65%) as well as over 85% of the 56,000 new HIV infections per year are among racial/ethnic minority populations (Centers for Disease Control and Prevention (CDC) 2008). Globally, of the 2.7 million adults and children newly infected with HIV in 2008, 70% were in sub-Saharan Africa and 10% in South and South-East Asia; in fact, only 3% of new cases occurred in the Western cultural regions of North America, Oceania, and Western and Central Europe (UNAIDS 2009).

We know from the mental health treatment literature that the inclusion of culturally competent practices in treatment, such as the incorporation of cultural values of clients or of ethnic matching between treatment providers and consumers, is associated with higher accessibility, increased likelihood of clients reporting satisfaction with interventions, and lower rates of premature termination (Sue 1998). A recent meta-analysis of mental health treatment studies comparing a culturally adapted intervention to a traditional intervention found moderate benefits of the culturally adapted treatments (average effect size $d = .45$ across 76 studies; Griner and Smith 2006).

Clinicians working with clients of color have long recognized the need to look beyond individual-focused treatment and to incorporate collectivist cultural schemas valuing relationship, interdependence, family hierarchy, obedience, resource sharing, and an overall emphasis on the role of family (Triandis 1995). Given the importance of family in the lives of ethnic minority individuals in the U.S. and most non-Western cultures, it is not surprising that family has become an important component of much therapeutic intervention and research with these populations.

There is growing research evidence to bolster clinicians' contentions that culturally informed family-based interventions are more efficacious than traditional family-based treatments. For example, a study of schizophrenic patients in Malaysia found that Culturally Modified Family Therapy was superior to Behavioral Family Therapy with respect to 1-year outcomes of medication adherence as well as family burden and overall psychosocial functioning (Razali et al. 2000). Similarly, Robbins et al. (2008) found that structural ecosystems therapy (SET) was more effective than a family process-only (FAM) intervention on drug-involved African American and Hispanic adolescents. While both approaches were based on brief strategic family therapy, SET involved intervening at ecological and culturally specific environmental levels. This line of research suggests more integrative and comprehensive family-based treatment that incorporate considerations of the family's cultural environment may be fruitful in future work on ART adherence.

10.11 Case Example of Family Issues in Adherence

Issues of disclosure, stigma, and medication adherence permeate all HIV care. These factors are also inter-related and must be considered at every encounter with a patient. Each family member's interaction with these factors must also be considered.

Adherence is not static but dynamic. Many factors affect the patient's adherence level. Some factors cause mild fluctuations and others cause a complete disruption. With new medications and once-daily regimens that may be more forgiving with regard to resistance, clinicians tend to focus on the major disruptions. Major disruptions are often stressors, which can be termed "interruptions." Examples include loss of a loved one, change in living arrangements, or acute illness. The family described above was able to overcome or minimize the interruptions and maximize their individual as well as family health.

Clinicians caring for children and adults with HIV work with limited evidence and often encounter a need for more research. As the HIV epidemic matures and the disease becomes more chronic, clinicians are gaining experience and coming to observe that greater family involvement is warranted. Traditionally, adult care is provided in the context of an individual with an acute illness – not a chronically ill person within a family context. On the other hand, pediatric health care providers automatically embed family into the care. Programs for children with special needs have paved the way for chronic illness care that incorporates family as partners (Jackson and Vessey 2000). The case example below demonstrates the success of family involvement related to adherence and illustrates the stages encountered in the Pyramid of Adherence.

The case is a 49-year-old woman with blood transfusion-related HIV infection. She lives with her HIV-negative husband and their 15-year-old daughter who has perinatally acquired HIV disease. She also has a 30-year-old daughter who is not HIV exposed or infected, with two young children, who live nearby. Her husband, and father of both children, runs the household, holding two jobs as a mechanic and janitor.

Both mother and child have good adherence rates (90%). However, the mother had refused the difficult-to-take protease inhibitors both for herself and her daughter until the latter was 13 years of age. On the basis of the available evidence, the mother was not convinced that the benefits outweighed the risks. The mother and child were on the same regimen for over 5 years.

Refusal of protease inhibitors changed when the mother was diagnosed with uterine cancer and her child's viral load was increasing and immune system was failing. Then the mother determined the benefits of protease inhibitors outweighed the risks. The mother also decided her child was ready for diagnosis disclosure. She disclosed her own IIIV status to both daughters.

The health care provider collaborated with the family to select the best regimen. The mother and child had little resistance to medications and therefore had many choices. They rearranged the medication delivery, changed the storage location (which no longer needed to be hidden), and asked for help from the father and the daughter living nearby. In a short period of time, the adherence rates were in the 90% range again, despite unpleasant side effects.

Then a crisis hit. The next year during the holidays, the father was diagnosed with HIV infection. The strain was similar to the mother's as they had had unprotected intercourse for over 10 years and thought they were safe. The father was coached by his daughter and wife on the medications, teaching him the "tricks of the trade." He was a fast learner and despite a 2-week adjustment period that was complicated by fatigue and nausea. The mother also asked the provider for help in discussing safe sex and relationships with her HIV-positive teenager. Once again the family achieved adherence rates in the 90%.

10.12   Conclusion

There are growing numbers of adults and children living with HIV worldwide. As their access to life-enhancing HIV medications increases, so will their need for support in optimizing adherence to their HIV medication regimens. Cross-sectional and other observational data point to multiple potential targets for interventions to promote adherence. Although seldom explicitly investigated, family factors often are shown to be influential in achieving optimal ART adherence.

In the case of pediatric HIV infection, family factors include caregiver psychosocial and material resources, knowledge and beliefs about the medications, and self-efficacy to support the child's adherence. The problematic use of alcohol and other drugs, non-disclosure of HIV infection, and poor relationship quality can impede adherence. There appears to be some appreciation on the part of researchers designing and evaluating interventions that family members and context must be considered, although specific research on exactly which process and attributes of family involvement matter most is lacking, as are methodologically sophisticated trials of efficacy. There is some evidence and consensus that effective support from family members should be practical and constant (Naar-King et al. 2006) and emanate from a family base that is organized and structured, with consistent routines that provide order and balance in the face of the disruptive influence of a chronic illness (Rotheram-Borus et al. 2010).

In contrast, research on ART adherence among adults mainly considers the individual living with HIV in isolation, decontextualized from family and partner. Research on barriers and facilitators of adherence largely ignores the potential impact of family structure and processes and significant others. Social support is consistently identified as being linked to adherence, but little work focuses on the persons most capable of providing ongoing, intensive, and comprehensive support, which are typically family members and partners. With the exception of one couples-based intervention (Remien et al. 2005) and one employing multisystemic family therapy (Feaster et al. 2010), there are practically no interventions for adults that capitalize on family relationship to promote adherence. Studies of home- and family-based interventions for HIV care overall may provide some direction for interventionists in this area. Future research in this area will be facilitated by the development of psychometrically sound instruments to assess and monitor family processes (Sacajiu et al. 2009; Davey et al. 2009), informational materials for family education, and clinical methods for intervention.

In sum, the field of adherence has viewed the individual living with HIV in isolation. Most persons infected with HIV are embedded in social and familial networks that must be navigated in terms of disclosure but that are important potential sources of social, emotional, and instrumental support for adherence. Only future work that considers these factors will have an impact on HIV treatment worldwide.

References

Akileswaran C, Lurie MN, Flanigan TP, Mayer KH. Lessons learned from use of highly active antiretroviral therapy in Africa. Clin Infect Dis. 2005;41(3):376–85.

Amico KR, Harman JJ, Johnson BT. Efficacy of antiretroviral therapy adherence interventions: a research synthesis of trials, 1996 to 2004. J Acquir Immune Defic Syndr. 2006;41(3):285–97.

Ammassari A, Trotta MP, Murri R, Castelli F, Narciso P, Noto P, et al. Correlates and predictors of adherence to highly active antiretroviral therapy: overview of published literature. J Acquir Immune Defic Syndr. 2002;31:S123–7.

Bangsberg DR, Hecht FM, Charlebois ED, Zolopa M, Holodniy L, Sheiner J, et al. Adherence to protease inhibitors, HIV-1 viral load, and development of drug resistance in an indigent population. AIDS. 2000;14(4):357–66.

Bangsberg DR, Perry S, Charlebois ED, Clark RA, Roberston M, Zolopa AR, et al. Non-adherence to highly active antiretroviral therapy predicts progression to AIDS. AIDS. 2001;15(9):1181–3.

Bangsberg DR, Ware N, Simoni JM. Adherence without access to antiretroviral therapy in sub-Saharan Africa? AIDS. 2006;20(1):140–1.

Beals KP, Wight RG, Aneshensel CS, Murphy DA, Miller-Martinez D. The role of family caregivers in HIV medication adherence. AIDS Care. 2006;18(6):589–96.

Berrien VM, Salazar JC, Reynolds E, McKay K. Adherence to antiretroviral therapy in HIV-infected pediatric patients improves with home-based intensive nursing intervention. AIDS Patient Care STDs. 2004;18:355–65.

Centers for Disease Control and Prevention. HIV prevalence estimates – United States 2006. MMWR Morb Mortality Wkly Rep. 2008;57:1073–6.

Chadoir SR, Fisher JD, Simoni JM. Understanding HIV/AIDS disclosure: a review and application of the disclosure processes Model. AIDS Behav. 2011;72(10):1618–29.

Davey MP, Foster J, Milton K, Duncan TM. Collaborative approaches to increasing family support for HIV positive youth. Fam Syst Health. 2009;27(1):39–52.

Ellis DA, Naar-King S, Cunningham PB, Secord E. Use of multisystemic therapy to improve antiretroviral adherence and health outcomes in HIV-infected pediatric patients: evaluation of a pilot program. AIDS Patient Care STDs. 2006;20(2):112–21.

Feaster DJ, Brincks AM, Mitrani VB, Prado G, Schwartz SJ, Szapocznik J. The efficacy of structural ecosystems therapy for HIV medication adherence with African American women. J Fam Psychol. 2010;24(1):51–9.

Gallant JE. Strategies for long-term success in the treatment of HIV infection. JAMA. 2000;283(10):1329–34.

García de Olalla P, Knobel H, Carmona A, Guelar A, López-Colomés JL, Caylà JA. Impact of adherence and highly active antiretroviral therapy on survival in HIV-infected patients. J Acquir Immune Defic Syndr. 2002;30(1):105–10.

Griner D, Smith TB. Cultural adapted mental health interventions: a meta-analytic review. Psychother Theor Res Pract Train. 2006;43(4):531–48.

Haberer J, Mellins C. Pediatric adherence to HIV antiretroviral therapy. Curr HIV/AIDS Rep. 2009;6(4):194–200.

Haynes RB, McKibbon KA, Kanani R. Systematic review of randomised trials of interventions to assist patients to follow prescriptions for medications. Lancet. 1996;348(9024):383–6.

Hogg RS, Anis A, Weber AE, O'Shaughnessy MV, Schecter MT. Triple-combination antiretroviral therapy in sub-Saharan Africa. Lancet. 1997;350(9088):1406.

Hosek SG, Harper GW, Rocco D. Predictors of medication adherence among HIV-infected youth. Psychol Health Med. 2005;10:166–79.

Ickovics JR, Meisler AW. Adherence in AIDS clinical trials: a framework for clinical research and clinical care. J Clin Epidemiol. 1997;50(4):385–91.

Ickovics JR, Wilson TE, Royce RA, Minkoff HL, Fernandez MI, Fox-Tierney R, et al. Prenatal and postpartum zidovudine adherence among pregnant women with HIV: results of a MEMS substudy from the Perinatal Guidelines Evaluation Project. J Acquir Immune Defic Syndr. 2002;30(3):311–5.

Jackson PL, Vessey J. Primary care of the child with chronic illness. 3rd ed. St Louis: Mosby; 2000.

Joint United Nations Programme on HIV/AIDS (UNAIDS). Global summary of the AIDS epidemic: December 2006. Retrieved from http://data.unaids.org/pub/EpiReport/2006/02-Global_Summary_2006_EpiUpdate_eng.pdf (2006). Cited 1 Mar 2011.

Joint United Nations Programme on HIV/AIDS (UNAIDS). Report on the global AIDS epidemic. Geneva, Switzerland: author. Retrieved from http:// www.unaids.org/en/Knowledge Centre/ HIVData/. GlobalReport/2008/2008_Global_report.asp (2008). Cited 1 Mar 2011.

Joint United Nations Programme on HIV/AIDS (UNAIDS). AIDS epidemic update December – 2009. Geneva, Switzerland: Author. Retrieved from: http:/www.unaids.org/en/dataanalysis/epi demiology/2009aidsepidemicupdate/ (2009). Cited 1 March 2011.

Leeper SC, Montague BT, Friedman JF, Flanigan TP. Lessons learned from family-centered models of treatment for children living with HIV: current approaches and future directions. J Int AIDS Soc. 2010;13 Suppl 2:S3.

Lyon ME, Trexler C, Akpan-Townsend C, Pao M, Shelden K, Fletcher J, et al. A family group approach to increasing adherence to therapy in HIV-infected youths: results of a pilot project. AIDS Patient Care STDs. 2003;17:299–308.

Lyon ME, Garvie PA, Kao E, Briggs L, He J, Malow R et al. An exploratory study of spirituality in HIV infected adolescents and their families: family centered advance care planning and medication adherence. J Adolesc Health. 2010; Advance online publication.

Marhefka SL, Koenig LJ, Allison S, Bachanas P, Bulterys M, Bettica L, et al. Family experiences with pediatric antiretroviral therapy: responsibilities, barriers, and strategies for remembering medications. AIDS Patient Care STDs. 2008;22(8):637–47.

Marks G, Gardner LI, Craw J, Crepaz N. Entry and retention in medical care among HIV-diagnosed persons: a meta-analysis. AIDS. 2010;24(17):2741–2.

Maslow AH. A theory of human motivation. Psychol Rev. 1943;50(4):370–96.

McDaniel SH, Campbell TL, Hepworth J, Lorenz A. Family-oriented primary care. 2nd ed. New York: Springer-Verlag; 2004.

Mellins CA, Kang E, Leu CS, Havens JF, Chesney MA. Longitudinal study of mental health and psychosocial predictors of medical treatment adherence in mothers living with HIV disease. AIDS Patient Care STDs. 2003;17(8):407–16.

Mills EJ, Nachega JB, Buchan I, Orbinski J, Attaran A, Singh S, et al. Adherence to antiretroviral therapy in sub-Saharan Africa and North America: a meta-analysis. JAMA. 2006;296(6): 679–90.

Müller AD, Bode S, Myer L, Stahl J, von Steinbüchel N. Predictors of adherence to antiretroviral treatment and therapeutic success among children in South Africa. AIDS Care. 2011;23(2): 129–38.

Murphy DA, Belzer M, Durako SJ, Sarr M, Wilson CM, Muenz LR. Longitudinal antiretroviral adherence among adolescents infected with human immunodeficiency virus. Arch Pediatr Adolesc Med. 2005;159(8):764–70.

Naar-King S, Arfken C, Frey M, Harris M, Secord E, Ellis D. Psychosocial factors and treatment adherence in paediatric HIV/AIDS. AIDS Care. 2006;18(6):621–8.

New MJ, Earp MJ, Dominguez KL, et al. Pediatric IMPACT: an intervention to promote adherence to antiretroviral medications in pediatric HIV. Unpublished paper presented at: the National HIV Prevention Conference, Atlanta, GA; 2005 June.

Newell ML, Coovadia H, Cortina-Boria M, Rollins N, Gaillard P, Dabis F. Mortality of infected and uninfected infants born to HIV-infected mothers in Africa: a pooled analysis. Lancet. 2004;364(9441):1236–43.

Palella FJ, Delaney KM, Moorman AC, Loveless MO, Fuhrer J, Satten GA, et al. Declining morbidity and mortality among patients with advanced human immunodeficiency virus infection. HIV Outpatient Study Investigators. N Engl J Med. 1998;338(13):853–60.

Paterson DL, Swindells S, Mohr J, Brester M, Vergis EN, Squier C, et al. Adherence to protease inhibitor therapy and outcomes in patients with HIV infection. Ann Intern Med. 2000;133(1):21–30.

Pearson CR, Micek MA, Simoni JM, Hoff PD, Matediana E, Martin DP, et al. Randomized control trial of peer-delivered, modified directly observed therapy for HAART in Mozambique. J Acquir Immune Defic Syndr. 2007;46(2):238–44.

Pequegnat W, Szapocznik J. Working with families in the era of HIV/AIDS. Thousand Oaks, CA: Sage Publications; 2000.

Peterson AM, Takiyah L, Finley R. Meta-analysis of trials of interventions to improve medication adherence. Am J Health Syst Pharm. 2003;60:657–65.

Pontali E. Facilitating adherence to highly active antiretroviral therapy in children with HIV infection: what are the issues and what can be done? Paediatr Drugs. 2005;7(3):137–49.

Razali SM, Hasanah CI, Khan UA, Subramaniam M. Psychosocial interventions for schizophrenia. J Ment Health. 2000;9(3):283–9.

Remien RH, Stirratt MJ, Dolezal C, Dognin JS, Wagner GJ, Carballo-Dieguez A, et al. Couple-focused support to improve HIV medication adherence: a randomized control trial. AIDS. 2005;19(8):807–14.

Robbins MS, Szapocznik J, Dillon FR, Turner CW, Mitrani VB, Feaster DJ. The efficacy of structural ecosystems therapy with drug-abusing/dependent African American and Hispanic American Adolescents. J Fam Psychol. 2008;22(1):51–61.

Rotheram-Borus MJ, Lee MB, Gwadz M, Draimin B. An intervention for parents with AIDS and their adolescent children. Am J Public Health. 2001;91:1294–302.

Rotheram-Borus MJ, Stein JA, Jiraphongsa C, Khumtong S, Lee SJ, Li L. Benefits of family and social relationships for Thai parents living with HIV. Prev Sci. 2010;11(3):298–307.

Sacajiu G, Raveis VH, Selwyn P. Patients and family care givers' experiences around highly active antiretroviral therapy (HAART). AIDS Care. 2009;21(12):1528–36.

Safren SA, Otto MW, Worth JL, Salomen E, Johnson W, Mayer K, et al. Two strategies to increase adherence to HIV antiretroviral medication: life-steps and medication monitoring. Behav Res Ther. 2001;39(10):1151–62.

Sandelowski M, Voils CI, Chang Y, Lee EJ. A systematic review comparing antiretroviral adherence descriptive and intervention studies conducted in the USA. AIDS Care. 2009;21(8):953–66.

Simoni JM, Davis ML, Drossman JA, Weinberg BA. Mothers with HIV/AIDS and their children: disclosure and guardianship issues. Women Health. 2000;31:39–54.

Simoni JM, Frick PA, Pantalone DW, Turner BJ. Antiretroviral adherence interventions: a review of current literature and ongoing studies. Top HIV Med. 2003;11(6):185–98.

Simoni JM, Pearson CR, Pantalone DW, Marks G, Crepaz N. Efficacy of interventions in improving highly active antiretroviral therapy adherence and HIV-1 RNA viral load. A meta-analytic review of randomized controlled trials. J Acquir Immune Defic Syndr. 2006;43 Suppl 1:S23–35.

Simoni JM, Montgomery A, Martin E, New M, Demas PA, Rana S. Adherence to antiretroviral therapy for pediatric HIV infection: a qualitative systematic review with recommendations for research and clinical management. Pediatrics. 2007;119(6):e1371–83.

Simoni JM, Pantalone DW, Plummer MD, Huang B. A randomized controlled trial of a peer support intervention targeting antiretroviral adherence and depressive symptomatology among HIV-positive men and women. Health Psychol. 2007;26:488–95.

Simoni JM, Amico RK, Pearson CR, Malow RM. Overview of adherence to antiretroviral therapies. In: Pope C, White RT, Malow R, editors. HIV/AIDS: global frontiers in prevention/intervention. New York: Taylor and Francis; 2008a. p. 191–200.

Simoni JM, Amico RK, Pearson CR, Malow RM. Strategies for promoting adherence to antiretroviral therapy: a review of the literature. Curr Infect Dis Rep. 2008b;10:515–21.

Simoni JM, Huh D, Frick PA, Pearson R, Andrasik MP, Dunbar PJ, et al. A randomized controlled trial of peer support and pager messaging to promote antiretroviral therapy adherence and clinical outcomes. J Acquir Immune Defic Syndr. 2009;52:465–73.

Steele RG, Nelson TD, Cole BP. Psychosocial functioning of children with AIDS and HIV infection: review of the literature from a socioecological framework. J Dev Behav Pediatr. 2007;28:58–69.

Sue S. In search of cultural competence in psychotherapy and counseling. Am Psychol. 1998;53:44–448.

Triandis H. Individualism and collectivism. Boulder, CO: Westview; 1995.

U.S. Food and Drug Administration – FDA. Antiretroviral drugs used in the treatment of HIV infection.Retrievedfrom:http://www.fda.gov/ForConsumers/byAudience/ForPatientAdvocates/HIVandAIDSActivities/ucm118915.htm.

Violari A, Cotton MF, Gibb DM, Babiker AG, Steyn J, Madhi SA, et al. Early antiretroviral therapy and mortality among HIV-infected infants. N Engl J Med. 2008;359(21):2233–44.

Vreeman RC, Wiehe SE, Pearce EC, Nyandiko WM. A systematic review of pediatric adherence to antiretroviral therapy in low- and middle-income countries. Pediatr Infect Dis J. 2008;27(8):686–91.

Weiser SD, Guzman D, Riley ED, Clark R, Bangsberg DR. Higher rates of viral suppression with nonnucleoside reverse transcriptase inhibitors compared to single protease inhibitors are not explained by better adherence. HIV Clin Trials. 2004;5(5):278–87.

Williams PL, Storm D, Montepiedra G, Nichols S, Kammerer B, Sirois P, et al. Predictors of adherence to antiretroviral medications in children and adolescents with HIV infection. Pediatrics. 2006;118:e1745–57.

World Health Organization. Global report: global summary of the AIDS epidemic. Retrieved from http://www.who.int/hiv/data/2009_global_summary.png (2009). Cited 2 March 2011.

World Health Organization. Table 4.1: number of adults and children (combined) receiving and needing antiretroviral therapy, and percentage coverage in low- and middle-income countries by region, December 2008 to December 2009. Retrieved from http://www.who.int/hiv/data/Table4.1_2010.png (2010). Cited 2 March 2011.

Wrubel J, Moskowitz JT, Richards TA, Prakke H, Acree M, Folkman S. Pediatric adherence: perspectives of mothers of children with HIV. Soc Sci Med. 2005;61:2423–33.

Young T, Busgeeth K. Home-based care for reducing morbidity and mortality in people infected with HIV/AIDS. Cochrane Database Syst Rev. 2010;1:CD005417.

Part III
Ethnic, Cultural, and Gender Issues in Families

Chapter 11
Family-Based HIV Prevention with African American and Hispanic Youth

Velma McBride Murry, Cady Berkel, Hilda Pantin, and Guillermo Prado

Abstract This chapter provides an overview of the HIV literature on African American and Hispanic adolescents in three areas: prevalence, etiology, and family-based preventive interventions. An extant research indicates that African American and Hispanic adolescents are at particularly high risk of engaging in HIV risky sexual behaviors. Culture and family processes play a salient role in the prevention of HIV risky sexual behaviors among both African Americans and Hispanics. Despite the elevated rates of HIV risky sexual behaviors and the importance of culture and family, there is a dearth of culturally specific family interventions designed to prevent HIV among these populations. The chapter also provides an overview of efficacious culturally specific family-based HIV preventive intervention for these populations and highlights some considerations for those interested in conducting family-based HIV prevention work with African American and Hispanic adolescents.

11.1 Prevalence of HIV Among African Americans and Hispanics

HIV infection is a serious public health concern in the United States (U.S.) and worldwide. It is estimated that there are over 1 million people living with HIV/AIDS in the U.S. alone (Centers for Disease Control and Prevention (CDC) 2006). Moreover, it is estimated that each year in the U.S. half of new sexually transmitted infections, including HIV, occur among people between the ages 15 and 24 (Weinstock et al. 2004). African Americans and Hispanics are particularly at risk, experiencing disproportionately high rates of HIV. For example, although African Americans represented 15% of the American adolescent population in 2007, they accounted for 63% of new HIV cases reported among persons aged 13–24 (Centers for Disease Control and Prevention (CDC) 2003). Similarly, although Hispanics

W. Pequegnat and C.C. Bell (eds.), *Family and HIV/AIDS: Cultural and Contextual Issues in Prevention and Treatment*, DOI 10.1007/978-1-4614-0439-2_11,
© Springer Science+Business Media, LLC 2012

represent 15% of the U.S. population, they account for 19% of people living with HIV in the U.S. Moreover, as the fourth and sixth leading cause of death among African Americans and Hispanics aged 25–34, respectively, HIV has become one of the most critical issues confronting African American and Hispanic youth today (National Center for Health Statistics 2006).

Among the most proximal risk factors for HIV infection is unprotected sexual behavior. In turn, the HIV risk from unprotected sex is potentiated by multiple partners and the use of drugs and alcohol (Santelli et al. 2000). African American and Hispanic youth have traditionally reported high rates of these risk behaviors (Centers for Disease Control and Prevention (CDC) 2007). Among adolescents surveyed in 2007, only 67.3% of African Americans and 61.5% of Hispanics reported using condoms during the last time they had sexual intercourse. Additionally, greater percentages of African American (27.6%) and Hispanic (17.3%) youth have had four or more partners than had the non-Hispanic Whites (11.5%). Finally, both Hispanic and African American youth report higher rates of lifetime drug use than do non-Hispanic White youth (Johnston et al. 2008). For example, 25.0% of Hispanic, 19.4% of Black, and 17.9% of non-Hispanic White eighth graders report using drugs in their lifetime (Johnston et al. 2002). These data underscore the importance of preventing these HIV risk behaviors among African American and Hispanic youth. To prevent these risk behaviors, it is important to identify the etiological and developmental processes that place African American and Hispanic youth at risk for engaging in HIV-related risk behaviors in adolescence and young adulthood.

11.2   Etiology of Risk and Protective Processes for HIV Risk Behaviors Among African American and Hispanic Youth

The risk and protective factors paradigm (Hawkins et al. 1992) is one of the most accepted frameworks for conceptualizing the determinants of adolescents' problematic behaviors, including HIV-related risk behaviors. Adolescents' interactions with their social contexts are important in determining whether they will engage in HIV risky sexual behaviors, including unprotected sexual behavior (see Buhi and Goodson 2007 for a review) and substance use (see Galae et al. 2004 for a review). Contemporary views of risk, such as Ecodevelopmental Theory (Szapocznik and Coatsworth 1999), take the multiple contexts influencing adolescent behavior, the interactions among these contexts, and the developmental trajectory of these contexts over time into consideration, as they influence each other and behaviors among youth. Our review of family-based HIV preventive intervention programs draws on theories explaining both risk and protective factors associated with adolescent behavior, as well as tenets of Bronfenbrenner and Morris's (1998) and Szapocznik and Coatsworth's (1999) conceptions of the ecology of development, and theories about the mechanism through which parents, identity formation, and social interactions forecast adolescent health behavior. We begin with a brief overview of the Ecodevelopmental Theory.

11.2.1 Ecodevelopmental Theory

11.2.1.1 Contexts

Ecodevelopmental Theory incorporates three integrated elements: (1) social ecological theory, (2) developmental theory, and (3) an emphasis on social interactions. The first element of ecodevelopmental theory, social ecological theory, draws from Bronfenbrenner's work on human development (Bronfenbrenner 1979, 1986). Bronfenbrenner organized the developmental factors influencing adolescents into multiple contexts according to their level of direct influence on individuals (i.e., macro-, exo-, meso-, and microsystems). Macrosystems are the broad societal factors and philosophical ideals that define a particular culture (e.g., cultural values and norms). Exosystems are the contexts that adolescents do not participate in directly, but this ecological level impacts important members of the adolescents' lives (e.g., parents' support systems). Mesosystems are comprised of interactions between important members of the different contexts in which the adolescents participate directly (e.g., parental monitoring of peer activities). Finally, microsystems are the contexts in which the adolescent participates directly (e.g., the family, peers, and school).

11.2.1.2 Developmental Theory

The second element of ecodevelopmental theory is derived from developmental theory and emphasizes systematic changes that occur among individuals across time as a function, both of their current social contexts, and the changes in social contexts that occur during individuals' entire lives. In other words, individuals and their social contexts are continually evolving and changing throughout the lifespan. For example, adolescent substance use is a risk factor of unsafe sexual behavior (Bailey et al. 1999; Boyer et al. 1999) that is influenced not only by the individuals' present social contexts, such as the amount of parental support during adolescence (Barrera and Li 1996; Oxford et al. 2001), but also by the family functioning throughout the individuals' childhood (Barnes et al. 1994).

11.2.1.3 Social Interactions

The third element of ecodevelopmental theory is social interactions such that encompass the relational patterns and direct interactions between individuals within and across the different contextual levels can increase risk and protective processes for substance use and unsafe sexual behavior (Garbarino and Abramowitz 1992; Szapocznik and Coatsworth 1999). For instance, parental support of their children can be predicted by the extent to which parents experience support from their own social contexts (Swick and Broadway 1997). Parental support of adolescents in turn affects the adolescent substance use and unsafe sexual behavior

(Miller et al. 1998; Perkins et al. 1998; Whitbeck et al. 1993). Especially important may be mesosystemic conflicts, in which Latino and African American parents have socialized their children to a specific set of values and expectations, which may differ from those values and expectations they confront in White-dominated institutions such as schools (Gonzales et al. 2004a).

11.3   Family-Based HIV Risk Reduction Programs

Family is among the most prominent contexts of ecodevelopmental theory (Perrino et al. 2002) and the most fundamental social system influencing human development (Bronfenbrenner 1979, 1986; Szapocznik and Coatsworth 1999). A substantive body of literature has demonstrated the critical role that families play in healthy development across all domains of adolescent adjustment (McAdoo 1997; Schwartz et al. 2007). Parental influence is important in Latino and African American cultures, whose traditional values emphasize the primacy of the family (Gonzales et al. 2008; Murry and Brody, 2004), making family-based prevention a relevant modality with these two groups. Studies on African American and Hispanic families have shown that the family environment serves a powerful protective role in buffering youth from engaging in high-risk behavior (e.g., through parents' caregiving practices) (Brody et al. 2001, 2002; Murry and Brody 1999). Supportive, communicative family environments reduce African American and Hispanic youths' risk of engaging in HIV risk behaviors (Murry and Brody 2002). A longitudinal study by Brody and colleagues (2000) found that African American youth who reported having conversations with their parents about sexually related issues were less influenced by their peers' actions and perceived peer norms for sexual behavior and less likely to engage in sexual risk behaviors. Among Hispanic youth, improvements in parent–adolescent communication have been found to be associated with subsequent decreases in HIV risk behaviors (Prado et al. 2007). Other family processes found to be negatively associated with HIV risk behaviors among African American and Hispanic youth include parental monitoring, family support, and racial/ethnic socialization (Murry and Brody 2002; Pantin et al. 2004; Prado et al. 2007; Murry et al. 2007). In addition, studies have shown that attachment to parents, parental monitoring, and family communication are stronger protective factors in deterring high-risk sexual behavior among African American youth than their European American youth counterparts (DiClemente et al. 2001; Miller et al. 1999; Perrino et al. 2000).

The etiological research on the role of family in the prevention of HIV risk behaviors has provided the impetus and basis for the development of family-centered preventive interventions (Pequenat and Szapocznik 2000). Family processes, including parenting practices, parent–adolescent communication, and racial/ethnic socialization, appear to be malleable targets of intervention and central in reducing adolescent sexual risk behaviors.

In the next section, we provide a brief overview of some important considerations in doing family-based HIV prevention work with both African American and Hispanic adolescents and give examples of how challenges have been met in the extant literature. In keeping with our focus on reviewing family-based HIV risk reduction programs, we target processes primarily at the microsystem level, with consideration given to other aspects of youths' environment that have implications for explaining youth's vulnerability to HIV infection.

11.4 Review of Efficacious Family-Based HIV Preventive Interventions for African American and Hispanic Youth

A search of the PsycInfo literature database using the terms "HIV or drug or alcohol or multiple partners or sex" and "prevention or preventive or intervention" and "family or parent" and "Hispanic, Latino, African American, or Black" from January 1985 through October 2008 was conducted to identify efficacious family-based HIV preventive interventions for Hispanic and African American youth. Included in this review are studies that met the following criteria: (1) randomized controlled trials (RCT), (2) adolescents aged 10–17, (3) primarily African American or Hispanic sample (i.e., 70% or greater) or reported separate results for either African Americans or Hispanics, and (4) intervention has an impact on one or more HIV risk behaviors (e.g., unprotected sex, substance use).

11.4.1 Programs for African American Adolescents

11.4.1.1 Strong African American Families

The only family-based HIV risk preventive intervention that has been efficacious in preventing alcohol use and sexual risk behaviors among rural African American adolescents is the Strong African American Families (SAAF) program (Brody et al. 2006; Murry et al. 2005, 2007). SAAF was developed via community involvement and over a decade of longitudinal research from within the same communities, thus, both the targeted outcomes and modifiable mediators originated from within the local context (Murry and Brody 2004). The SAAF program consists of 2-hour sessions that take place for seven consecutive weeks. After a meal catered by local African American providers, caregivers and children attend concurrent breakout sessions and then join together for the last hour for a large discussion. Parent sessions focus on both general (e.g., monitoring and communication with children about sex) and racially specific (e.g., racial socialization) parenting practices via videotaped vignettes and group discussions designed to foster social support. Adolescent sessions focus on topics such as dealing with difficult situations (e.g., racism), images of risk behaviors, and peer pressure resisting strategies via games and activities. Family sessions reinforce the messages from parent and adolescent session and build mutual understanding and communication.

The SAAF program was evaluated by randomizing counties in the rural South to either the SAAF condition or a minimum-control condition in which parents were mailed information about early adolescent development, stress management, and techniques to promote exercise among youth. The researchers followed up with families for 52 months and tested the mediating mechanisms of the program with Structural Equation Modeling. Findings suggest that participating in SAAF evoked increases in regulated-communicative parenting and in youth intrapersonal protective processes (racial identity, self-esteem, self-regulation, and positive self-image). SAAF-induced effects on parenting behavior deterred not only precursors to risk behavior such as risk-related attitudes, future orientation, self-regulatory capacity, and resistance efficacy, but also immediate HIV-related risk behavior, including early onset of substance use and sexual intercourse and alcohol use trajectories (Brody et al. 2004, 2005; Gerrard et al. 2007; Gibbons et al. 2007).

11.4.1.2 Parents Matter!

The Parents Matter! Program (PMP) was designed to reduce sexual risk behavior and its consequences, including HIV, other STDs, and pregnancy for African American youth by fostering communication and positive parenting skills with parents (Dittus et al. 2004). Surface structure of the program reflected the importance of cultural relevance as it was infused with African proverbs, African American actors, and media reference (Murry et al. 2004). Furthermore, because facilitators were also African American parents, they were able to adapt the program by incorporating specific examples from the community and using colloquial language. Finally, it was recognized that "Many African American parents are reluctant to participate in programs that they believe challenge their authority to raise their children according to their own personal and cultural standards" (Murry et al. 2004, p. 91). Thus, parents were encouraged to impart messages to children that reflected their personal values for their family (Long et al. 2004).

The evaluation of PMP consisted of an RCT with three conditions: enhanced intervention, single-session intervention, and a general health intervention as an attention-control condition (Ball et al. 2004). The enhanced intervention version was the full program of five 2.5-hour sessions with two annual boosters ($N=378$). The brief version offered the same content, but was delivered in 2.5 hours using lecture format, with none of the social support building discussions ($N=379$). The general health intervention was the same format as the brief version, but focused on how children could reduce their risk for preventable health problems such as obesity and cardiovascular disease ($N=366$). Findings suggested that participating in the five session enhanced intervention was associated with adolescent decreases in sexual risk behavior (Forehand et al. 2007). However, the single-session intervention was not a substantial improvement over the control condition. Authors surmised that repeated exposure to interactive intervention activities is required for reducing African American adolescents' sexual risk behavior.

11.4.1.3 CHAMP Family Program

The CHAMP Family Program was designed in close collaboration with community members, who played major roles in the program's design, implementation, and evaluation to reduce HIV risk among urban African American adolescents (McKay et al. 2004). As with other family-based interventions, CHAMP was designed as a multiple family group format. This delivery format was thought to be especially useful in increasing social support and mutual aid, creating strategies to deal with common problems, and reducing the stigma associated with talking about sensitive issues (McBride et al. 2007). Families meet for 20 minutes to discuss the topic of that night's meeting and then break out for 45-minutes concurrent parent and child sessions. In youth sessions, participants learn and role-play peer pressure scenarios and communication with parents. The parent sessions focus on monitoring, social support, problem solving, and communication with young people about sensitive topics. At the conclusion of each meeting, parents and children reconvene to make an action plan for their home practice activities.

CHAMP was evaluated with a pretest–posttest design which included a no-treatment comparison group from the CHAMP longitudinal study (McKay et al. 2004). Results from parents demonstrated a positive increase in family decision making relative to the comparison group, as did comfort in communicating about sensitive topics with their children. Among adolescents, children in the intervention group were less often exposed to mixed-gender settings without parental supervision (McBride et al. 2007). Youth in the intervention condition reported higher family conflict, perhaps because the intervention encouraged them to communicate more with their parents about sensitive topics. In addition, CHAMP has demonstrated effects on externalizing behaviors. Moreover, the CHAMP Family Program has been adapted in several other contexts, including HIV + youth (McKay et al. 2007), South Africa (Bell et al. 2008), and Trinidad and Tobago (Baptiste et al. 2007), with positive results.

11.4.1.4 Keepin' It R.E.A.L.!

The Keepin' It R.E.A.L.! Program targeted sexual risk reduction for African American adolescents (mostly sons) and their mothers (DiIorio et al. 2006). The program had two conditions, one based on social cognitive theory (SCT) and the other was a life skills program (LSK) based on problem behavior theory, which promotes the idea that the problem behaviors co-occur due to an underlying problem or condition. Both conditions met for seven sessions over 14 weeks for 2 hours each session. In the SCT condition, mothers and adolescents attended joint sessions together for four of those sessions, and were separate for the remaining three. Sessions included information about reducing HIV transmission, general communication skills, as well as specific communication about sex, values, decision making, and peer influence. In the LSK condition, mothers and adolescents attended separate sessions, except for portions of the first and last sessions where they met together. Mothers participated in a stress reduction activity at the beginning of each session. They then discussed personal experiences related to the session's topic and learned strategies based on a Freirean approach. Adolescents were given a stress reduction activity at the beginning of each meeting and then discussed a specific risk behavior. Community service activities were also part of the LSK condition, as was an overnight trip to a Historically Black College or University. Both the SCT and LSK conditions were highly interactive and home practice exercises were assigned at each meeting.

Keepin' It R.E.A.L.! was evaluated in an RCT with the two described intervention conditions (SCT: $N = 194$; LSK: $N = 187$) and a control condition ($N = 201$) that received a 1-hour training on HIV prevention. Mothers in the SCT condition increase their HIV knowledge at a rate double that of the LSK and control conditions and were more likely to report recent conversations with their children about sex. Mothers in the SCT and LSK conditions reported a greater level of intent and comfort about discussing sex with their children than in the control group. Adolescents in all conditions demonstrated significant increases in sexual behavior over time, as well as self-efficacy and outcome expectations for abstinence. SCT and control conditions increased HIV knowledge as twice the rate of LSK. Higher percentages of sexually active adolescents in the SCT and LSK conditions reported condom use and intentions to end their sexual activity until they were older.

In addition, a father and son program was developed based on the SCT approach, which was similar in format and content to the mothers' program (DiIorio et al. 2007). It was also evaluated with a randomized cluster design comparing effects of the SCT condition ($N = 141$) with a control condition focusing on nutrition and exercise ($N = 132$). Fathers in the SCT condition reported more communication and greater intent to communicate. Adolescents in the SCT condition reported less sexual behavior and more condom use for those who were sexually active. Increased condom use was a more robust finding than abstinence, despite being addressed in only one of the program sessions. Authors suggest that for African American male adolescents, condom use may be a more acceptable HIV prevention strategy than abstinence.

11.4.1.5   Parents Who Care

Parents Who Care target reductions in substance use and delinquency and delays in sexual debut among White and African American adolescents (Haggerty et al. 2007). The intervention lasts for seven 2-h sessions which include parent, child, and family components. It is based on the social development model and targets bonding to prosocial institutions, especially to the family. Parents Who Care was evaluated based on an RCT (African American, $N = 163$; White, $N = 168$) with three conditions, group-based, self-administered with telephone support (completed within 10 weeks), and a no-treatment control (Haggerty et al. 2007). African American adolescents in either the self-administered or group-based version were roughly 70% less likely to initiate sexual behavior/substance use as compared to controls. In the group-based version, they were significantly less likely to initiate sexual behavior than in either of the other two groups. Neither of these findings held for White adolescents.

11.4.1.6 ImPACT

ImPACT was designed to increase monitoring and communication between African American parents and their adolescents to reduce the risk of HIV. The program is unique in structure in that rather than being group-based, program facilitators bring the program to families' homes (Stanton et al. 2000). The single-session curriculum, guided by social-cognitive theory, consists of a 22-minute video shown to both parents and youth, followed by condom use skills practice and role playing. ImPACT has been evaluated in two RCTs. In the first, results of the intervention group were compared to a control group who received the "Goal for IT!!" intervention, which promotes education and career training using the same format as the ImPACT intervention (Stanton et al. 2000). Assessments were collected at pretest, 2 months and 6 months post-intervention ($N=237$). Participation in ImPACT increased parents' awareness of their children's participation in substance use and having a dating partner. In addition, condom use skills were higher among intervention than in control participants. A second evaluation study examined the additive benefits of ImPACT on the adolescent only program, *Focus on Kids* (FOK) (Stanton et al. 2004). Out of 817 families receiving FOK, 496 also participated in ImPACT. Significant additive benefits were found for consistent condom use and reductions in substance use among adolescents participating in FOK.

11.4.1.7 Mother/Daughter HIV Risk Reduction Program

Mother/Daughter HIV Risk Reduction (MDRR) program was designed to reduce HIV risk behavior among low income, urban African American adolescent females through mothers' involvement by increasing daughters' HIV knowledge and self-efficacy and intent to refuse sex (Dancy et al. 2006). The program was developed in collaboration with mothers in the community and was based on social cognitive theory, theory of planned behavior, and "community-other-mothers," a concept derived from Black Feminist Theory. After attending 12-week training, mothers teach the program curriculum to their daughters in groups over six weekly sessions. Mothers choose which sections of the program they are most comfortable for teaching. The program includes interactive games and skills practice approaches.

The program was evaluated using an RCT design ($N=262$) with two control conditions: the Mother/Daughter Health Promotion (MDHP) curriculum ($N=62$), which promotes healthy eating and exercise, and the Health Expert HIV Risk Reduction (HERR) curriculum ($N=97$), which is similar to MDRR, but health experts facilitate the program directly, rather than training mothers to implement it. Results from data collected 2 months post-intervention demonstrated that knowledge, self-efficacy, and reported sexual behavior in the two HIV conditions differed significantly from the general health condition, indicating that mothers were just as effective as professional health educators in teaching HIV-related content to their daughters. Because of mothers' continuing relationship with their daughters, long-term follow-up data are required to determine if maternal delivery may have more lasting effects than those obtained from professional health educators.

11.4.2 Programs for Latino Adolescents

11.4.2.1 Familias Unidas

Familias Unidas is an efficacious preventive intervention for Hispanic youth. Familias Unidas, which is based on Ecodevelopmental Theory (Pantin et al. 2004), promotes four major family processes: (1) positive parenting, (2) parent–adolescent communication, (3) parental involvement, and (4) family support (Pantin et al. 2003; Prado et al. 2007), all of which are protective against substance use and unsafe sexual behavior. Consistent with Hispanic cultural expectations, Familias Unidas places parents in positions of leadership and expertise in helping to prevent problematic outcomes in their adolescents.

Familias Unidas has been evaluated in two separate RCTs, and a third and a fourth are ongoing. In the first RCT, Pantin and colleagues (2003) found that Familias Unidas was efficacious (in a sample of 167 Hispanic youth), relative to a no-intervention control group, in (1) increasing parental involvement, parent–adolescent communication, and parental support for the adolescent; and in (2) reducing adolescent behavior problems, a risk factor for drug use and HIV risk behaviors. Results also indicated that increases in parental investment were related to decreases in behavior problems. In the second RCT, Prado and colleagues (2007) evaluated the efficacy of Familias Unidas relative to a family-centered HIV preventive intervention and a family-centered adolescent cardiovascular health intervention over a 3-year period of time. The results of the study found that over time Familias Unidas was efficacious in reducing illicit drug use relative to the cardiovascular preventive intervention. Familias Unidas was also found to be efficacious in reducing cigarette use over time, when compared with both the HIV preventive intervention and the cardiovascular preventive intervention. Finally, Familias Unidas was efficacious in reducing unprotected sexual behavior and preventing the incidence of sexually transmitted diseases. The effects of Familias Unidas on smoking and illicit drug were mediated by improvements in family functioning. Improvements in positive parenting (reward contingencies offered by parents) and in parent–adolescent communication explained some of the effects of intervention condition on cigarette and illicit drug use.

11.4.2.2 ¡Cuídate!

¡Cuídate! is a program to increase parent–child communication about sex in Mexican families (Villarruel et al. 2008). The theory of planned behavior was combined with a focus on Mexican cultural values, including familism and religiosity, in the design of the program. Familism was utilized as a motivational impetus to frame the importance of talking with children about sex. The influence of religiosity on decision making about sexual behavior was considered (e.g., whether or not to teach condom use in addition to abstinence). The 6-hour program was conducted with separate sessions for parents and adolescents on two consecutive Saturdays. The intervention group ($n=404$) was provided with information about the prevention of HIV and pregnancy as well as support for general and sexual communication with children. The control group ($n=317$) received a 6-hour general health intervention, which also emphasized the principal role of parents in determining adolescents' health, but did not discuss parent–child communication. Both groups were assigned homework to complete with their adolescents. Participants in the intervention group reported more communication, communication about sex, and comfort in communication than parents in the control group. Moreover, this effect was mediated by the perceived utility of communication about sex, attitudes of the adolescent, family, and church related to communication about sex, and parents' comfort in discussing sex with adolescents. Effects were not moderated by familism, religiosity of either gender of parents or children.

11.4.2.3 Bridges to High School/Puentes a la Secundária

Bridges to High School/Puentes a la Secundária is a family-based program intended to improve mental health and prevent dropout among Mexican American adolescents (Gonzales et al. 2004b); however, it also appears to have reduced adolescents' sexual risk taking (Germán 2009). Content and structural elements of Bridges/Puentes were based on: (1) qualitative interviews and focus groups with Mexican-origin families including Spanish- and English-speaking parents who were born in the United States (U.S.) born or Mexico, (2) key informant interviews with school personnel and service providers and (3) longitudinal research on risk and protective processes within the same communities (Dumka et al. 1998; Gonzales et al. 2007). The program's nine weekly sessions and two home visits targeted parenting, child coping, family cohesion, and school involvement (Gonzales et al. 2007).

Bridges/Puentes was evaluated via an RCT with 555 families from four middle schools in Phoenix (Gonzales et al. 2007). A recent dissertation study found that the targeted mediators of mental health and school engagement also extended to sexual risk behavior, such that intervention-induced changes in appropriate discipline reduced the likelihood of early intercourse (Germán 2009). The program's success may be attributable to the incorporation of traditional Mexican cultural values such as familism at all levels of the program (Dillman Carpentier et al. 2007). Familism values were promoted through both program content (cohesiveness, co-parenting, adolescent family support-seeking) and structure (recruiting multiple caregivers, joint sessions with parents and children) (Gonzales et al. 2007). Traditional values were used as a motivational tool to encourage parents and children to internalize and incorporate elements of the program into regular practice. For example, the program emphasized parents that families are an important source of strength to support the school success of their children. For children, it was emphasized that doing well in school helped their families in times of stress and reflected well on their families. The incorporation of traditional values resulted in salience of the program for Spanish-speaking and less acculturated families, who reported higher satisfaction and who participated more than their English-speaking and more acculturated counterparts (Dillman Carpentier et al. 2007).

11.5 Considerations in Conducting Family-Based HIV Prevention Work with Both African American and Hispanic Adolescents

On the basis of the microsystem of the Ecodevelopmental Theory, our review provides support that parenting, family processes, cultural, and strength-based approaches are the most efficacious preventive interventions for Hispanic and African American youth (Szapocznik 2006; Prado et al. 2008). Parental monitoring, parental involvement, communication self-efficacy, general communication skills, and communication about sex are parenting processes that have been targeted by programs to modify child-level mechanisms, including HIV risk behaviors (DiIorio et al. 2006, 2007; Dittus et al. 2004; Forehand et al. 2007; Haggerty et al. 2007; Klein et al. 2005). As is evident from this list of mechanisms, family-based preventive interventions serving African Americans or Hispanics have, for the most part, targeted the same types of child and parent-level mediators as those targeting White families, perhaps because the theories guiding many programs are not racially specific and may be limited in their ability to consider cultural or structural factors (Gentry et al. 2005). Although these universal parent- and child-level mediators do appear to have effects on behavior change (e.g., Forehand et al. 2007), it is also beneficial to consider program outcomes and mediators that may be specific to the populations of interest (Stanton et al. 2006) such as acculturation to the American culture for Hispanics (Gonzales et al. 2007) and racial socialization for African Americans (Murry et al. 2007). Understanding the strengths and needs of a local context is the foundation of a culturally specific family intervention (Cross et al. 1989). Consulting with community members in the early stages of program design has been advocated, as it may identify community needs and strengths that could otherwise be overlooked by researchers (Dumka et al. 1998). Because cultural groups differ in their values, they also differ in terms of what they would consider a successful program (LaFrance 2004). Preventive interventions that do not include cultural components often fail to gain community support and, as a result, the targeted populations are less likely to participate (Murry et al. 2004). Targeting problems and supporting strengths identified by the community as relevant will produce more relevant and meaningful outcomes.

11.5.1 Formative Research

Another key consideration when developing family preventive interventions is the use of focus groups to inform intervention design. For example, in preparation for the Strong African American Families (SAAF) program, an HIV family preventive intervention, and for Familias Unidas, a family preventive intervention, community representatives identified sexual risk behavior and substance use as causes for concern among local parents (Murry and Brody 2004). In addition, for the SSAF program, parents highlighted strengths that were relevant for both the "surface structure" and the "deep structure" of the program (Resnicow et al. 2000). In terms of surface structure, an emphasis on the benefits of the Black church in protecting young people resulted in a local pastor being featured as one of the narrators of the program video. The fact that teaching children to be proud of their heritage, while simultaneously acknowledging racism, was seen as another of the community's most valuable assets resulted in racial socialization becoming ingrained in the deep structure of the program, by serving a primary role in the program's theoretical model. Indeed, empirical evidence showed that racial socialization played a major role in reducing sexual risk behavior in the long-term follow-up (Murry et al. 2007). During focus groups for the development of the Familias Unidas intervention, parents highlighted the role of acculturation to the American culture as an important reason why their youth were engaging in problem behaviors. Consequently, Familias Unidas was developed to address very well-defined cultural risk and protective processes such as parent–child acculturation gaps and other acculturation stressors.

11.5.2 Underserved Populations

A third consideration when developing family-based preventive interventions is that African Americans and Hispanics have been underrepresented in family preventive intervention programs (Beadnell et al. 2003; Brown et al. 2000). The result is that not only are these populations not receiving the services afforded to others, but evaluation results do not incorporate their "lived" experiences. Programs validated based on White, middle class samples lack ecological validity and may not generalize to other groups (Rowland and Wampler 1983). To be effective in reducing disparities, culturally competent program content must be paired with recruitment, and retention strategies that ensure the disproportionately affected populations have access to the program (Dumka et al. 1995; Murry and Brody 2004).

A review of the literature suggests that partnering with local communities is also the most effective way to engage participants (Anderson et al. 2002). Community buy-in motivates and sustains program engagement (Castro et al. 2004; Ross and Williams 2002). For groups that have been historically mistreated, approval from community leaders can foster a sense of trust (Brach and Fraser 2000), a crucial part of engagement with disenfranchised groups. Some programs have employed community liaisons/facilitators extensively to serve as a bridge between researchers and participants for recruitment, maintaining up-to-date contact information, adding credibility, and serving as safe outlet for participant concerns (Armistead et al. 2004; Murry and Brody, 2004). Murry and Brody (2004) and Prado and colleagues (2006) attribute their retention rates of over 90% to support from their community liaisons and their abilities to join and engage with the participating families. At the implementation level, strategies have been developed which aim to increase participant engagement, including matching participants and facilitators on race and/or other important cultural characteristics (e.g., language), as well as fostering positive group process, and training experiences are designed to ensure that liaisons/facilitators are not only complete but culturally prepared for program delivery (Armistead et al. 2004; Forehand et al. 2007; Murry and Brody 2004).

11.6   Conclusions

This chapter has reviewed the literature on the prevalence and etiology of HIV risk behaviors in African American and Hispanic youth and efficacious family-based HIV preventive interventions for these youth. Family-based HIV prevention programs for African American and Hispanic adolescents should target both universal parent and child mediators, while simultaneously giving attention to the needs and strengths of the cultural and community contexts. Community representatives can provide vital information that should be incorporated into both the surface and deep structure of the program content. A culturally competent program, however, is necessary but not sufficient to decrease disparities in the realm of HIV prevention. For family-based interventions with demonstrated efficacy such as those reviewed here, there is a need to move from tests of efficacy to effectiveness to broad dissemination and implementation (Bell et al. 2007). In addition, strategies that incorporate community involvement and create supportive relationships must be in place to support the continued attendance and engagement of program participants, a critical precursor to achieving outcomes. Finally, although family-based interventions have potential, this approach is limited by the fact that behavior is confined and molded by context (Barrow et al. 2008; Bronfenbrenner 1979, 1986). We must begin to consider more comprehensive intervention efforts that not only increase sources of resilience for adolescents, but also reduce the stressors to which African American and Hispanic adolescents and their families are exposed (Berkel et al. 2010).

References

Anderson EA, Kohler JK, Lettiecq BL. Low-income fathers and "responsible fatherhood" programs: a qualitative investigation of participants' experiences. Fam Relat. 2002; 51(2):148–55.

Armistead LP, Clark H, Barber CN, Dorsey S, Hughley J, Favors M, et al. Participant retention in the parents matter! program: strategies and outcome. J Child Fam Stud. 2004;13(1): 67–80.

Bailey SL, Pollock NK, Martin CS, Lynch KG. Risky sexual behaviors among adolescents with alcohol use disorders. Journal of Adolescent Health. 1999;25:179–81.

Ball J, Pelton J, Forehand R, Long N, Wallace SA. Methodological overview of the parents matter! program. J Child Fam Stud. 2004;13(1):21–34.

Baptiste D, Voisin DR, Smithgall C, Martinez DDC, Henderson G. Preventing HIV/AIDS among Trinidad and Tobago teens using a family-based program: preliminary outcomes. Soc Work Ment Health. 2007;5(3–4):333–54.

Barnes GM, Farrell MP, Banerjee S. Family influences on alcohol abuse and other problem behaviors among Black and White adolescents in a general population sample. Journal of Research on Adolescence. 1994;4:183–201.

Barnes GM, Reifman AS, Farrell MP, Uhteg L, Dintcheff BA. Longitudinal effects of parenting on alcohol misuse among adolescents. Alcoholism: Clinical and Experimental Research. 1994;18:507.

Barrera MR, Li SA. The relation of family support to adolescents' psychological distress and behavior problems. In G. R. Pierce, B. R. Sarason, I. G. Sarason, G. R. Pierce, B. R. Sarason, I. G. Sarason (Eds.), Handbook of social support and the family (pp. 313–343). New York, NY US: Plenum Press. Retrieved from EBSCOhost; 1996.

Barrow RY, Berkel C, Brooks LC, Groseclose SL, Johnson DB, Valentine JA. Traditional STD prevention and control strategies: adaptation for African American communities. Sex Transm Dis. 2008;35(12):S30–9.

Beadnell B, Baker SA, Knox K, Stielstra S, Morrison DM, DeGooyer E, et al. The influence of psychosocial difficulties on women's attrition in an HIV/STD prevention programme. AIDS Care. 2003;15(6):807–20.

Bell CC, Bhana A, McKay MM, Petersen I. A commentary on the triadic theory of influence as a guide for adapting HIV prevention programs for new contexts and populations: the CHAMP-South Africa story. Soc Work Ment Health. 2007;5(3–4):241–67.

Bell CC, Bhana A, Petersen I, McKay MM, Gibbons R, Bannon W, et al. Building protective factors to offset sexually risky behaviors among black youths: a randomized control trial. J Natl Med Assoc. 2008;100(8):936–44.

Berkel C, Knight GP, Zeiders KH, Tein J-Y, Roosa MW, Gonzales NA, et al. Discrimination and adjustment for Mexican American adolescents: a prospective examination of the benefits of culturally-related values. J Res Adolesc. 2010;20(4):893–915.

Boyer CB, Tschann JM, Shafer M. Predictors of risk for sexually transmitted diseases in ninth grade urban high school students. Journal of Adolescent Research. 1999;14(4):448–65.

Brach C, Fraser I. Can cultural competency reduce racial and ethnic health disparities? A review and conceptual model. Med Care Res Rev. 2000;57 (Suppl 1):181–217.

Brody GH, Ge X, Katz J, Arias I. A longitudinal analysis of internalization of parental alcohol-use norms and adolescent alcohol use. Appl Dev Sci. 2000;4(2):71–9.

Brody GH, Ge X, Conger RD, Gibbons FX, Murry VM, Gerrard M. The influence of neighborhood disadvantage, collective socialization, and parenting on African American children's affiliation with deviant peers. Child Dev. 2001;72(4):1231–46.

Brody GH, Dorsey S, Forehand R, Armistead L. Unique and protective contributions of parenting and classroom processes to the adjustment of African American children living in single-parent families. Child Dev. 2002;73:274–86.

Brody GH, Murry V, McNair L, Chen Y, Gibbons FX, Gerrard M, Wills T. Linking Changes in Parenting to Parent-Child Relationship Quality and Youth Self-Control: The Strong African American Families program. Journal of Research on Adolescence. 2005;15(1):47–69.

Brody GH, Murry V, Gerrard M, Gibbons FX, Molgaard V, McNair L, Neubaum-Carlan E. The Strong African American Families program: Translating Research Into Prevention Programming. Child Development. 2004;75(3):900–17.

Brody GH, Murry VM, Gerrard M, Gibbons FX, McNair L, Brown AC, et al. The Strong African American Families program: prevention of youths' high-risk behavior and a test of a model of change. J Fam Psychol. 2006;20:1–11.

Bronfenbrenner U. The ecology of human development. Cambridge, MA: Harvard University Press; 1979.

Bronfenbrenner U. Ecology of the family as a context for human development: research perspectives. Dev Psychol. 1986;22(6):723–42.

Bronfenbrenner U. Morris PA. The ecology of developmental processes. In W. Damon & R. M. Lerner (Eds.), Handbook of child psychology, Vol. 1: Theoretical models of human development (5th ed., pp. 993–1023). New York: John Wiley and Sons, Inc; 1998.

Brown BA, Long HL, Gould H, Weitz T, Milliken N. A conceptual model for the recruitment of diverse women into research studies. J Womens Health Gend Based Med. 2000;9(6):625–32.

Buhi ER, Goodson P. Predictors of adolescent sexual behavior and intention: a theory-guided systematic review. The Journal of adolescent health : official publication of the Society for Adolescent Medicine. 2007;40(1):4–21.

Castro FG, Barrera M, Martinez CR. The cultural adaptation of prevention interventions: resolving tensions between fidelity and fit. Prev Sci. 2004;5(1):41–5.

Centers for Disease Control and Prevention (CDC). HIV/AIDS surveillance by race/ethnicity. 2003. Available via: http://www.cdc.gov/hiv/graphics/minority.htm. Cited 4 Mar 2011.

Centers for Disease Control and Prevention (CDC). Divisions of HIV/AIDS prevention. 2006. Available at: http://www.cdc.gov/hiv/stats.htm.

Centers for Disease Control and Prevention (CDC). Divisions of HIV/AIDS prevention. 2007. Available at: http://www.cdc.gov/hiv/stats.htm.

Cross TL, Bazron BJ, Dennis KW, Isaacs MR. Towards a culturally competent system of care: a monograph on effective services for minority children who are severely emotionally disturbed, vol I. Washington, DC: National Technical Assistance Center for Children's Mental Health, Georgetown University Child Development Center; 1989.

Dancy BL, Crittenden KS, Talashek M. Mothers' effectiveness as HIV risk reduction educators for adolescent daughters. J Health Care Poor Underserved. 2006;17(1):218–39.

DiClemente RJ, Wingood GM, Crosby RA, Cobb BK, Harrington K, Davies SL. Parent-adolescent communication and sexual risk behaviors among African American adolescent females. J Pediatr. 2001;139:407–12.

DiIorio C, Resnicow K, McCarty F, De AK, Dudley WN, Wang DT, et al. Keepin' It R.E.A.L.!: results of a mother-adolescent HIV prevention program. Nurs Res. 2006;55(1):43–51.

DiIorio C, McCarty F, Resnicow K, Lehr S, Denzmore P. REAL men: a group randomized trial of an HIV prevention intervention for adolescent boys. Am J Public Health. 2007;97(6):1084–9.

Dillman Carpentier F, Mauricio AM, Gonzales NA, Millsap RE, Meza CM, Dumka L, et al. Engaging Mexican origin families in a school-based preventive intervention. J Prim Prev. 2007;28(6):521–46.

Dittus PJ, Miller KS, Kotchick BA, Forehand R. Why parents matter! the conceptual basis for a community-based HIV prevention program for the parents of African American youth. J Child Fam Stud. 2004;13(1):5–20.

Dumka LE, Roosa MW, Michaels ML, Suh KW. Using research and theory to develop prevention programs for high risk families. Fam Relat. 1995;44(1):78–86.

Dumka LE, Gonzales NA, Wood JL, Formoso D. Using qualitative methods to develop contextually relevant measures and preventive interventions: an illustration. Am J Community Psychol. 1998;26(4):605–37.

Forehand R, Armistead L, Long N, Wyckoff SC, Kotchick BA, Whitaker D, et al. Efficacy of a parent-based sexual-risk prevention program for African American preadolescents. Arch Pediatr Adolesc Med. 2007;161(12):1123–9.

Galea S, Nandl A, Vlahov D. The social epidemiology of substance use. Epidemiol Rev 2004;26:36–52.

Garbarino JA, Abramowitz RH. The Ecology of Human Development. Pp. 11–33 in Children and Families in the Social Environment, J. Garbarino, Ed. New York, NY: Aldine de Gruyter; 1992.

Gentry QM, Elifson K, Sterk C. Aiming for more relevant HIV risk reduction: a Black Feminist perspective for enhancing HIV intervention for low-income African American women. AIDS Educ Prev. 2005;17(3):238–52.

Germán M. An experimental test of parental influences on risky sexual behaviors among Mexican-origin adolescents. Unpublished Dissertation, Arizona State University, Tempe, AZ; 2009.

Gerrard M, Gibbons FX, Brody GH, Murry V, Cleveland MJ, Wills TA. A theory-based dual-focus alcohol intervention for preadolescents: The Strong African American Families program. Psychology of Addictive Behaviors. 2006;20(2):185–95.

Gibbons FX, Reimer RA, Gerrard M, Yeh H, Houlihan AE, Cutrona C, Brody G. Rural-urban differences in substance use among African-American adolescents. The Journal of Rural Health. 2007;23(Suppl 1):22–8.

Gonzales NA, Knight GP, Birman D, Sirolli AA. Acculturation and enculturation among Latino youth. In: Maton KI, Schellenbach CJ, Leadbeater BJ, Solarz AL, editors. Investing in children, youth, families, and communities: strengths-based research and policy. Washington DC: American Psychological Association; 2004a. p. 285–302.

Gonzales NA, Dumka LE, Deardorff J, Carter SJ, McCray A. Preventing poor mental health and school dropout of Mexican American adolescents following the transition to junior high school. J Adolesc Res. 2004b;19(1):113–31.

Gonzales NA, Dumka LE, Mauricio AM, Germán M. Building bridges: Strategies to promote academic and psychological resilience for adolescents of Mexican origin. In: Lansford JE, Deater-Deckard K, Bornstein MH, editors. Immigrant families in contemporary society. New York: Guilford Press; 2007. p. 268–86.

Gonzales NA, Germán M, Kim SY, George P, Fabrett FC, Millsap R, et al. Mexican American adolescents' cultural orientation, externalizing behavior and academic engagement: the role of traditional cultural values. Am J Community Psychol. 2008;41:151–64.

Haggerty KP, Skinner ML, MacKenzie EP, Catalano RF. A randomized trial of parents who care: effects on key outcomes at 24-month follow-up. Prev Sci. 2007;8(4):249–60.

Hawkins JD, Catalano RF, Miller JY. Risk and protective factors for alcohol and other drug problems in adolescence and early adulthood: Implications for substance abuse prevention. PSYCHOLOGICAL BULLETIN. 1992;112(1):64–105.

Johnston-Briggs BD, Liu J, Carter-Pokras O, Barnet B. Effect of partner relationship on motivation to use condoms among adolescent mothers. Journal of the National Medical Association. 2008;100(8):929–35.

Klein JD, Sabaratnam P, Pazos B, Auerbach MM, Havens CG, Brach MJ. Evaluation of the parents as primary sexuality educators program. J Adolesc Health. 2005;37(3 Suppl 1):S94–9.

LaFrance J. Culturally competent evaluation in Indian country. New Directions Eval. 2004;102:39–50.

Long N, Austin B-J, Gound MM, Kelly AO, Gardner AA, Dunn R, et al. The parents matter! program interventions: content and the facilitation process. J Child Fam Stud. 2004;13(1):47–65.

McAdoo HP. Black families. Thousand Oaks, CA: Sage; 1997.

McBride CK, Baptiste D, Traube D, Paikoff RL, Madison-Boyd S, Coleman D, et al. Family-based HIV preventive intervention: child level results from the CHAMP family program. Soc Work Ment Health. 2007;5(1–2):203–20.

McKay MM, Chasse KT, Paikoff R, McKinney LD, Baptiste D, Coleman D, et al. Family-level impact of the CHAMP family program: a community collaborative effort to support urban families and reduce youth HIV risk exposure. Fam Process. 2004;43(1):79–93.

McKay M, Minott D, Block M, Miranda C, Mellins C, Petterson J, et al. Adapting a family-based HIV prevention program for HIV-infected preadolescents and their families: youth, families and health care providers coming together to address complex needs. Soc Work Ment Health. 2007;5(3–4):355–78.

Miller K, Levin ML, Whitaker DJ, Xu X. Patterns of condom use among adolescents: The impact of maternal-adolescent communication. American Journal of Public Health. 1998;88: 1542–44.

Miller KS, Forehand R, Kotchick BA. Adolescent sexual behavior in two ethnic minority samples: the role of family variables. J Marriage Fam. 1999;61:85–98.

Murry VM, Brody GH. Self-regulation and self-worth of Black children reared in economically stressed, rural, single mother-headed families: the contribution of risk and protective factors. J Fam Issues. 1999;20(4):458–84.

Murry VM, Brody GH. Racial socialization processes in single-mother families: Linking maternal racial identity, parenting, and racial socialization in rural, single-mother families with child self-worth and self-regulation. In: McAdoo HP, editor. Black children: social, educational, and parental environments. Thousand Oaks, CA: Sage; 2002. p. 97–115.

Murry VM, Brody GH. Partnering with community stakeholders: engaging rural African American families in basic research and The Strong African American Families preventive intervention program. J Marital Fam Ther. 2004;30(3):271–83.

Murry VM, Kotchick BA, Wallace S, Ketchen B, Eddings K, Heller L, et al. Race, culture, and ethnicity: implications for a community intervention. J Child Fam Stud. 2004;13(1):81–99.

Murry VM, Brody GH, McNair LD, Luo Z, Gibbons FX, Gerrard M, et al. Parental involvement promotes rural African American youths' self-pride and sexual self-concepts. J Marriage Fam. 2005;67(3):627–42.

Murry VM, Berkel C, Brody GH, Gerrard M, Gibbons FX. The Strong African American Families program: longitudinal pathways to sexual risk reduction. J Adolesc Health. 2007;41(4):333–42.

National Center for Health Statistics. Centers for Disease Control, HIV/AIDS Youth Risk Surveillance Report, 2006. *MMWR* 2006:1–131.

Oxford M, Oxford ML, Harachi TW, Catalano RF, Abbott RD. Preadolescent predicors of substance initiation: A test of both the direct and medicated effect of family social control factors on deviant peer associations and substance initiation. The American Journal of Drug and Alcohol Abuse. 2001;27:599–616.

Pantin H, Coatsworth D, Feaster DJ, Newman FL, Briones E, Prado G, Szapocznik J. Familias Unidas: The Efficacy of an Intervention to Increase Parental Investment in Hispanic Immigrant Families. Prevention Science. 2003;4:189–201.

Pantin H, Schwartz SJ, Sullivan S, Prado G, Szapocznik J. Ecodevelopmental HIV prevention programs for Hispanic adolescents. American Journal of Orthopsychiatry. 2004;74(4):545–58.

Perkins DF, Luster T, Villarruel FA, Small S. An Ecological, Risk-Factor Examination of Adolescents' Sexual Activity in Three Ethnic Groups. Journal of Marriage and the Family. 1998;60:660–73.

Perrino T, González-Soldevilla A, Pantin H, Szapocznik J. The role of families in adolescent HIV prevention: a review. Clin Child Fam Psychol Rev. 2000;3(2):81–96.

Prado G, Pantin H, Schwartz S, Lupei N, Szapocznik J. Predictors of engagement and retention in a family-centered substance abuse and HIV preventive intervention for Hispanic adolescents. Journal of Pediatric Psychology. 2006;31(9):874–90.

Prado G, Pantin H, Briones E, Schwartz S, Feaster D, Huang S, Szapocznik J. A randomized controlled trial of a family-centered intervention in preventing substance use and HIV risk behaviors in Hispanic adolescents. Journal of Consulting and Clinical Psychology. 2007; 75:914–26.

Prado G, Szapocznik J, Schwartz S, Maldonado-Molina M, Pantin H. Drug abuse prevalence, etiology, prevention, and treatment in Hispanic adolescents: A Cultural Perspective. Journal of Drug Issues. 2008;22:5–36.

Resnicow K, Soler R, Braithwaite RL, Ahluwalia JS, Butler J. Cultural sensitivity in substance use prevention. J Community Psychol. 2000;28(3):271–90.

Ross MW, Williams ML. Effective targeted and community HIV/STD prevention programs. J Sex Res. 2002;39(1):58–62.

Rowland SB, Wampler KS. Black and White mothers' preferences for parenting programs. Fam Relat. 1983;32(3):323–30.

Santelli JS, Lindberg LD, Abma J, McNeely CS, Resnick M. Adolescent sexual behavior: estimates and trends from four nationally representative surveys. Fam Plann Perspect. 2000;32:156–67.

Schwartz SJ, Pantin H, Coatsworth JD, Szapocznik J. Addressing the challenges and opportunities for today's youth: toward an integrative model and its implications for research and intervention. J Prim Prev. 2007;28(2):117–44.

Stanton B, Harris C, Cottrell L, Li X, Gibson C, Guo J, et al. Trial of an urban adolescent sexual risk-reduction intervention for rural youth: a promising but imperfect fit. J Adolesc Health. 2006;38(1):55.e25–36.

Stanton BF, Cole M, Galbraith J, Li XM, Pendleton S, Cottrel L, et al. Randomized trial of a parent intervention: parents can make a difference in long-term adolescent risk behaviors, perceptions, and knowledge. Arch Pediatr Adolesc Med. 2004;158(10):947–55.

Stanton BF, Li X, Galbraith J, Cornick G, Feigelman S, Kaljee L, et al. Parental underestimates of adolescent risk behavior: a randomized, controlled trial of a parental monitoring intervention. J Adolesc Health. 2000;26(1):18–26.

Swick KJ, Broadway F. Parental efficacy and successful parent involvement. Journal of Instructional Psychology. 1997;24(1):69–75.

Szapocznik J, Coatsworth JD. An ecodevelopmental framework for organizing the influences on drug abuse: A developmental model of risk and protection. In M.. Glantz & C. R. Hartel (Eds.), Drug abuse: Origins and interventions (pp. 331–366). Washington, DC: American Psychological Association; 1999.

Villarruel AM, Cherry CL, Cabriales EG, Ronis DL, Zhou Y. A parent-adolescent intervention to increase sexual risk communication: results of a randomized controlled trial. AIDS Educ Prev. 2008;20(5):371–83.

Weinstock H, Berman S, Cates W Jr. Sexually transmitted diseases among American youth: incidence and prevalence estimates, 2000. Perspect Sex Reprod Health. 2004;36(1):6–10.

Whitbeck LESB, Conger RD, Kao MY. The Influence of Parental Support, Depressed Affect, and Peers on the Sexual Behaviors of Adolescent Girls. Journal of Family Issues. 1993;14:261.

Chapter 12
Parents as Agents of HIV Prevention for Gay, Lesbian, and Bisexual Youth

Brian Mustanski and Joyce Hunter

Abstract Young men who have sex with men (MSM) account for the majority of HIV infections among young people in the United States and young women who have sex with women and men can also become infected with HIV. While family-based approaches have been established for other groups of youth, very few have been developed and tested with sexual minority youth. This chapter reviews evidence for the feasibility of developing family-based programs for these youth as well some of the factors that should be incorporated into such an approach.

12.1   Introduction

In the early years of HIV/AIDS, prior to the current pandemic, little was known about how the HIV virus spread, nor could we have envisioned the many challenges HIV would present on gay, lesbian, and bisexual (GLB) people. This chapter focuses on the role of families in preventing HIV among GLB youth.

The term "GLB" is used to represent the population of youth that are same-sex attracted, engage in same-sex behavior, or use GLB identity labels, while acknowledging that these are not entirely overlapping constructs in the same youth on a single occasion or across development (Savin-Williams and Ream 2007). The GLB abbreviation is used except where the data suggest a finer distinction is necessary. For example, difference between non-gay identified men who have sex with men (MSM) and gay men. It should be noted that the state of the science on HIV prevention among GLB youth is largely based on epidemiological research among young MSM, as there has been less research on family factors, prevention approaches, and risk among young women. It is also critical to note that most

W. Pequegnat and C.C. Bell (eds.), *Family and HIV/AIDS: Cultural and Contextual Issues in Prevention and Treatment*, DOI 10.1007/978-1-4614-0439-2_12,
© Springer Science+Business Media, LLC 2012

GLB adolescents and young adults are healthy (Mustanski et al. 2007), grow up to be resilient, and lead productive lives, with many having families of their own (Hunter and Baer 2007).

While rates of HIV infections continue to rise fastest among young MSM of color (Centers for Disease Control and Prevention (CDC) 2008), the virus has also spread to other segments of the population, including young women, whose sexual and drug behaviors put them at risk. While lesbians are thought to be the group least vulnerable to HIV infection, some have been infected since the early days of the epidemic. It is important to examine the risk and vulnerability of both lesbians and bisexual women, the reality of their HIV risk, and the contexts in which they are vulnerable (Hunter and Alexander 1996; Gomez 1995).

12.2 Young Men and HIV

Recent data from the National HIV/AIDS Reporting System indicated that male-to-male transmission accounts for almost 80% of HIV diagnoses among men ages 16–19 (Rangel et al. 2006). Since 2001, young MSM account for more new infections than young women across all forms of exposure. However, unlike young women whose rates are declining, and older gay men where rates are level, increases of up to 14% annually have been reported among young MSM (Hall et al. 2007; Rangel et al. 2006). The limited available prevalence data among urban, young MSM suggest an even more alarming picture. The Center for Disease Control and Prevention (CDC) 1994–1998 Young Men's Survey of Urban Young MSM ages 15–22 in seven US cities found an overall HIV prevalence of 7.2% (Valleroy et al. 2000). As in other groups, HIV/AIDS disproportionately impacts racial and ethnic minority young MSM, especially Latino/Hispanic (Loue 2006; Warren et al. 2007) and Black MSM. The data from the Young Men's Survey revealed that White young MSM (ages 15–22) had an overall HIV prevalence of 3.3%, but Black and Latino/Hispanic young MSM had much higher rates, 14.1% and 7%, respectively (Valleroy et al. 2000). There is a limited understanding of the factors that underlie racial disparities in HIV among young MSM, although some differences in risk factors have been identified (Celentano et al. 2005; Harawa et al. 2004; Mustanski et al. 2008; Sifakis et al. 2007; Warren et al. 2007).

Despite the increasing rate of HIV infection among young MSM, there has not been commensurate increase in attention to the HIV prevention needs of these youth. The majority of adolescent HIV prevention programs in the published literature are focused on heterosexual youth (Harper 2007). A recent meta-analysis of HIV behavioral interventions targeting MSM did not report a single randomized control trial (RCT) where the mean age was less than 23 years (Herbst et al. 2005), and the CDC's HIV/AIDS Prevention Research Synthesis Team stated that there is a significant gap in HIV prevention programs targeting young MSM (Lyles et al. 2007). Scientifically sound preventive interventions are needed for high-risk young men. These programs cannot be modifications of programs developed for older MSM or heterosexual adolescents. Young MSM are impacted by different cultural and contextual factors (Garofalo and Harper 2003; Harper 2007; Rosario et al. 2006).

12.3 Young Lesbian and Bisexual Women and HIV

HIV among lesbians and bisexual women is a hidden health issue. Sexual and other risk behaviors of young lesbian and bisexual women make them vulnerable, and it is important to consider prevention in the context of their families. In New York City (NYC), the Gay Men's Health Crisis (GMHC) Women's Institute serves an active client base, with 23% of GMHC's HIV-positive clients being women (GMHC served 2,698 clients in 2008). Within the Women's Institute, the Lesbian AIDS Project (LAP), founded in 1992, was created to address the HIV prevention and care needs of lesbians, bisexual women, and "women who have sex with women" (WSW), regardless of their self-identification. Specific outreach has been to women of color in NYC who have sex with women. The program currently serves 85 active female clients per year through regular services and activities, and the majority are African American, Caribbean-American, or Latina living in high HIV-prevalence areas of NYC. Other large cities in the US have similar populations (Hill 2006).

Few studies report specifically on lesbians or bisexual women who have sexual relationships with both men and women. Researchers tend to combine them in their studies (Baernstein et al. 2006).

While female-to-female sexual contact may be a less efficient route of HIV transmission when compared to male/male or male/female sexual contact, we know from experience with cases in this population that WSW do engage in high-risk HIV-related behaviors and do become infected with HIV. Some WSW use injection drugs and may share needles and some lesbians and bisexuals have had sexual histories with HIV-positive men and/or injection drug users (Gomez 1995).

There is an assumption that if a young woman is pregnant, she is heterosexual. Hunter and Alexander (1996) found that young lesbians have risk for becoming pregnant. In the US, large-scale population-based studies have been conducted in high schools, with similar findings. Four of the 52 states have included questions about sexual orientation and sexual behavior in their Adolescent Health Surveys with high school students. Results of Minnesota's Adolescent Health Survey (1987, 2005) found that lesbian and bisexual young women were twice as likely to be teen parents as their heterosexual counterparts. In Seattle high schools, results from the Teen Health Risk Behavioral Survey in 1995 found that GLB youth were two times more likely than their heterosexual peers to have been pregnant or impregnated someone (24% versus 12%). Similar results were documented in Massachusetts and Vermont (Blake et al. 2001; Saewyc 2006).

12.4 Family Influences on GLB Youth

In many ways, HIV is a family disease. Across racial/ethnic groups, the family is a key influence on youths' sexual socialization, sexual values, sex roles, sexual attitudes, and sexual behavior (Perrino et al. 2000). Looking at the numerous influences on the health and sexual risk behaviors of GLB youth, we examine the family dynamics and social contexts. Lack of family support will influence a youth's sexual identity and behavior. Often parents do not have accurate knowledge or information to help their adolescent children through the confusing process of maturation (Ryan and Hunter 2001). There are many challenges as young people enter adolescence and become sexual beings. While becoming independent of their parents, adolescents develop their self-concept, personal identity, social skills, and social support networks based on their gender, family, and cultural, racial, and ethnic reference points (Hunter et al. 2006). During this period, youth are susceptible to peer influences, putting them at risk for drug use that can lead to unsafe sexual behaviors. Parents are not always able to understand or support young people who come out as gay, lesbian, or bisexual or behave in ways that deviate from "traditional" behavioral norms (e.g., dating, dress).

Youth of color face additional stresses and challenges in integrating their sexual, cultural, racial, and ethnic identities (Tremble et al. 1989). Cultural, racial, and ethnic identities are being formed at early ages, prior to a person becoming aware of sexual feelings, including same-sex feelings. This is especially true for girls, who often appear to be more willing than boys to adapt to adult's expectations (Santrock 2008). Thus, young people who may be GLB have little support for developing their identity in healthy ways. Lesbian, gay, and bisexual youth of color interact with their family's cultural, racial, and ethnic context, mainstream society's expectations, and, if they are aware of them, GLB community norms (Hunter and Schaecher 1995). Gomez (1995) noted that this need to manage more than one stigmatized identity increases the adolescent's level of vulnerability and stress. Thus, openly identifying themselves as gay, lesbian, or bisexual may jeopardize acceptance by their family and their cultural, racial, and ethnic community. Cultural, racial, and ethnic groups may experience a social cultural dissonance (Chan 1989; Hunter and Schaecher 1995), resulting in stress generated from belonging to two different cultures. Various cultural, ethnic, and racial values and norms may conflict with European-American values and norms, and this may inhibit a person from disclosing or coming out to family members. These conflicting values can have a negative effective on one's personal potential. Thus, lesbian, gay, and bisexual youth of color confront a tricultural experience – membership in their cultural, racial, and ethnic community, the GLB communities, and the larger society (Hunter and Schaecher 1995). Further, the manner in which they manage issues of acculturation could isolate them and put them at risk for alienation from support systems.

The proper focus should not be youth's culture, race, or ethnic identity or their sexual orientation, but rather their risk behaviors (Rosario et al. 1999). Observations from the LAP Program suggest that WSW of color in NYC experience a number of environmental adversities that may drive risk and confound expectations that influence their lives. For example, in the US, many young women of color live in low socioeconomic areas of cities.

12.5   Disclosure of Sexual Orientation to Parents

Family-based HIV prevention strategies have not been extensively developed for gay and bisexual youth. This lack may be due to an assumption that parents are unaware or rejecting of their children's homosexual or bisexual orientation and, therefore, uninterested in intervention efforts (Garofalo et al. 2008). Personal narratives and small studies of gay and bisexual youth and their parents conducted in the 1980s emphasized poor communication about and parental rejection of sexual orientation, as well as verbal and physical abuse upon disclosure (D'Augelli and Hershberger 1993; Remafedi 1987; Savin-Williams 1989b).

Recent studies of GLB youth find greater openness about sexual orientation (Floyd and Bakeman 2006), more frequent and earlier disclosure of sexual orientation to parents (D'Augelli et al. 2005; Garofalo et al. 2008; Savin-Williams 2005), and more positive parental reactions (D'Augelli et al. 2005; Garofalo et al. 2008). These changes may reflect a historical trend toward increased social acceptance of non-heterosexual orientations. In a recent study of 15–19-year-old GLB youth, 66% reported that their parents were aware of their sexual orientation. Among male youth, 55% of mothers and 48% of fathers reacted positively or very positively to disclosure (D'Augelli et al. 2005). In a study of urban ethnically diverse GLB youth ages 16–24, male participants connected to both parents reported that 83% of mothers and 70% of fathers knew their sexual orientation and of those, 84% and 74% of mothers and fathers, respectively, were accepting or tolerant (Garofalo et al. 2008). Caucasian youth were more likely to have disclosed to their mother or father, and to be accepted by their father, than either African American or Latino youth. Mother's acceptance did not differ significantly by racial or ethnic group. These results confirm previous findings of differences in disclosure and parental acceptance by race and ethnicity (Dube and Savin-Williams 1999; Rosario et al. 2004) and further indicate that despite these differences, rates of disclosure/acceptance are relatively high across all groups.

Among GLB youth, disclosure to parents and parental reactions must be considered both in terms of their status and timing. Status refers to the extent to which a youth has or has not disclosed their sexual orientation. "Coming out" to others is an ongoing process that includes dropping hints, disclosing attractions, disclosing a GLB identity, and introducing parents to a same-sex significant other. Timing refers to the age at which these disclosures occur. Considering the interaction between timing and status is critical, as the effects of disclosure may vary with age. For example, coming out to parents may be more difficult at younger ages when children are financially dependent on their parents and rejection could result in being kicked out of the home. Disclosure to parents may also be more difficult during later adulthood when parents have become accustomed to considering their adult child to be heterosexual or to not discussing the subject. In fact, there may not be any "right time" to come out to parents; instead, it depends on a mixture of developmental, logistical, and relational concerns.

Most parents eventually accept their child's homosexual or bisexual orientation, but initial reactions are often negative, including disbelief, denial, silence, grief, or guilt (D'Augelli et al. 2005; Savin-Williams 2001). Initial negative parental reactions to disclosure are common and coincide with a period of increased vulnerability for risk behavior among GLB youth. These reactions reflect a predominant view of homosexuality/bisexuality as a "problem," and thus, disrupt parents' "idealized" view of their child and his/her future. Negative reactions are common among parents without access to information to counteract misconceptions of homosexuality and/or gay or bisexual individuals. When a child identifies as GLB, parents face multiple challenges: (1) adapting to their child's sexual orientation; (2) adapting their own identity as a parent of a gay or bisexual child; and (3) adapting parenting roles and expectations for a child with psychological, social, and developmental challenges. Gay and bisexual youth are vulnerable to psychological distress and increased victimization following disclosure (D'Augelli et al. 2005). In addition, parents' initial emotional turmoil may persist and result in emotional detachment and/or abdication of active parenting (Saltzburg 2004). Because youth are disclosing at earlier ages (Floyd and Bakeman 2006), many still live in the parental home and are likely to be directly impacted by parental reactions for sustained periods of time.

Among young MSM, there is evidence that parental influences are significantly related to HIV risk. In our Project Q study, 14% of the young MSM reported an HIV-positive serostatus. Controlling for age, race, and ethnicity, a composite measure of family connectedness reduced the odds of an HIV infection by 30% (Garofalo et al. 2008). LaSala (2007) found, in a sample of 35 parents of 30 gay male youth (ages 16–25), that parents of 83% of the youth regularly discuss safer sex with their sons in order to influence their behavior. Of these youth, 57% reported that their relationship with their parents influenced their decision to practice safer sex. Thus, recent trends reflecting greater disclosure of sexual orientation to parents, greater acceptance by parents, and parental influence on gay youth's sexual behavior support the feasibility and significance of family-based interventions to prevent risky sexual behavior among GLB youth.

In addition to influencing risk for HIV, there is reason to believe that family-based approaches are promising for addressing other health issues linked to HIV risk among GLB youth, such as substance use and mental health (Mustanski et al. 2011). Parental attitudes and acceptance of sexual orientation influence youth psychological well-being, which is associated with both substance abuse and sexual risk across ethnic/racial groups. Research has demonstrated that parental acceptance or rejection shapes an adolescent's views of self.

Negative attitudes toward homosexuality are related to higher religiosity, social conservatism, and lower socioeconomic status (Herek and Gonzalkez-Rivera 2006; Herek and Society for the Psychological Study of Lesbian and Gay Issues 1998). Less frequent disclosure and more frequent parental rejection of ethnic minority GLB youth may reflect more negative views of homosexuality among African Americans and Latinos (Pew Hispanic Center and Pew Forum on Religion and Public Life 2007).

Among GLB youth, positive parental attitudes and parent–child relationship satisfaction are associated with higher self-esteem and fewer depressive symptoms (Mustanski et al. 2011; Savin-Williams 1989b). One study found that GLB young adults who reported higher levels of family rejection during adolescence were 8.4 times more likely to report having attempted suicide, 5.9 times more likely to report high levels of depression, 3.4 times more likely to use illegal drugs, and 3.4 times more likely to report having engaged in unprotected sexual intercourse compared with peers from families that reported no or low levels of family rejection (Ryan et al. 2009).

The effect of parental attitudes on youth psychological well-being may be mediated by self-acceptance. Parental acceptance of sexual orientation is related to self-acceptance of one's own sexual orientation, particularly for youth who value parents as integral to their own self-worth (Savin-Williams 1989a). An affirmative sexual minority identity is related to self-esteem and psychological adjustment (Hershberger and D'Augelli 1995), regardless of ethnicity (Rosario et al. 2004). Effects of parental support may also change across development. For example, Mustanski and colleagues (2011) found an interaction between age and parental support in predicting psychological distress; the positive effects of parental support significantly decreased from age 16 to 24 (Mustanski et al. 2011). This finding suggests that late adolescence may be a critical developmental period for delivering a family-based program in order to maximize effectiveness.

12.6 Interventions for GLB Youth and Their Families

12.6.1 Feasibility of a Family-Based HIV Prevention Program for GLB Youth

Conducting family-based HIV prevention programs necessitates that parents participate in the program. Little research exists to demonstrate the feasibility of such an approach with GLB youth. LaSala (2007) was able to recruit a small sample of parents and their gay sons ($N = 30$ families) to participate in qualitative interviews about family relationships and HIV risk. In a longitudinal study of 246 GLB youth ages 16–20 at baseline (e.g., Mustanski et al. 2010; Mustanski 2011), participants were asked if they would be willing to allow investigators to contact their parents (either or both) for research-related purposes (i.e., "Do you think that you would consent for us to contact your mother/father?"). Among participants under age 18, 81% were living with parents, 83% were in contact with their mothers, and 64% with their fathers (Mustanski 2011). Of the youth in contact with each parent, 53% felt neutral to positive about the researchers contacting mothers, 41% felt neutral to positive about contacting fathers, and 66% said they would likely consent to the researchers contacting at least one parent. Frequency of unprotected vaginal or anal sex in the last 6 months did not differ significantly by willingness to involve parents in research. While these data do not indicate actual success with involving parents in a family-based prevention program, they do suggest that the many GLB youth would be willing to have their parents contacted to participate in research. These findings help dispel the concern that only those youth who are low risk would be willing to participate in such a program.

Experience also suggests that a family-based HIV prevention program would be of interest to many parents of gay and bisexual children. The authors of this chapter have given numerous presentations to groups of Parents and Friends of Lesbians and Gays (PFLAG), and parents often talk about being concerned about the HIV status of their GLBT children. Few if any of the parents report having specific HIV risk prevention training and many expressed feeling ill-equipped to address risk with their children. Parents desired an intervention to provide them with skills to address risk with their children and felt that many parents would attend such an educational program. Many parents express a sentiment along the lines of, "I am not sure all parents would want to come to a PLAG meeting, but many of the parents who told me they would not attend [a PLAG meeting] have expressed worry about HIV. These parents care about the health of their sons and would come to something like this if they thought it would help keep their sons from becoming infected." This sentiment suggests that a desire to keep their children healthy may trump some parents' negative attitudes toward homosexuality.

Because of the complexities, many community-based organizations (CBOs) that serve GLB youth reach out to parents with caution. Professionals cannot assume that young people have come out to their parents or that it would be safe to do so. In Dr. Hunter's experience as a clinician and clinical supervisor at a youth-serving CBO, it is important to first gain the trust of the young person and know enough about the youth's relationship with their family members before suggesting bringing families in. When youth want their family members involved in their process of coming out, parents are brought in on a case-by-case basis. In these situations, a family therapy approach with a strong psycho-educational emphasis is indicated to address and resolve relationship issues within the family.

12.6.2   Challenges to Delivering a Family-Based HIV Prevention Program

The lack of formative research is a barrier to developing and delivering family-based HIV prevention programs targeting the needs of GLB youth and their families. There have been few research efforts to engage these families in a systemic way and little is known about the issues that might arise in recruiting them. Research suggests that the current generation of GLB youth is coming out to their parents in their teens and that most parents are accepting. However, there are still many youth who are not out or parents who are not accepting and these parents may be most in need of the program. The second barrier to delivering an intervention is the ability to engage parents from racial and ethnic groups that tend to have more negative attitudes toward homosexuality. Young men from these groups (e.g., African Americans, Latinos) also show the highest prevalence of HIV. Research on how to most effectively engage such families in prevention programs should be made a priority. Fortunately, CBOs have been operating for decades and have developed grass-roots approaches to reaching parents and other relatives of GLB people. These CBOs could serve as key collaborators in the development and dissemination of family-based HIV prevention programs (Hunter and Baer 2007).

12.7 Conclusions and Implications

In summary, insufficient attention has been applied to develop and validate prevention programs targeting the unique needs of GLB youth and their families. As with other youth, research suggests that parents of GLB youth can serve as a strong positive influence on health risks, including HIV. Yet, family-based approaches to preventing HIV and substance use and promoting mental health have not been developed and tested. Efforts to develop such programs should be supported given their potential to address many of the health disparities experienced by young GLB youth.

In order to improve community health outcomes for this population, community norms and attitudes related to GLB youths' sexual behaviors must change. Because of the increased complexity of their lives and where the epidemic is thriving, special attention needs to be focused on young gay and bisexual men of color. To combat dynamics of racism, sexism, poverty, and fears of female sexuality, developing and implementing culturally compelling large-scale community interventions aimed at cultivating resiliency is a critical HIV prevention strategy.

Basic research on GLB youth and families is needed to inform the development of needed family-based HIV prevention programs. Our review of the literature suggests such programs are likely feasible and have great potential to address not only HIV prevention, but other related health issues that disproportionately affect these young people (i.e., mental illness, substance use). Working with families, schools (including school-based clinics that also outreach to out-of-school youth), and social services agencies would be conducive to an integrated response to preventing HIV in young people. Parents of GLB youth can be agents of change.

Acknowledgements Dr. Mustanski would like to acknowledge the support of NIMH for supporting Project Q (PI: Garofalo; R03MH070812) and the American Foundation for Suicide Prevention, William T Grant Foundation, and David Bohnett Foundation for supporting Project Q2 (PI: Mustanski). He would also like to acknowledge the collaborations of Drs. Garofalo, Donenberg, Kuhns, and his research staff in the IMPACT Program, including Erin Emerson, Steve Garcia, Louisa Bigelow, Michael Newcomb, and Katherine Samuels. Thanks to all of the youth who have participated in the research described here and for the youth services provided by Howard Brown Health Center.

Dr. Hunter would like to acknowledge the Hetrick-Martin Institute for their continuing work with LGBT youth in New York City.

References

Baernstein A, Bostwick WB, Carrick KR, Dunn PM, Goodman KW, Hughes TL, et al. Lesbian and bisexual women's public health. In: Shankle MD, editor. The handbook of lesbian, gay, bisexual, and transgender public health: a practitioner's guide to service. New York: Harrington Park Press; 2006. p. 87–109.

Blake SM, Ledsky R, Lehman T, Goodenow C, Sawyer R, Hack T. Preventing sexual risk behaviors among gay, lesbian, and bisexual adolescents: the benefits of gay-sensitive HIV instruction in schools. Am J Public Health. 2001;91(6):489–93.

Centers for Disease Control and Prevention (CDC). Trends in HIV/AIDS diagnoses among men who have sex with men – 33 states, 2001–2006. MMWR Morb Mortality Wkly Rep. 2008;57(25):681–6.

Celentano DD, Sifakis F, Hylton J, Torian LV, Guillin V, Koblin BA. Race/ethnic differences in HIV prevalence and risks among adolescent and young adult men who have sex with men. J Urban Health. 2005;82(4):610–21.

Chan CS. Issues of identity development among Asian-American lesbians and gay men. J Counsel Dev. 1989;68:16–20.

D'Augelli AR, Hershberger SL. Lesbian, gay, and bisexual youth in community settings: personal challenges and mental health problems. Am J Community Psychol. 1993;21(4): 421–48.

D'Augelli AR, Grossman AH, Starks MT. Parents' awareness of lesbian, gay, and bisexual youths' sexual orientation. J Marriage Fam. 2005;67(2):474–82.

Dube EM, Savin-Williams RC. Sexual identity development among ethnic sexual-minority male youths. Dev Psychol. 1999;35(6):1389–98.

Floyd FJ, Bakeman R. Coming-out across the life course: implications of age and historical context. Arch Sex Behav. 2006;35(3):287–96.

Garofalo R, Harper GW. Not all adolescents are the same: addressing the unique needs of gay and bisexual male youth. Adolesc Med. 2003;14(3):595–611, vi.

Garofalo R, Mustanski B, Donenberg G. Parents know and parents matter; is it time to develop family-based HIV prevention programs for young men who have sex with men? J Adolesc Health. 2008;43(2):201–4.

Gomez C. Lesbians at risk for HIV: the unresolved debate. In: Herek GM, Green B, editors. AIDS, identity, and community: the HIV epidemic and lesbians and gay men, vol. 2. Thousand Oaks, CA: Sage; 1995. p. 19–30.

Hall HI, Byers RH, Ling Q, Espinoza L. Racial/ethnic and age disparities in HIV prevalence and disease progression among men who have sex with men in the United States. Am J Public Health. 2007;97(6):1060–6.

Harawa NT, Greenland S, Bingham TA, Johnson DF, Cochran SD, Cunningham WE, et al. Associations of race/ethnicity with HIV prevalence and HIV-related behaviors among young men who have sex with men in 7 urban centers in the United States. J Acquir Immune Defic Syndr. 2004;35(5):526–36.

Harper GW. Sex isn't that simple: culture and context in HIV prevention interventions for gay and bisexual male adolescents. Am Psychol. 2007;62:806–13.

Herbst JH, Sherba RT, Crepaz N, Deluca JB, Zohrabyan L, Stall RD, et al. A meta-analytic review of HIV behavioral interventions for reducing sexual risk behavior of men who have sex with men. J Acquir Immune Defic Syndr. 2005;39(2):228–41.

Herek GM, Gonzalkez-Rivera M. Attitudes toward homosexuality among U.S. residents of Mexican descent. J Sex Res. 2006;43(2):122–35.

Herek GM, Society for the Psychological Study of Lesbian and Gay Issues. Stigma and sexual orientation: understanding prejudice against lesbians, gay men, and bisexuals. Thousand Oaks, CA: Sage Publications; 1998.

Hershberger SL, D'Augelli AR. The impact of victimization on the mental health and suicidality of lesbian, gay, and bisexual youths. Dev Psychol. 1995;31(1):65–74.

Hill M. Lesbian AIDS project, GMHC. Interview. New York: GMHC; 2006.

Hunter J, Alexander P. Women who sleep with women. In: Ankrah M, Long LD, editors. Women's experiences with HIV/AIDS: an international perspective. New York: Columbia University Press; 1996. p. 43–55.

Hunter J, Baer J. HIV prevention and care for gay, lesbian, bisexual and transgender youths: "best practices" from existing programs and policies. In: Meyer IH, Northridge ME, editors. The health of sexual minorities: public health perspectives on lesbian, gay, bisexual and transgender populations. New York: Springer; 2007. p. 653–92.

Hunter J, Schaecher R. Gay and lesbian adolescents, Encyclopedia of social work, vol. 19. Washington, DC: NASW Press; 1995.

Hunter J, Cohall A, Mallon G, Moyer MB, Riddel J. Health Care Delivery and Public Health Related to GLBT Youth and Young Adults. In: Shankle MD, Mallon D, editors. The handbook of lesbian, gay, bisexual and transgender public health: a practitioner's guide to services. New York: Routledge; 2006. p. 221–45.

LaSala MC. Parental influence, gay youths, and safer sex. Health Soc Work. 2007;32(1):49–55.

Loue S. Preventing HIV, eliminating disparities among Hispanics in the United States. J Immigr Minor Health. 2006;8(4):313–8.

Lyles CM, Kay LS, Crepaz N, Herbst JH, Passin WF, Kim AS, et al. Best evidence interventions: findings from a systematic review of HIV behavioral interventions for US populations at high risk, 2000–2004. Am J Public Health. 2007;97(1):133–43.

Minnesota Department of Health (1987. 2005 Report on Minnesota adolescents: STD, HIV, and pregnancy. Minneapolis: Minnesota Department of Health; 2005.

Mustanski B. Ethical and regulatory issues with conducting sexuality research with LGBT adolescents: a call to action for a scientifically informed approach. Arch Sex Behav. 2011;40(1):189–99.

Mustanski B, Garofalo R, Herrick A, Donenberg G. Psychosocial health problems increase risk for HIV among urban young men who have sex with men: preliminary evidence of a syndemic in need of attention. Ann Behav Med. 2007;34(1):37–45.

Mustanski B, Stauffer A, Garofalo R. At the intersection of HIV/AIDS disparities: young African American men who have sex with men. In: Johnson W, editor. The social work and social justice response to the African American male. Oxford, UK: Oxford Press; 2008.

Mustanski BS, Garofalo R, Emerson EM. Mental health disorders, psychological distress, and suicidality in a diverse sample of lesbian, gay, bisexual, and transgender youths. Am J Public Health. 2010;100(12):2426–32.

Mustanski B, Newcomb M, Garofalo R. Mental health of lesbian, gay, and bisexual youth: a developmental resiliency perspective. J Gay Lesbian Soc Serv. 2011;23(2):204–25.

Perrino T, Gonzalez-Soldevilla A, Pantin H, Szapocznik J. The role of families in adolescent HIV prevention: a review. Clin Child Fam Psychol Rev. 2000;3(2):81–96.

Pew Hispanic Center, and Pew Forum on Religion and Public Life. Changing faiths: Latinos and the transformation of American religion. Washington, DC: Pew Research Center; 2007.

Rangel MC, Gavin L, Reed C, Fowler MG, Lee LM. Epidemiology of HIV and AIDS among adolescents and young adults in the United States. J Adolesc Health. 2006;39(2):156–63.

Remafedi G. Adolescent homosexuality: psychosocial and medical implications. Pediatrics. 1987;79(3):331–7.

Rosario M, Mahler K, Hunter J, Gwadz M. Understanding the unprotected sexual behaviors of gay, lesbian, and bisexual youths: an empirical test of the cognitive environmental model. Health Psychol. 1999;18(3):272–80.

Rosario M, Schrimshaw EW, Hunter J. Ethnic/racial differences in the coming out process of lesbian, gay, and bisexual youths: a comparison of sexual identity development over time. Cultur Divers Ethnic Minor Psychol. 2004;10(3):215–28.

Rosario M, Schrimshaw EW, Hunter J. A model of sexual risk behaviors among young gay and bisexual men: longitudinal associations of mental health, substance abuse, sexual abuse, and the coming-out process. Aids Educ Prev. 2006;18(5):444–60.

Ryan C, Hunter J. Clinical issues with youth. In: A provider's guide to substance abuse treatment for lesbian, gay, bisexual, and transgender individuals. Washington, DC: Center for Substance Abuse Treatment/SAMHSA (CSAT); 2001. p. 99–103.

Ryan C, Huebner D, Diaz RM, Sanchez J. Family rejection as a predictor of negative health outcomes in white and Latino lesbian, gay, and bisexual young adults. Pediatrics. 2009;123(1):346–52.

Saewyc E. Pregnancy among lesbian, gay, and bisexual adolescents: influences of stigma, sexual abuse and sexual orientation. In: Omoto AM, Kurtzman HS, editors. Sexual orientation and mental health: examining identity and development in lesbian, gay, and bisexual people, Contemporary perspectives on lesbian, gay, and bisexual psychology, xi. Washington, DC: American Psychological Association; 2006 (p. 95–116). 323 pp. doi: 10.1037/11261-005.

Saltzburg S. Learning that an adolescent child is gay or lesbian: the parent experience. Soc Work. 2004;49(1):109–18.

Santrock JW. Adolescence. 12th ed. New York: McGraw-Hill; 2008. p. 287–9.

Savin-Williams RC. Coming out to parents and self-esteem among gay and lesbian youths. J Homosex. 1989a;18(1–2):1–35.

Savin-Williams RC. Parental influences on the self-esteem of gay and lesbian youths: a reflected appraisals model. J Homosex. 1989b;17(1–2):93–109.

Savin-Williams RC. Mom, dad, I'm gay: how families negotiate coming out. 1st ed. Washington, DC: American Psychological Association; 2001.

Savin-Williams RC. The new gay teenager. Cambridge, MA: Harvard University Press; 2005.

Savin-Williams RC, Ream GL. Prevalence and stability of sexual orientation components during adolescence and young adulthood. Arch Sex Behav. 2007;36(3):385–94.

Sifakis F, Hylton JB, Flynn C, Solomon L, Mackellar DA, Valleroy LA, et al. Racial disparities in HIV incidence among young men who have sex with men: the Baltimore Young Men's Survey. J Acquir Immune Defic Syndr. 2007;46(3):343–8.

Tremble B, Schneider M, Appathurai C. Growing up gay or lesbian in a multicultural context. J Homosex. 1989;17(3–4):253–67.

Valleroy LA, MacKellar DA, Karon JM. HIV prevalence and associated risks in young men who have sex with men: Young Men's Survey Study Group. JAMA. 2000;284:198–204.

Warren JC, Fernandez MI, Harper GW, Hidalgo MA, Jamil OB, Torres RS. Predictors of unprotected sex among young sexually active African American, Hispanic, and White MSM: the importance of ethnicity and culture. AIDS Behav. 2007;12(3):459–68.

Chapter 13
Family-Based HIV-Prevention for Adolescents with Psychiatric Disorders

Geri R. Donenberg, Larry Brown, Wendy Hadley, Chisina Kapungu, Celia Lescano, and Ralph DiClemente

Abstract Family factors are influential in both HIV/AIDS-risk behavior and mental illness, and thus, families can be a critical resource in HIV/AIDS prevention efforts, especially for young people with psychiatric problems. Surprisingly few HIV-risk reduction programs capitalize on the strengths of families to prevent risk behavior while simultaneously addressing mental health. This chapter reviews current research on the association of mental health, HIV/AIDS-risk behavior, and behavioral interventions with special emphasis on the role of families in improving health outcomes for young people. Given the paucity of available empirically validated family-based interventions, we describe an innovative and highly promising program for teens with in mental health treatment based on the Social-Personal Framework of HIV/AIDS-risking mental health issues.

13.1 Linkages Between Mental Health and HIV/AIDS

Mental health has many important linkages with HIV/AIDS (Brown et al. 1997a, 2010; Donenberg et al. 2001; Donenberg and Pao 2005; Treisman and Angelino 2004; Tubman et al. 2003). Mental illness is related to high rates of risky sexual behavior and drug use (Donenberg and Pao 2005), poor health promotion, inconsistent and untimely medication adherence, and limited and less-sustained effects of behavioral interventions (Cournos et al. 2005; Mehta et al. 1997; Wagner et al. 2004). Untreated mental health problems diminish safe sex decision making and are barriers to HIV prevention (Brooks-Gunn and Paikoff 1997; Donenberg and Pao 2005). Although improved mental health augments physical health, HIV/AIDS behavioral interventions have been inconsistent and lagged behind when it comes to addressing mental health issues.

W. Pequegnat and C.C. Bell (eds.), *Family and HIV/AIDS: Cultural and Contextual Issues in Prevention and Treatment*, DOI 10.1007/978-1-4614-0439-2_13,
© Springer Science+Business Media, LLC 2012

Family factors are influential in both HIV/AIDS-risk behavior and mental illness, and thus, families can be a critical resource in HIV/AIDS prevention efforts (Donenberg et al. 2006), especially for young people with psychiatric problems. Surprisingly few HIV-risk reduction programs capitalize on the strengths of families to prevent risk behavior while simultaneously addressing mental health. This chapter reviews current research on the association of mental health, HIV/AIDS-risk behavior, and behavioral interventions with special emphasis on the role of families in improving health outcomes for young people. Given the paucity of available empirically validated family-based interventions, we describe an innovative and highly promising program for teens with in mental health treatment based on the Social-Personal Framework of HIV/AIDS-risk (Donenberg and Pao 2005).

The mechanisms linking mental health and HIV/AIDS are diverse and multi-level, and they reflect a complex mix of social, psychological, economic, structural, and interpersonal relationship influences. Still, most health behavior change theories (e.g., Theory of Reasoned Action, Health-Belief Model; Fishbein 1980) implicate individual factors (Donenberg and Pao 2005) and emphasize person-level behavior change. These models often require a level of intellectual maturity and stability that are undeveloped in many youth, especially teens with mental health problems. For example, teen sexual behavior is frequently unplanned, spontaneous, and not the result of careful decision making (Fantasia 2008; Kirby et al. 1994), particularly for troubled youth who tend to be impulsive and self-destructive (Brown et al. 1997b; Frances et al. 1985). Many youth in psychiatric care do not understand how to avoid risky situations and lack important skills to promote healthy behavior (e.g., sexual communication skills, assertiveness, refusal skills) (Donenberg and Pao 2005; Henggeler et al. 1992; Kipke et al. 1998). Teens in psychiatric care engage in the same risky behaviors as their peers, but they do so at higher rates (Donenberg and Pao 2005); they use condoms less consistently, have more sexual partners, and report more frequent sexual activity.

13.2 Framework for Developing Preventions for Troubled Adolescents and Their Families

The Social-Personal Framework (Donenberg and Pao 2005) provides an alternative approach to understanding risk taking that underscores the importance of individual, psychosocial, and contextual risk mechanisms, while also addressing the role of cognitive factors typically included in health behavior theories (e.g., HIV/AIDS knowledge, attitudes, beliefs). The Social-Personal Framework has been used to guide multiple HIV-prevention studies as well as the development of several innovative HIV/AIDS prevention interventions for youth in mental health care (see below). The framework emphasizes personal attributes, family context, and peer and partner relationships as predictors of adolescent risk taking (see Fig. 13.1). For a full description of the framework, please see Donenberg and Pao (2005).

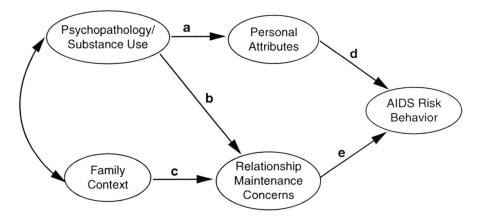

Fig. 13.1 Social-personal theoretical framework (adapted from Donenberg and Pao 2005)

13.2.1   Personal Attributes

Increasing accurate information about HIV/AIDS transmission and prevention, enhancing perceptions of personal vulnerability, and improving self-efficacy for safer sex behavior are important HIV/AIDS prevention goals. Unfortunately, improving HIV/AIDS knowledge is necessary but insufficient to stem high-risk behavior (Aruffo et al. 1994; DiClemente et al. 1993; DiClemente et al. 1996b; Donenberg et al. 2005; Hingson et al. 1990a; Keller et al. 1988; Mustanski et al. 2006; Rolf et al. 1991; Sikand et al. 1996). Greater perception of vulnerability, motivation to prevent transmission, intention to practice safe sex, and condom use self-efficacy are needed to increase safer sex among youth and adults (Donenberg and Pao 2005; Fisher and Fisher 1995; Santelli et al. 2004; Sterk et al. 2004; St. Lawrence et al. 1998).

Impulsivity, impaired problem solving, poor negotiation skills, and limited social and self-efficacy skills are factors common in troubled teens that hamper their ability to use accurate knowledge and good intentions to implement safe sex behavior (Brown et al. 1997b; Carey et al. 1997; Di Scipio 1994; Donenberg and Pao 2005; Mustanski et al. 2006). Many teens with psychiatric problems lack the self-confidence and interpersonal and social skills (assertiveness, effective communication) necessary to negotiate safe sex practices (Brown et al. 1997a; Carey et al. 1997). Similarly, good emotion regulation in the face of distress (e.g., managing one's fear of potential rejection by a partner because of asking to use a condom) (Lescano et al. 2007) may help reduce risk behaviors (DiClemente et al. 2001a), but many youths in psychiatric care exhibit poor affect regulation. Emotion dysregulation has been tied to multiple problem behaviors, e.g., suicide attempts, depression, substance use, negative family interactions, and HIV/AIDS risk (DiClemente et al. 2001a, b; Fritsch et al. 2000; MacLean et al. 2000; Sheeber et al. 2000, 2001). Fortunately, HIV attitudes, beliefs, and skills are amenable to intervention, and emotion regulation can be influenced through learning and modeling, especially in a therapeutic context (Cicchetti et al. 1995).

13.2.2 Family Context

Parents and families play a major role in adolescents' sexual values, attitudes, and behavior (Crosby and Miller 2002; Perrino et al. 2000). The family is the primary source of sexual socialization for children (Fisher and Feldman 1998; Perrino et al. 2000). Parental influence may be indirect, facilitating or hindering teens' acquisition of HIV/AIDS knowledge, attitudes, and prevention skills, or direct through communication and modeling about risk, sex, and prevention (Donenberg et al. 2011; Kotchick et al. 2001; Miller et al. 2000; Repetti et al. 2002; Somers and Paulson 2000). Four areas of family functioning are consistently related to youths' sexual risk taking and attitudes: affective characteristics (warmth, support, hostility), instrumental characteristics (monitoring, supervision, control), parent–adolescent communication, and parental attitudes and behavior.

13.2.2.1 Affective Characteristics of Families

Affective characteristics (warmth, support, hostility) play a critical role in youths' intimate relationships (Chodorow 1974, 1978; Stevens 2002; Surrey 1983) and sexual experience (Miller and Fox 1987; Miller et al. 2001; Donenberg et al. 2003). Close family relationships, parental involvement, positive parenting, and parental support predict more consistent condom use, less exposure to risky situations, and later sexual debut among teens (Aronowitz et al. 2005; Chewning and Van Koningsveld 1998; Danziger 1995; Donenberg et al. 2011; Hindelang et al. 2001; Jaccard et al. 1998; Jones and Philliber 1983; Longmore et al. 2001; Meschke et al. 2002; Moore and Chase-Lansdale 2001; O'Donnell et al. 2008; Resnick et al. 1997; Upchurch et al. 1999). Family availability, support, connectedness, and cohesion are related to reduced sexual experience, less risky sexual behavior, and fewer health-risk behaviors among youth (Benda and DiBlasio 1994; Biglan et al. 1990; Crosby et al. 2001; DiBlasio and Benda 1990; Emerson et al. under review; Fisher and Feldman 1998). Greater satisfaction with the mother–child relationship is associated with later sexual debut, less frequent sexual activity, and more consistent teen contraceptive use. Thus, families can be powerful collaborators in the prevention of mental health problems and HIV/AIDS (Donenberg et al. 2006).

13.2.2.2 Instrumental Characteristics of Families

Likewise, instrumental characteristics (monitoring, supervision, permissiveness) are related to teens' sexual debut, intercourse frequency, risky sexual behavior, number of partners, pregnancy, and condom use (Donenberg et al. 2011; Li et al. 2000; Metzler et al. 1994; Romer et al. 1994, 1999). Parental monitoring limits opportunities for teen sexual activity (Paikoff 1995) and is linked to fewer behaviors that cooccur with risky sex, including drug and alcohol use (Bahr et al. 1998; Flannery et al. 1994; Thomas et al. 2000) and delinquency (Ary et al. 1999; Dishion and Patterson 1993; Gorman-Smith et al. 1996). More parental permissiveness and less parental availability are implicated in more frequent sexual behavior, risky sex, and substance use among youth (Davis and Friel 2001; DiClemente et al. 2001b; Mounts 2001; Werner and Silbereisen 2003). For troubled teens, more parental monitoring and supervision, and less permissiveness (Donenberg et al. 2002; Wilson et al. 2001) are related to reduced sexual risk, but the associations are stronger for girls than boys (Donenberg et al. 2002). Recent evidence suggests that for these teens, parental monitoring moderates the relationship between the quality of family communication and sexual risk behavior among African American but not Caucasian and Hispanic families (Nappi et al. 2009). Namely, African American parents who reported open family sexual communication and frequent monitoring had adolescents who reported less sexual risk behavior.

13.2.2.3 Parental Communication with Youth

Parent–teen communication that is open, receptive, and comfortable is linked to reduced sexual experience and risky sexual behavior in teens (Donenberg et al. 2011; Dutra et al. 1999; East 1996; Fisher 1987; Handelsman et al. 1987; Kastner 1984; Lock and Vincent 1995; Miller et al. 1998a, b, c, 2000; Moore et al. 1986; Whitaker et al. 1999). Parent–teen sexual communication that precedes first sex predicts condom use at debut (Miller and Whitaker 2001; O'Sullivan et al. 2001). Parent–teen discussions about sexual behavior and AIDS, especially with parents who are knowledgeable, open, and comfortable, are associated with more consistent condom use (Miller et al. 2007). Closeness between the parent and teen provides the context needed for youth to adopt parental values and engage in productive conversations about sex. Closeness also predicts greater confidence of the adolescent in talking to parents about sexual issues. Greater parental confidence in talking to teens about sex and the belief that talking will produce a positive outcome, are associated with parents and teens actually engaging in such conversations (DiIorio et al. 2000). When teens perceive their parents as trustworthy and accessible, they are more likely to have discussions about sex (Guilamo-Ramos et al. 2006). Barriers to parent–child sexual discussions are parental discomfort, embarrassment, and a lack of confidence in discussing these sexual topics (Aronowitz et al. 2007; Jaccard et al. 2000; Pluhar et al. 2006; Rosenthal et al. 1998). Youth who discuss sex with parents feel more confident talking to their partners and do so more frequently. They also are less influenced by risky peers (Hutchinson and Cooney 1998; Shoop and Davidson 1994). For youth in psychiatric care, both talking about condoms with parents and the quality of parent–teen communication about HIV/AIDS is related to more consistent condom use (Wilson & Donenberg, 2004;

Hadley et al. 2009) and less sexual risk-taking. Thus, increasing parental comfort and skills to discuss HIV/AIDS effectively with teens should promote safer sex.

13.2.3   Peer and Partner Relationships

Peers and romantic partners become increasingly important during adolescence and they influence youths' sexual development and behavior (Brooks-Gunn and Paikoff 1993; Hofferth and Hayes 1987; Townsend 2002). Three areas of peer and partner relationships that are especially salient for adolescent sexual risks are: (1) peer norms, (2) partner relationship concerns, and (3) partner communication. The desire for conformity peaks during adolescence (Costanzo and Shaw 1966), and peers are an important source of sexual information (DiIorio et al. 1999; Handelsman et al. 1987). Teens' sexual behavior often reflects perceptions of peer norms, including decisions to use birth control and condoms, and the timing of sexual initiation (Brown et al. 1992; Corsaro and Eder 1990; Cvetkovitch and Grote 1980; Doljanac and Zimmerman 1998; Fisher et al. 1992; Kinsman et al. 1998; Prinstein et al. 2003; Rodgers and Rowe 1993; Whitaker and Miller 2000). In one study, positive peer norms about abstinence were the single best predictor of delayed sexual initiation among middle school students (Santelli et al. 2004). Negative peer influence has been strongly associated with risky sex among youths in outpatient psychiatric care and appears to mediate links between psychopathology and risk (Donenberg et al. 2001). Moreover, peer influence is highly correlated with alcohol and drug use (Donenberg et al. 2001), which is associated with more risky sexual behavior. For youth in psychiatric care, whose interpersonal relationships are typically strained, the need for peer acceptance may supersede other concerns (e.g., risk of HIV/AIDS). However, there is evidence that strong parent attachment may mitigate negative peer influence for troubled youth (Emerson et al. under review).

Romantic relationships are often accompanied by intense fears of rejection and abandonment (Welsh et al. 2003). Responsible sexual behavior, such as abstinence or condom use, is a potential source of conflict with and even rejection by romantic partners (Eyre et al. 1998). Desire for intimacy, love, and affiliation has been linked to sexual behavior among both boys and girls (Ott et al. 2004; Sanderson and Cantor 1995) and is a primary reason for first sexual intercourse (Rodgers 1996). Eyre et al. (1998) found that adolescent girls believed that asking a partner to use a condom would endanger the feeling of trust between partners. Pressure to maintain relationships in order to meet intimacy needs may be particularly powerful for youths in psychiatric care, because they tend to have strained, conflictual, and unsupportive relationships with family, peers, and partners (Brown et al. 1997a; Seefeldt et al. 2003). These teens may respond less assertively to partner pressure in order to avoid disconnection (Donenberg et al. 2001; Welsh et al. 2003) and to maintain affiliation, closeness, and intimacy (Cochran and Mays 1989; Downey and Feldman 1996). Practicing prevention may avoided if it risks partner rejection or disapproval by peers, whereas engaging in risk behavior may enhance peer approval and/or secure a partner's love and commitment.

Sexual communication between teenage partners is critical for safer sex behavior, but teens often have difficulty communicating assertively and negotiating safe sex practices (Crosby et al. 2003; Hutchinson and Cooney 1998; Whitaker et al. 1999). In fact, 50% of youth do not discuss contraception or STIs with their partners before initiating sex (Manlove et al. 2007), because they feel uncomfortable discussing sex and contraception (Shoop and Davidson 1994; Widman et al. 2006). Communication between teenage sexual partners is associated with less sexual risk-taking, more HIV prevention self-efficacy, fewer partners, more consistent condom use (Hutchinson and Cooney 1998; Tschann and Adler 1997; Whitaker et al. 1999), asking partners to use condoms (Dancy and Berbaum 2005), more contraceptive use (Widman et al. 2006), and more precautions against HIV (Biglan et al. 1990; Catania et al. 1989; DiClemente 1991; Rickman et al. 1994; Shoop and Davidson 1994; Whitaker et al. 1999). Teens who express a desire to use condoms to their partner are more likely to use them, and youths who discuss their sexual history have fewer partners. Adolescents who feel confident about initiating safer sex discussions with a partner are also more likely to use a condom and/or resist pressures to engage in high-risk sex in real sexual encounters (St. Lawrence 1993). Teens in psychiatric care may be less likely to talk to partners, because they are especially vulnerable to rejection, fear relationship loss (Donenberg and Pao 2005), and lack self-assertion skills (Brown et al. 1997a, b). Moreover, these youth often lack critical interpersonal and social skills (assertiveness, effective communication) to negotiate safe sex.

In summary, there is substantial research that supports a broad Social–Personal framework of HIV/AIDS risk among youths with mental health problems. This model offers several directions for HIV-prevention programs designed to reduce transmission behaviors, and it underscores the need for preventive interventions to address a multitude of factors that affect risk. Specifically, programs that incorporate families and address teens' broader social context have the potential to produce more positive and sustained outcomes. Yet, few family-based adolescent HIV/AIDS prevention interventions address mental health. In the remainder of this chapter, we will use Project STYLE, an innovative and promising program designed for families and youth with mental health issues, as an example of an efficacious intervention based on the Social–Personal Framework. Project STYLE is an example of how strengthening families can be a useful force to decrease HIV risk among youth in mental health treatment.

13.3 Strengthening Today's Youth Life Experience (Project STYLE)

Project STYLE is the first family-based HIV/AIDS prevention program designed specifically for families whose adolescents are in mental health treatment. Project STYLE was conducted with parents and their male and female 13–18-year-olds,

Table 13.1 Project STYLE intervention overview

	Adolescent topics	Parent topics
Module 1		
Learning about HIV/STDs; parent–teen communication	Introduction and ground rules	Introduction and ground rules
	General HIV and STD information	General HIV and STD information
	Personal vulnerability to HIV and STDs	Adolescent development
	Parent, peer, and partner assertive communication	Parent–teen assertive communication
Module 2		
Parent–teen communication; identify and manage risky situations and behaviors	Parent–teen communication about sex	Parent–teen communication about sex
	Identify, personalize, and manage risky situations and behaviors	Parental monitoring
	Affect management	Affect management
	Healthy relationships	Being a more assertive parent
Module 3		
Condom skills; parent–teen communication about sexual values	Condom use skills	Condom use skills
	Parent, peer, and partner communication about HIV and STD risk behaviors	Increase comfort level when talking about sex

who were recruited from psychiatric hospitals and outpatient mental health centers in three cities of the United States: Providence, Rhode Island, Atlanta, Georgia, and Chicago, Illinois. Ethnic, racial, economic, and behavioral differences among youth across the three cities provided a unique opportunity to reach diverse youths with a range of psychiatric problems.

Consistent with earlier research, youths reported high rates of risky sexual behavior; 56.3% reported ever having oral, anal, and/or vaginal sex. Sexually active teens reported condom use 40% of the time, with a mean number of 6.4 unprotected sexual acts in the last 90 days, and 12% reported ever having an STI. Urine screening for Chlamydia, Gonorrhea, and Trichomonas at randomization revealed a baseline rate of 19% of sexually active teens with one or more of these STIs, a much higher than expected prevalence for youth not in Family Planning/STI treatment settings. Substance use was also high; 40% of teens reported using alcohol and/or marijuana five out of the last 30 days. Retention rates were excellent for this mental health sample at 3 months (91%), 6 months (88%), and 12 months (85%).

For a full list of topics covered in the prevention program, see Table 13.1. Each of three modules had specific goals. In module 1, the goals were to (1) establish group rules and norms, (2) build a sense of group membership to motivate participation, (3) increase parents' and teens' knowledge and awareness of HIV/AIDS, other STIs, risk behaviors, and modes of transmission, (4) underscore the dangers of high-risk behavior and the benefits of practicing safe sex, and (5) improve general communication skills between parents and adolescents. With parents, we presented information about typical adolescent development, and with teens, we emphasized their sense of personal vulnerability to HIV/AIDS/STI infections and highlighted the utility and benefits of good parent–teen communication.

In module 2, we focused heavily on parent–adolescent communication. Parents and teens exchanged general feedback about good and bad communication styles, and they practiced talking to each other about sexual topics. With parents, we also discussed effective, consistent, and appropriate parental monitoring, the need to manage their own affective arousal in response to teens' behavior, and the unique challenges associated with teenage mental illness (e.g., greater risk taking, HIV risks linked to mental health problems, need for increased monitoring). We taught assertive communication strategies and emphasized the importance of comfortable and effective discussions about sex, sexual relationships, and sexual partners with their teens. Each parent created a personalized monitoring plan and identified how to use affect management strategies facilitate effective parenting. With the goal of improving communication patterns, rather than resolving long-standing conflicts, parents and teens discussed these plans in front of the entire group. After feedback on their communication styles, parents and teens again discussed the issues while focusing on improving their communication.

During module 2 with the teens, we also taught assertive communication skills with peers and families, particularly in high-risk situations where teens may worry about rejection or the desire to maintain relationships over safer sex behavior. We discussed strategies to manage their own affective arousal during stressful situations and ways to recognize and choose healthy peer and partner relationships. Youths were taught to identify risky people, places, and situations, and they developed personalized risk plans to increase safe behavior.

Module 3 was designed to build safer sex skills and reinforce effective parent–teen communication about personal values. The goals for parents and teens were to (1) increase knowledge about and comfort using condoms through repeated practice, and (2) practice new communication strategies while confidently expressing personal values about sexual behavior.

13.3.1 Family-Based HIV Prevention Intervention Content

The content and design of the family-based condition was derived from several important theoretical assumptions and empirical evidence and specifically tailored for youth in mental health treatment. While many of these adaptations and principles apply to all families in challenging circumstances, they are of particular relevance for families with youth with mental health concerns.

13.3.1.1 Talking About Sex Is a Mastery Experience

Families in psychiatric care typically engage in ineffective communication during stressful discussions (Donenberg and Weisz 1997). Learning and practicing how to talk about difficult topics, like sex, with guidance from professionals provides families with a mastery experience. Parents reported anxiety about talking with their teens about sex, but these discussions were rarely the major focus of family conflict. Although nervous and tentative about sexual discussions, the communication patterns were less entrenched and emotionally charged than other issues (e.g., factors leading to recent suicide attempts) and, thus, more amenable to change. The opportunity offered in Project STYLE normalized family members' anxiety about sexuality discussions and helped them to regulate the negative affect that often accompanies these conversations. As families observed and critiqued one another during these discussions, there was a chance to build skills, provide, and receive emotional support, and take in nonjudgmental feedback to improve communication styles.

13.3.1.2   Parent/Adolescent Mutual Understanding

Parent/adolescent mutual understanding fosters a more positive relationship, which is essential to develop in families with mental health issues. The curriculum was designed, in part, to increase parents and adolescents' mutual understanding and tolerance for one another. Families in psychiatric care often have coercive interactions (Patterson 1982) and may lack empathy for each other's perspective due to personal distress and traumas. In Project STYLE, parents and teens "stepped" into one another's shoes and learned how it feels to be on the other side in a difficult parent/teen discussion. Parents learned recent scientific evidence on adolescent brain development and received feedback from other parents about their teen's behavior. This feedback normalized the challenges of parenting a teenager, particularly one with mental illness, and provided support for the conflicts and struggles they confront on a daily basis. Likewise, adolescents were challenged to consider how parents should respond to risky situations, the barriers parents experience in trying to assist and advise their teens, and the importance of parental monitoring and supervision to keep them safe. These activities helped to establish the empathy that is necessary to establish and maintain collaborative relationships.

13.3.1.3   Collaborative Communication

Collaborative communication enhances family relationships and reduces adolescent risk, especially for youth in mental health care. The intervention emphasized collaborative communication throughout the program, by first having the facilitators model it with each other and with the participants and next by activities designed to increase collaboration between the participants. The use of vignettes and role plays, consistent feedback, and in-depth discussions provided an overall sense that "we are in this together." This same sense of collaborative communication was extended to the parent–teen relationship. For example, at the beginning of the workshop, parents and teens were asked to discuss a conflict in their relationship that was identified by both of them as problematic. Many parents began the discussion by lecturing their teens, and as is typical of youth, teens responded with silence and withdrawal. During the intervention, however, group leaders encouraged and fostered collaborative communication between family members and taught parents and adolescents strategies for positive, respectful, and assertive communication with one another. The relevance of collaboration in achieving mutual goals (i.e., staying safe, maintaining calm within the family, getting what you want) was emphasized. By the end of the workshop, many family members reported a new understanding and appreciation of how to talk to each other.

13.3.1.4 Acquiring and Practicing New Skills

Acquiring and practicing new skills is essential to mastery and risk reduction. Project STYLE taught new skills, such as assertive communication, condom use, and affect regulation, and then engaged participants in numerous exercises to practice them, including role-plays, games, and other activities. We brought family members together to try out new behaviors with one another in a "real-life" situation. They discussed a conflict in their relationship while attempting to use emotion regulation strategies and using collaborative verbal and nonverbal assertive communication. Practice and application of new skills to a variety of circumstances was especially important for families with mental health issues because of long-standing ineffective behavioral patterns. We assigned homework to practice new skills, and we used the booster sessions to reinforce gains and to problem solve barriers to adherence.

13.4 Summary

HIV/AIDS is related to psychiatric disorders in complex and varied ways that require interventions that go beyond targeting individual-level factors of adolescents. Families are critical in helping youth with mental disorders to navigate the HIV-risk environment. This chapter describes the issues that families and youth face, and uses Project STYLE, an innovative and tailored HIV prevention program for parents and youths with psychiatric disorders as an example. Current prevention efforts show not only positive short-term outcomes but also significant decay over time. For youth, families can be important collaborators in risk reduction efforts by delivering prevention messages long after the formal program ends. Project STYLE is an example of a family-based program with strong theoretical underpinnings that illustrates a promising new intervention for parents and youths with psychiatric disorders. Preliminary outcome data reveal safer sex behavior among troubled teens as a result of the program. Future data analyses will examine the long-term effects of Project STYLE on adolescent risk taking, with special attention to the sustainability of positive outcomes over time.

Acknowledgments This research was supported by NIMH (R01MH63008). We gratefully acknowledge the administrators and clinical staff at the psychiatric hospitals and outpatient mental health clinics in Chicago, Providence, and Atlanta. We also thank the research staff, parents, and adolescents without whom this research could not have been completed. All correspondence should be sent to Geri R. Donenberg, Institute for Juvenile Research, Department of Psychiatry, University of Illinois at Chicago (M/C 747), 1747 W. Roosevelt Road, Rm. 155, Chicago, Illinois 60608. E-mail: gdonenberg@psych.uic.edu.

References

Aronowitz T, Rennells RE, Todd E. Heterosocial behaviors in early adolescent African American girls: the role of mother-daughter relationships. J Fam Nurs. 2005;11:122–39.

Aronowitz T, Todd E, Agbeshie E, Rennells R. Attitudes that affect the ability of African American preadolescent girls and their mothers to talk openly about sex. Issues Ment Health Nurs. 2007;28:7–20.

Aruffo J, Gottlieb A, Webb R, Neville B. Adolescent psychiatric inpatients: alcohol use and HIV risk-taking behavior. Psychosoc Rehabil J. 1994;17:150–6.

Ary DV, Duncan TE, Biglan A, Metzler CW, Noell JW, Smolkowski K. Development of adolescent problem behavior. J Abnorm Child Psychol. 1999;27:141–50.

Bahr SJ, Maughan SL, Marcos AC, Li B. Family, religiosity, and the risk of adolescent drug use. J Marriage Fam. 1998;60:979–92.

Benda BB, DiBlasio FA. An integration of theory: adolescent sexual contacts. J Youth Adolesc. 1994;23:403–20.

Biglan A, Metzler C, Wirt R, Ary D, Noel J, Oochs L, et al. Social and behavioral factors associated with high-risk behavior among adolescents. J Behav Med. 1990;13:245–61.

Brooks-Gunn J, Paikoff RL. Sex is a gamble, kissing is a game: adolescent sexuality and health promotion. In: Millstein SG, Petersen AC, Nightingale EO, editors. Promoting the health of adolescents: New directions for the twenty-first century. New York: Oxford University Press; 1993. p. 180–208.

Brooks-Gunn J, Paikoff R. Sexuality and developmental transitions during adolescence. In: Schulenberg J, Maggs JL, Hurrelmann K, editors. Health risks and developmental transitions during adolescence. New York: Cambridge University Press; 1997. p. 190–219.

Brown LK, DiClemente RJ, Park T. Predictors of condom use in sexually active adolescents. J Adolesc Health. 1992;13:651–7.

Brown LK, Danovsky MB, Lourie KJ, DiClemente RJ, Ponton LE. Adolescents with psychiatric disorders and the risk of HIV. J Am Acad Child Adolesc Psychiatry. 1997a;36:1609–17.

Brown LK, Reynolds LA, Lourie K. A pilot HIV prevention program for adolescents in a psychiatric hospital. Psychiatr Serv. 1997b;48:531–3.

Brown LK, Hadley W, Stewart A, Lescano CM, Whitely L, Donenberg G, et al. Psychiatric disorders and sexual risk among adolescents in mental health treatment. J Consult Clin Psychol. 2010;78(4):590–7.

Carey MP, Carey KB, Kalichman SC. Risk for human immunodeficiency virus (HIV) infection among persons with severe mental illnesses. Clin Psychol Rev. 1997;17:271–91.

Catania JA, Dolcini MM, Coates TJ, Kegeles SM, Greenblatt RM, Puckett S, et al. Predictors of condom use and multiple partnered sex among sexually-active adolescent women: implications for AIDS-related health interventions. J Sex Res. 1989;26(4):514–24.

Chewning B, Van Koningsveld R. Predicting adolescents' initiation of intercourse and contraceptive use. J Appl Soc Psychol. 1998;28:1245–85.

Chodorow N. Family structure and feminine personality. In: Rosaldo MZ, Lamphen L, editors. Women, culture, and society. Stanford, CA: Stanford University Press; 1974. p. 43–66.

Chodorow N. Mothering, object-relations, and the female oedipal configuration. Fem Stud. 1978; 4:137–58.

Cicchetti D, Akerman B, Izard C. Emotions and emotion regulation in developmental psychopathology. Dev Psychopathol. 1995;7:1–10.

Cochran SD, Mays VM. Women and AIDS-related concerns: roles for psychologists in helping the worried well. Am Psychol. 1989;44:529–35.

Corsaro WA, Eder D. Children's peer cultures. Annu Rev Sociol. 1990;16:197–220.

Costanzo PR, Shaw ME. Conformity as a function of age level. Child Dev. 1966;37:967–75.

Cournos F, McKinnon K, Wainberg M. What can mental health interventions contribute to the global struggle against HIV/AIDS? World Psychiatry. 2005;4:135–41.

Crosby R, Miller K. Family influences on adolescent females' sexual health. In: Wingwood G, DiClemente R, editors. Handbook of women's sexual and reproductive health. New York, NY: Kluwer Academic/Plenum Publishers; 2002. p. 113–27.

Crosby RA, DiClemente RJ, Wingwood GM, Cobb BK, Harrington K, Davies SL, et al. HIV/STD-protective benefits of living with mothers in perceived supportive families: a study of high-risk African American female teens. Prev Med. 2001;33:175–8.

Crosby R, DiClemente R, Wingwood G, Salazar L, Harrington K, Davies SL, et al. Identification of strategies for promoting condom use: a prospective analysis of high-risk African American female teens. Prev Sci. 2003;4:263–70.

Cvetkovitch G, Grote B. Psychological development and the social problem of teenage illegitimacy. In: Chilman C, editor. Adolescent pregnancy and childbearing: findings from research. Washington, DC: US Department of Health and Human Services; 1980. p. 15–41.

Dancy B, Berbaum M. Condom use predictors for low-income African American women. West J Nurs Res. 2005;27:28–44.

Danziger SK. Family life and teenage pregnancy in the inner-city: experiences of African American youth. Child Youth Serv Rev. 1995;17:183–202.

Davis EC, Friel LV. Adolescent sexuality: disentangling the effects of family structure and family context. J Marriage Fam. 2001;63:669–81.

Di Scipio WJ. Sex, drugs, and AIDS: issues for hospitalized emotionally disturbed youth. Psychiatr Q. 1994;65:149–55.

DiBlasio FA, Benda BB. Adolescent sexual behavior: multivariate analysis of a social learning model. J Adolesc Res. 1990;5:449–66.

DiClemente RJ. Predictors of HIV-preventive sexual behavior in a high-risk adolescent population: the influence of perceived peer norms and sexual communication on incarcerated adolescents' consistent use of condoms. J Adolesc Health. 1991;12:385–90.

DiClemente RJ, Brown LK, Beausoleil NI, Lodico MM. Comparison of AIDS knowledge and HIV-related sexual risk behaviors among adolescents in low and high AIDS prevalence communities. J Adolesc Health. 1993;14:231–6.

DiClemente RJ, Lodico M, Grinstead OA, Harper G, Rickman RL, Evans PE, et al. African-American adolescents residing in high-risk urban environments do use condoms: correlates and predictors of condom use among adolescents in public housing developments. Pediatrics. 1996a;98:269–78.

DiClemente RJ, Ponton LE, Hansen WB. New directions for adolescent risk prevention and health promotion research and interventions. In: DiClemente RJ, Hansen WB, Ponton LE, editors. Handbook of adolescent health risk behavior. New York City: Plenum Press; 1996b. p. 413–20.

DiClemente RJ, Wingood GM, Crosby RA, Sionean C, Brown LK, Rothbaum B, et al. A prospective study of psychological distress and sexual risk behavior among black adolescent females. Pediatrics. 2001a;108:1–6.

DiClemente RJ, Wingood GM, Crosby RA, Sionean C, Cobb BK, Harrington K, et al. Parental monitoring: association with adolescents' risk behaviors. Pediatrics. 2001b;107:1363–8.

DiIorio C, Kelley M, Hockenberry-Eaton M. Communication about sexual issues: mothers, fathers, and friends. J Adolesc Health. 1999;24:181–9.

DiIorio C, Denzmore P, Resnicow K, Rogers-Tillman G, Wang DT, Dudley WN, et al. Keepin' It R.E.A.L.!: a mother-adolescent HIV prevention program. In: Pequagnat W, Szapocznik J, editors. Working with families in the era of HIV/AIDS. Thousand Oaks, CA: Sage; 2000.

Dishion TJ, Patterson GR. Antisocial behavior: using a multiple gating strategy. In: Singer MI, Singer LT, Anglin TM, editors. Handbook for screening adolescents at psychological risk. New York City: Lexington Books; 1993. p. 375–99.

Doljanac RF, Zimmerman MA. Psychological factors and high-risk sexual behavior: race differences among urban adolescents. J Behav Med. 1998;21:451–67.

Donenberg G, Pao M. Youths and HIV/AIDS: psychiatry's role in a changing epidemic. J Am Acad Child Adolesc Psychiatry. 2005;44:728–47.

Donenberg G, Weisz J. Experimental task and speaker effects on parent-child interactions of aggressive and depressed/anxious children. J Abnorm Child Psychol. 1997;25:367–87.

Donenberg G, Emerson E, Bryant F, Wilson H, Weber-Shifrin E. Understanding AIDS-risk behavior among adolescents in psychiatric care: links to psychopathology and peer relationships. J Acad Child Adolesc Psychiatry. 2001;40:642–53.

Donenberg GR, Wilson H, Emerson E, Bryant FB. Holding the line with a watchful eye: the impact of perceived parental permissiveness and parental monitoring on risky sexual behavior among adolescents in psychiatric care. AIDS Educ Prev. 2002;14:138–57.

Donenberg GR, Bryant FB, Emerson E, Wilson HW, Pasch KE. Tracing the roots of early sexual debut adolescents in psychiatric care. J Am Acad Child Adolesc Psychiatry. 2003;42:594–608.

Donenberg GR, Schwartz R, Emerson E, Wilson HW, Bryant FB, Coleman G, et al. Applying a cognitive-behavioral model of HIV risk to youths in psychiatric care. AIDS Educ Prev. 2005;17:200–16.

Donenberg G, Paikoff R, Pequegnat W. Introduction to the special section on families, youth, and HIV: family-based intervention studies. J Pediatr Psychol. 2006;31(9):869–73.

Donenberg G, Emerson E, Mackesy-Amiti M. Sexual risk among African American girls: psychopathology and mother-daughter relationships. J Consult Clin Psychol. 2011;79(2):153–8.

Downey G, Feldman S. The implications of rejection sensitivity for intimate relationships. J Pers Soc Psychol. 1996;70:1327–43.

Dutra R, Miller KS, Forehand R. The process and content of sexual communication with adolescents in two-parent families: associations with sexual risk-taking behavior. AIDS Behav. 1999;3:59–66.

East PL. The younger sisters of childbearing adolescents: their attitudes, expectations, and behaviors. Child Dev. 1996;67:267–82.

Emerson E, Donenberg G, Wilson H. Health protective effects of attachment among African American girls in psychiatric care. Under review.

Eyre S, Hoffman V, Millstein S. The gamesmanship of sex: a model based on African American adolescent accounts. Med Anthropol Q. 1998;12:67–489.

Fantasia H. Concept analysis: sexual decision-making in adolescence. Nurs Forum. 2008;43:80–90.

Fishbein M. A theory of reasoned action: some applications and implications. Nebr Symp Motiv. 1980;27:65–116.

Fisher TD. Family communication and the sexual behavior and attitudes of college students. J Youth Adolesc. 1987;16:481–95.

Fisher L, Feldman S. Familial antecedents of young adult health risk behavior: a longitudinal study. J Fam Psychol. 1998;12:66–80.

Fisher WA, Fisher JD. Understanding and promoting AIDS-preventative behavior: insights from the theory of reasoned action. Health Psychol. 1995;14:255–64.

Fisher JD, Misovich SJ, Fisher WA. The impact of perceived social norms on adolescents' AIDS-risk behavior and prevention. In: DiClemente RJ, editor. Adolescents and AIDS: a generation in Jeopardy. Beverly Hills, CA: Sage; 1992. p. 117–36.

Flannery DJ, Vazsonyi AT, Torquati J, Fridrich A. Ethnic and gender differences in risk for early adolescent substance abuse. J Youth Adolesc. 1994;23:195–213.

Frances R, Wikstrom T, Alcena V. Contracting AIDS as a means of committing suicide. Am J Psychiatry. 1985;142:656.

Fritsch S, Donaldson D, Spirio A, Plummer B. Personality characteristics of adolescent suicide attempters. Child Psychiatry Hum Dev. 2000;29:219–35.

Gorman-Smith D, Tolan PH, Zelli A, Huesmann LR. The relation of family functioning to violence among inner-city minority youth. J Fam Psychol. 1996;10:115–29.

Guilamo-Ramos V, Jaccard J, Dittus P, Bouris AM. Parental expertise, trustworthiness, and accessibility: parent-adolescent communication and adolescent risk behavior. J Marriage Fam. 2006;68:1229–46.

Hadley W, Brown LK, Lescano CM, Kell H, Spalding K, DiClemente R, et al. Parent-adolescent sexual communication: discussing condoms matters. AIDS Behav. 2009;13:997–1004.

Handelsman CD, Cabral RJ, Weisfeld GE. Sources of information and adolescent sexual knowledge and behavior. J Adolesc Res. 1987;2:455–63.

Henggeler S, Melton G, Rodrigue J. Pediatric and adolescent AIDS: research findings from the social sciences. CA, Sage: Newbury Park; 1992.

Hindelang RL, Dwyer WO, Leeming FC. Adolescent risk-taking behavior: a review of the role of parental involvement. Curr Probl Pediatr. 2001;31:67–83.

Hingson R, Strunin L, Berlin B. Acquired immunodeficiency syndrome transmission: changes in knowledge and behaviors among teenagers, Massachusetts statewide surveys, 1986 to 1988. Pediatrics. 1990a;85:24–9.

Hingson RW, Strunin L, Berlin BM, Heeren T. Beliefs about AIDS, use of alcohol and drugs, and unprotected sex among Massachusetts adolescents. Am J Public Health. 1990b;80:295–9.

Hofferth SL, Hayes CD. Risking the future: adolescent sexuality, pregnancy, and childbearing, vol. 2. Washington, DC: National Academy Press; 1987.

Hutchinson MK, Cooney TM. Patterns of parent-teen sexual risk communication: implications for intervention. Fam Relat. 1998;47:185–94.

Jaccard J, Dittus PJ, Gordon VV. Parent-adolescent congruency in reports of adolescents sexual behavior and in communications about sexual behavior. Child Dev. 1998;69:247–61.

Jaccard J, Dittus P, Gordon VV. Parent-teen communication about premarital sex: factors associated with the extent of communication. J Adolesc Res. 2000;15:187–208.

Jones JB, Philliber S. Sexually active but not pregnant: a comparison of teens who risk and teens who plan. J Youth Adolesc. 1983;12:235–51.

Kastner LS. Ecological factors predicting adolescent contraceptive use: implications for intervention. J Adolesc Health Care. 1984;5:79–86.

Keller SE, Schleifer SJ, Bartlett JA, Johnson RL. The sexual behavior of adolescents and risk of AIDS. JAMA. 1988;260:3586.

Kinsman S, Romer D, Furstenberg F, Schwartz D. Early sexual initiation: the role of peer norms. Pediatrics. 1998;102:1185–92.

Kipke M, Boyer C, Hein K. An evaluation of an AIDS risk reduction education and skills training (ARREST) program. J Adolesc Health. 1998;14:533–9.

Kirby D, Short L, Collins J, Rugg D, Kolbe L, Howard M, et al. School-based programs to reduce sexual risk behaviors: a review of effectiveness. Public Health Rep. 1994;109:339–60.

Kotchick BA, Shaffer A, Miller KS, Forehand R. Adolescent sexual risk behavior: a multi-system perspective. Clin Psychol Rev. 2001;21:493–519.

Lescano C, Brown L, Miller P, Puster K. Distress concerning condom use: do feelings matter? J Prev Interv Community. 2007;33:51–62.

Li X, Feigelman S, Stanton B. Perceived parental monitoring and health risk behaviors among urban low-income African-American children and adolescents. J Adolesc Health. 2000;27:43–8.

Lock SE, Vincent ML. Sexual decision-making among rural adolescent females. Health Values: J Health Behav Educ Promot. 1995;19:47–58.

Longmore MA, Manning WD, Giordano PC. Preadolescent parenting strategies and teens' dating and sexual initiation: a longitudinal analysis. J Marriage Fam. 2001;63:322–35.

MacLean MG, Paradise MJ, Cauce AM. Substance use and psychological adjustment in homeless adolescents: a test of three models. Am J Community Psychol. 2000;27:405–27.

Manlove J, Ryan S, Franzetta K. Contraceptive use patterns across teens' sexual relationships: the role of relationships, partners, and sexual histories. Demography. 2007;44:603–21.

Mehta S, Moore RD, Graham NMH. Potential factors affecting adherence with HIV therapy AIDS. AIDS. 1997;11:1665–70.

Meschke LL, Bartholomae S, Zentall SR. Adolescent sexuality and parent adolescent processes: promoting healthy teen choices. J Adolesc Health. 2002;31:264–79.

Metzler CW, Noell J, Biglan A, Ary D, Smolkowski K. The social context for risky sexual behavior among adolescents. J Behav Med. 1994;17:419–38.

Miller BC, Fox GL. Theories of adolescent heterosexual behavior. J Adolesc Res. 1987;2:269–82.

Miller KS, Whitaker DJ. Predictors of mother-adolescent discussions about condoms: implications for providers who serve youth. Pediatrics. 2001;108:E28.

Miller BC, Norton MC, Fan X, Christopherson CR. Pubertal development, parental communication, and sexual values in relation to adolescent sexual behaviors. J Early Adolesc. 1998a;18:27–52.

Miller K, Kotchick B, Dorsey S, Forehand R, Ham AV. Family communication about sex: what are parents saying and are their adolescents listening? Fam Plann Perspect. 1998b;30:218–35.

Miller KS, Levin ML, Whitaker DJ, Xu X. Patterns of condom use among adolescents: the impact of mother-adolescent communication. Am J Public Health. 1998c;88:1542–4.

Miller KS, Forehand R, Kotchick BA. Adolescent sexual behavior in two ethnic minority groups: a multi-system perspective. Adolescence. 2000;35:313–33.

Miller BC, Benson B, Galbraith KA. Family relationships and adolescent pregnancy risk: a research synthesis. Dev Rev. 2001;21:1–38.

Miller K, Fasula A, Dittus P, Wiegand R, Wyckoff S, McNair L. Barriers and facilitators to maternal communication with preadolescents about age-relevant sexual topics. AIDS Behav. 2007;13(2):365–74.

Moore M, Chase-Lansdale P. Sexual intercourse and pregnancy among African American adolescent girls in high poverty neighborhoods: the role of family and perceived community involvement. J Marriage Fam. 2001;63:1146–57.

Moore KA, Peterson JL, Furstenberg FF. Parental attitudes and the occurrence of early sexual activity. J Marriage Fam. 1986;48:777–82.

Mounts NS. Young adolescents' perceptions of parental management of peer relationships. J Early Adolesc. 2001;21:92–122.

Mustanski B, Donenberg G, Emerson E. I can use a condom, i just don't: the importance of motivation to prevent HIV in adolescents seeking psychiatric care. AIDS Behav. 2006;10:753–62.

Nappi C, Thakral C, Kapungu C, Donenberg GR, DiClemente R, Brown L. Parental monitoring as a moderator of the effect of family sexual communication on sexual risk behavior among adolescents in psychiatric care. AIDS Behav. 2009;13:1012–20.

O'Donnell L, Stueve A, Duran R, Myint-U A, Agronick G, San Doval A, et al. Parenting practices, parents' underestimation of daughters' risks, and alcohol and sexual behaviors of urban girls. J Adolesc Health. 2008;42:496–502.

O'Sullivan LF, Meyer-Bahlburg HFL, Watkins B. Mother-daughter communication about sex among urban African American and Latino families. Journal of Adolescent Research. 2001;16: 269–292.

Ott M, Millstein S, Halpern-Felsher B. Positive motivations for sex among male and female teens. J Adolesc Health. 2004;34:150.

Paikoff RL. Early heterosexual debut: situations of sexual possibility during the transition to adolescence. Am J Orthopsychiatry. 1995;65:389–401.

Patterson G. Coercive family processes. Eugene, OR: Castalia Publishing Company; 1982.

Perrino T, Gonzalez-Soldevilla A, Pantin G, Szapocznik J. The role of families in adolescent HIV prevention: a review. Clin Child Fam Psychol Rev. 2000;3:81–96.

Pluhar E, Jennings T, DiIorio C. Getting an early start: communication about sexuality among mothers and children 6–10 years old. J HIV/AIDS Prev Child Youth. 2006;7:7–35.

Prinstein M, Meade C, Cohen G. Adolescent oral sex, adolescent peer popularity, and perceptions of best friends' sexual behavior. J Pediatr Psychiatry. 2003;28:243–9.

Repetti RL, Taylor SE, Seeman TE. Family social environments and the mental and physical health of offspring. Psychol Bull. 2002;128:330–66.

Resnick MD, Bearman PS, Blum RW, Bauma KE, Harris KM, Jones J, et al. Protecting adolescents from harm: findings from the national longitudinal study on adolescent health. JAMA. 1997;278:823–32.

Rickman RL, Lodico M, DiClemente RJ, Morris R, Baker C, Huscroft S. Sexual communication is associated with condom use by sexually active incarcerated adolescents. J Adolesc Health. 1994;15:383–8.

Rodgers J. Sexual transitions in adolescence. In: Graber J, Brooks-Gunn J, Peterson A, editors. Transitions through adolescence: interpersonal domains and context. Mahwah, NJ: Erlbaum; 1996. p. 85–110.

Rodgers JL, Rowe DC. Social contagion and adolescent sexual behavior: a developmental and EMOSA model. Psychol Rev. 1993;100:479–510.

Rolf J, Nanda J, Baldwin J, Chandra A, Thompson L. Substance misuse and HIV/AIDS risks among delinquents: a prevention challenge. Int J Addict. 1991;25:533–59.

Romer D, Black M, Ricardo I, Feigelman S, Kaljee L, Galbraith J, et al. Social influences on the sexual behavior of youth at risk for HIV exposure. Am J Public Health. 1994;84:977–85.

Romer D, Stanton B, Galbraith J, Feigelman S, Black MM, Li X. Parental influence on adolescent sexual behavior in high-poverty settings. Arch Pediatr Adolesc Med. 1999;153:1055–62.

Rosenthal DA, Feldman SS, Edwards D. Mum's the word: mother's perspective on communication about sexuality with adolescents. J Adolesc. 1998;21:727–43.

Sanderson C, Cantor N. Social dating goals in late adolescence: implications for safer sexual activity. J Pers Soc Psychol. 1995;68:1121–34.

Santelli JS, Kaiser J, Hirsch L, Radosh A, Simkin L, Middlestadt S. Initiation of sexual intercourse among middle school adolescents: the influence of psychosocial factors. J Adolesc Health. 2004;34:200–8.

Seefeldt T, Florsheim P, Benjamin L. Psychopathology and relational dysfunction among adolescent couples: the structural analysis of social behavior as an organizing framework. In: Florsheim P, editor. Adolescent romantic relations and sexual behavior: theory, research, and practical implications. Mahwah, NJ: Erlbaum; 2003. p. 163–84.

Sheeber L, Allen N, Davis B, Sorensen E. Regulation of negative affect during mother-child problem solving interactions: adolescent depressive status and family processes. J Abnorm Child Psychol. 2000;28:467–79.

Sheeber L, Hops H, Davis B. Family processes in adolescent depression. Clin Child Fam Psychol Rev. 2001;4:19–35.

Shoop DM, Davidson PM. AIDS and adolescents: the relation of parent and partner communication to adolescent condom use. J Adolesc. 1994;17:137–48.

Sikand A, Fisher M, Friedman SB. AIDS knowledge, concerns, and behavioral changes among inner-city high school students. J Adolesc Health. 1996;18:325–8.

Somers CL, Paulson SE. Students' perceptions of parent-adolescent closeness and communication about sexuality: relations with sexual knowledge, attitudes, and behaviors. J Adolesc. 2000;23:629–44.

St. Lawrence J. African-American adolescents' knowledge, health-related attitudes, sexual behavior, and contraceptive decisions: implications for the prevention of adolescent HIV infection St. J Consult Clin Psychol. 1993;61:104–12.

St. Lawrence J, Eldridge G, Reitman D, Little C, Shelby M, Brasfield T. Factors influencing condom use among African American women: implications for risk reduction interventions. Am J Community Psychol. 1998;26:7–28.

Sterk C, Klein H, Elifson K. Predictors of condom-related attitudes among at-risk women. J Womens Health. 2004;13:676–88.

Stevens JW. Smart and sassy: the strengths of inner-city black girls. New York: Oxford University Press; 2002.

Surrey JL. The self-in-relation: a theory of women's development. In: Jordan JV, Kaplan AG, Miller JB, Stiver IP, Surrey JL, editors. Women's growth in connection. New York: Guilford; 1983. p. 51–66.

Thomas G, Reifman A, Barnes GM, Farrell MP. Delayed onset of drunkenness as a protective factor for adolescent alcohol misuse and sexual risk taking: a longitudinal study. Deviant Behav. 2000;21:181–210.

Townsend TG. The impact of self-components on attitudes towards sex among African American preadolescent girls: the moderating role of menarche. Sex Roles. 2002;47:11–20.

Treisman GJ, Angelino AF. The psychiatry of AIDS: a guide to diagnosis and treatment. Baltimore, MD: Johns Hopkins University Press; 2004. p. 217.

Tschann J, Adler N. Sexual self-acceptance, communication with partner, and contraceptive use among adolescent females: a longitudinal study. J Adolesc Res. 1997;7:413–30.

Tubman JG, Gil AG, Wagner EF, Artigues H. Patterns of sexual risk behaviors and psychiatric disorders in a community sample of young adults. J Behav Med. 2003;26:473–500.

Upchurch D, Aneshensel C, Sucoff C, Levy-Storms L. Neighborhood and family contexts of adolescent sexual activity. J Marriage Fam. 1999;61:920–33.

Wagner GJ, Kanouse DE, Koegel P, Sullivan G. Adherence to HIV antiretrovirals among persons with serious mental illness. In: Laurence J, editor. Medication Adherence in HIV/AIDS. Larchmont, NY: Mary Ann Liebert, Inc; 2004. p. 295–302.

Welsh D, Grello C, Harper M. When love hurts: depression and adolescent romantic relationships. In: Florsheim P, editor. Adolescent romantic relations and sexual behavior: theory, research and practical implications. Mahwah, NJ: Erlbaum; 2003. p. 185–212.

Werner NE, Silbereisen RK. Family relationship quality and contact with deviant peers as predictors of adolescent problem behaviors: the moderating role of gender. J Adolesc Res. 2003;18:454–80.

Whitaker DJ, Miller KS. Parent-adolescent discussions about sex and condoms: impact on peer influences of sexual risk behavior. J Adolesc Res. 2000;15:251–73.

Whitaker DJ, Miller KS, May DC, Levin ML. Teenage partners' communication about sexual risk and condom use: the importance of parent-teenager discussions. Fam Plann Perspect. 1999;31:117–21.

Widman L, Welsh D, McNulty J, Little K. Sexual communication and contraceptive use in adolescent dating couples. J Adolesc Health. 2006;39:893–9.

Wilson H, Donenberg G. Quality of parent communication about sex and its relationship to mentally ill adolescents' risky sexual behavior. J Child Psychol Psychiatry. 2004;45:387–95.

Wilson H, Emerson E, Donenberg G. Risky sexual behavior in clinically disturbed girls: which relationships matter – parents, peers, or partners? Annual NIMH international research conference on the role of families in preventing and adapting to HIV/AIDS, Los Angeles, CA; 2001.

Part IV
Implementing Family Systems
Evidence-Based Prevention

Chapter 14
Adaptation of Interventions for Families Affected by HIV

**Mary Jane Rotheram-Borus, Sung-Jae Lee, Bita Amani,
and Dallas Swendeman**

Abstract HIV infection affects families, not only individuals. HIV brings a set of predictable challenges that impact the family's daily routines, social status, and resources. Persons living with HIV (PLH), their partners, children, and extended family must meet the challenges. This chapter demonstrates how we adapted an evidence-based intervention (EBI) for Families Affected by HIV (FAH) to subgroups with different transmission risks, cultural heritages, and organizations of their health systems. Family interventions in the USA, Thailand, and South Africa are described.

A set of standardized functions are shared across each of the adapted EBI: It (1) provides a framework to assign the meaning of HIV family-based programs; (2) helps families apply key health information to one's life; (3) builds cognitive, affective, and behavioral self-management skills; (4) addresses environmental barriers to implementing health behaviors; and (5) provides tools to develop ongoing social and community support. Based on counseling models, individual, small group, multiple family group, and community activities have been the delivery formats for interventions for FAH. Each meeting has a similar sequence of activities: sharing compliments and successes, introducing new information, brainstorming and problem solving how to apply the information to one's life, practicing the implementation, setting a goal, and sharing compliments among the attendees. To implement these intervention routines, the interactions are highly structured; the leaders must be able to elicit and manage effectively the attendees' feelings, thoughts, and behaviors; and a strong bond must be formed among the attendees to sustain behavior change. Four levels of context are highlighted for adapting family-based interventions (country, local institutions, local communities, and families).

W. Pequegnat and C.C. Bell (eds.), *Family and HIV/AIDS: Cultural and Contextual Issues in Prevention and Treatment*, DOI 10.1007/978-1-4614-0439-2_14,
© Springer Science+Business Media, LLC 2012

14.1   Introduction

The global need for comprehensive family-based HIV interventions exceeds our current capacities to design, deliver, and diffuse programs that are both effective and relevant to local communities. Given the increase in global health funding, from 5.6 billion in 1990 to 21.8 billion in 2007 (Ravishankar et al. 2009), new models of intervention design and adaptation are needed to quicken the adoption and adaptation processes. Increasing capacity and responsibility must be placed with service providers, community leaders, and families affected by HIV (FAH). Evidence-based interventions (EBI) share a set of common factors, processes, and principles that can be adapted locally in order to implement culturally sensitive programs. Family-based interventions provide opportunities to intervene early in the life course, build social support and skills that prevent HIV, promote health broadly throughout life, and overcome stigma that is a significant barrier to HIV-identified service utilization.

HIV infection affects families, not only individuals. Families are the basic social unit of most societies. Surviving is contingent upon the family members internally banding together to support each other. HIV radiates among family members: sexual partners infect each other and mothers infect their children. If illness causes unemployment to one family member, no one in the family eats. When a neighbor knows one family member has HIV, the stigma is assigned to all members. Isolation is familial, not personal. Interventions providing understanding, knowledge, skills, and support are needed for each family member, tailored to the challenges and developmental capacities of the person.

In countries with generalized epidemics and subgroups with generalized epidemics (e.g., gay men and injecting drug users), the communities of families are needed to support each other. In South Africa, the country with the highest number of HIV-infected persons globally, 40% of a family's monthly income comes from its neighbors (Bhana and Pattman 2009). If one family fails to share resources with their peers, the non-sharing family's survival will be threatened the next time their family is in need: their neighbors will not share with them. Therefore, when a devastating and life-threatening infectious disease affects one member of a family, the entire network is impacted.

We will present in this chapter examples of countries facing epidemics only among persons at very high risk based on various factors, including occupation (i.e., sex workers), sexual orientation, and risk history. The USA, for instance, has subpopulations with a higher risk and prevalence of HIV than the overall population (El-Sadr et al. 2010). In South Africa, the babies of pregnant HIV+ women are potentially the easiest to protect from transmission: perinatal HIV has been an area with huge and dramatic prevention breakthroughs. Yet, the infection rate of babies of HIV+ mothers is about 23% at 2 years and another 12% die by 5 years of age (Rollins et al. 2007). Finally, villagers in rural Thailand, a Buddhist country, are affected across three and four generations when extended family members reside together in a household with an HIV+ individual (Knodel 2008).

We propose a set of concrete steps to enable adaptation and diffusion of EBI for FAH. The factors and processes that are universal across all EBI also apply to interventions for FAH. We will demonstrate the points with family-based programs in three countries and with subgroups that are at risk, then highlight the four levels of family-based interventions, and propose that successful adaptation and diffusion of interventions require addressing each of these levels. Drawing upon our experience in these three countries, we will describe our adaptation and diffusion of our interventions aimed at increasing families' capacity to cope effectively with HIV in the USA, South Africa, and Thailand.

14.2 Common Challenges Facing Families Affected by HIV

There are common challenges for persons living with HIV, which consistently involve their families: (1) to reduce transmission acts, as about 33–50% continue sexual risk acts (Crepaz and Marks 2002; Rotheram-Borus et al. 2001; Kalichman 2000), and substance abuse, as greater than 70% of substance abusers relapse over time (Abdul-Quader et al. 2002); (2) to increase health maintenance behaviors, since 70% utilize and 66% adhere to HAART, with inconsistent adherence to medical regimens and appointments, and assertiveness with providers; (3) to decrease mental health symptoms and disorders, as up to 70% of people affected by HIV attend mental health counseling (Rotheram-Borus et al. 2001, 2004, 2006; Benotsch and Kalichman 2001; Crepaz and Marks 2001) and mental health problems are associated with lower adherence and increased transmission risks (Remien and Rabkin 2001); and (4) to maintain positive social relationships, particularly within the family, and in the face of stigma, HIV-related challenges of disclosure, and to adapt to ever-changing profile of risk and protective behaviors. The advances in treatment suggest that parents now face the long-term challenges of routinely following strict health care regimens that accompany chronic disease maintenance (Rotheram-Borus and Miller 1998).

14.2.1 Adherence to Health Regimens

The health challenges facing persons living with HIV vary based on the stage of illness, the age and gender of the family members, and the organization of health care services that often precipitate iatrogenic effects. Since 1996, HIV has increasingly become a chronic disease (Swendeman et al. 2009). Antiretroviral therapies (ART) are available for persons living with HIV, and this has extended the length and the quality of life to be more than 20 years (http://www.aids.org/atn). Yet, among the 1.2 million persons living with HIV in the USA, most African–Americans and Latinos do not get an HIV diagnosis until about 1 year before they are diagnosed with AIDS (Crepaz et al. 2007). Among those who do know their status, half do not seek treatment in the first 3 years after an HIV diagnosis, and this rate has not changed significantly since 1998 (Wolitski et al. 2008). There is a strong need to identify HIV+ persons as soon as possible after infection, and to link persons living with HIV to care, once they are diagnosed.

Families' health challenges vary substantially based on the organization of health care in the country. Similar to the USA, many of the health systems in the developing world are organized to deliver services to age- and gender-segregated subgroups. Approximately 26% of pregnant women in low- and middle-income countries are tested for HIV during pregnancy (http://www.who.int/hiv/topics/mtct/data/en/index1.html), even though vertical transmission can be lowered to less than 2% (European Collaborative Study 2005). When pregnant women are identified as HIV+ during pregnancy, they then face the challenge of informing their sexual partner (or not) about their serostatus (Rotheram-Borus et al. 2011). If couples or families are tested for HIV, this challenge does not emerge (Mubangizi et al. 2000), yet, almost no HIV testing is provided to families or couples. The focus is on individual rights, rather than family adjustment to HIV. This characterizes HIV testing in the USA, South Africa, Thailand, and India. When family-based HIV testing was implemented, 80% of family members were tested for HIV and received their results (Kellerman and Essajee 2010).

Inconsistent adherence to medical regimens and appointments, and assertiveness with care providers are consistent challenges for FAH (Benotsch and Kalichman 2001; Crepaz and Marks 2001). There is substantial data from the literature on adherence, that is, family involvement in planning for adherence to ART leads to significantly higher adherence rates (Pearson et al. 2006). Therefore, the greater the family involvement throughout the continuum of care, the easier implementation of services will be for FAH.

14.2.2   Maintaining Mental Health

Early in the epidemic, rates of clinical disorder were high. In our family program in New York City in the mid 1990s, 70% of parents with HIV attended mental health counseling (Rotheram-Borus et al. 1997, 2001, 2003) and 84% reported enough symptoms to be considered seriously disturbed. Among the children of FAH, 39% reported anxiety disorders, 20% depressive disorders, and 46% any disorder (Rice et al. 2009). Parents and children's mental health symptoms are highly correlated, as would be expected. Adolescents, in particular, may copy their parents' styles of coping with stress (Lester et al. 2009). Mothers were faced with balancing their illness and managing various life stressors (i.e., medication adherence, health care providers, economic and housing pressures, finances, single parenthood, and partner, child, and family relational problems). Teens were faced with the challenges of living with an ill parent (i.e., worry and questions about parental illness, focusing on individual lives despite parental illness, and parentification). Even with a public social and health care safety net, families in the developed world required long-term emotional and informational support in coping with stressors.

Yet, 10 years later in the USA in 2004, FAH did not have significant mental health symptoms; when HIV is a chronic illness and families have access to health care, there are far fewer negative consequences from HIV (Rice et al. 2009). FAH report few problem behaviors related to physical health, mental health, or sexual or drug transmission acts. In fact, FAH reported lower rates of alcohol use and family conflict than did a matched sample of non-HIV-affected families. A randomized controlled trial of 339 mothers and 259 of their school-age children in FAH was randomly assigned to receive an intervention of 16 sessions in a cognitive-behavioral, small-group format; or standard services as the control condition. Compared to mothers in FAH in the control condition, mothers in the intervention FAH were significantly more likely to monitor their own health, and their children were more likely to decrease drug use than children in FAH in the control condition. Interventions remain useful, but the much lower levels of distress and problems in the FAH in Los Angeles from 2002 to 2006 suggest the dramatic changes associated with HIV becoming a chronic disease with ready access to treatment in the USA.

14.2.3   Reducing Sexual and Drug Transmission Acts

After learning that one is seropositive, between half to two-thirds of HIV+ persons reduce their transmission acts (Rotheram-Borus and Miller 1998). Parent's substance abuse has an immediate impact on youth's substance use, but the impact decreases when parents stop using. Active parental use of hard drugs was related to increased adolescent emotional distress, depression, anxiety, and difficult peer relationships. Higher rates of substance use were reported in children whose parents used marijuana. This suggested that the teens' behaviors were influenced by parental modeling. The dysfunctional adolescent symptoms improved and were more similar to the experience of children of nonuser parents when parents refrained from actively using hard drugs (Rotheram-Borus et al. 2009a).

14.2.4   Social Relationships

Custody planning was initially perceived as an important issue for FAH in the USA during the early to mid-1990s as AIDS was a terminal illness with none or few available treatments. Other sessions focused on parents telling their "story of HIV" and identifying the meaning of HIV in their life. A significant number of the parent and teen sessions were focused on sadness, anger, and fear related to AIDS. Although one session addressed looking at the future, there was no emphasis on concrete long-term life goals. Instead, the sessions focused on looking at the future by examining "unfinished business," past pain, guilt, and forgiveness, and freeing themselves of their wants. Similarly, the individual teen sessions emphasized mother's legacy, coping with new custody arrangements, stigma, loss, and grief. If parents died, 16 sessions were delivered to new caregivers and adolescents, which focused on grief, bereavement, and setting new life goals. Since the advent of effective treatments for HIV infection, the interventions for FAH shifted focus on social relationships toward building and maintaining social support for coping with HIV as a chronic illness.

14.3   Adaptation of HIV Family Interventions in Los Angeles, South Africa, and Thailand

The situational challenges facing HIV-affected families are universal. One possible strategy to address these challenges is through the common factors and processes that cut across all EBI. Based on our research analyzing manuals from EBI, we proposed five factors that successful EBI for HIV prevention have in common: (1) establish a framework to understand behavior change; (2) convey issue-specific and population-specific information necessary for healthy actions; (3) build cognitive, affective, and behavioral self-management skills; (4) address environmental barriers to implementing health behaviors; and (5) provide tools to develop ongoing social and community support for healthy actions (Rotheram-Borus et al. 2009b).

14.4   Adaptation of HIV Family Interventions in the USA: New York City and Los Angeles

From 1993 to 1994, 307 eligible families (420 adolescent children and 307 parents living with HIV (PLH)) were recruited from the Division of AIDS Services in New York City, reflecting 84% of all traceable referrals of persons with AIDS. Of these, 134 mothers living with HIV (MLH) died about 28 months after recruitment, leaving 169 MLH alive. Over 6 years, we retained more than 85% of the parents and youth with at least one annual assessment. Assessments were conducted every 3 months for 2 years and then at 6-month intervals ($n = 17$ assessments), providing stable estimates of families' changes over 8 years. Half were randomly assigned to an intervention condition and half received the standard New York City intensive services from the Division of AIDS.

Focus groups, pilot work, and previous research informed the intervention design. Based on social cognitive theories, we based the intervention on the principle that people change slowly over time in relationships, taking small steps with opportunities and rewards (Bandura 1994). An extensive, detailed manual containing the specific goals, activities, and scripts for each session is available at http://chipts.ucla.edu. The intervention consisted of three modules totaling 24 sessions: (1) adapting to serostatus (including disclosure and custody issues); (2) stopping risk behaviors; and (3) bereavement. The sessions were delivered on 12 Saturdays in a centralized location in New York City that included two meals and childcare.

The parents were predominantly African–American and Latino injecting drug users and partners of injecting drug users. Most parents had histories of polydrug use, many had been jailed and treated in inpatient drug rehabilitation facilities, and 70% were diagnosed as HIV+ when presenting with an AIDS-defining illness and being hospitalized. The parents had many symptoms of depression: 84% reported enough symptoms to be concerned about a case of mental disorder (Derogatis et al. 1974). Only about half had a recent sexual partner, 3% had more than one sexual partner, and 50% had bartered sex at some point. About 75% of the parents and youth attended the intervention.

By 2 years after recruitment, the intervention adolescents and parents reported significantly fewer problem behaviors and less emotional distress than those in the standard care condition. Coping skills were significantly higher among intervention youth, and parents had significantly more positive social support in the intervention condition, compared to standard care condition. Over 4 years following the delivery of a coping skills intervention, fewer adolescents became teenage parents and fewer parents were drug dependent in the intervention compared to those in the control condition (Rotheram-Borus et al. 2009a). Intervention parents also tended to relapse less often into substance abuse and coped with a passive-withdrawal style less often. Adolescent conduct problems and parental problem behaviors tended to be lower in the intervention condition over 4 years compared to the standard care condition. At 6 years, offspring of teenagers in the intervention condition tended to have significantly higher IQ and home environment scores than offspring in the standard care condition (Rotheram-Borus et al. 2006). Adolescents also were more likely to be employed and to have better romantic relationships than the young people in the control condition.

HIV-affected populations, treatment options, and delivery systems have changed dramatically in the last 10 years, which has shifted the predictable, HIV-related challenges that impact MLH and their children. From 2002 to 2006, we randomized 339 mostly Latino and African–American MLH and 159 of their school-age children in Los Angeles, CA, to either (1) an efficacious small-group, 16-session intervention adapted to the new challenges or (2) a control condition. In addition, a neighborhood control of 159 non-HIV-affected mothers and children was also recruited, with 78% retention for follow-up assessments at 6, 12, and 18 months later. At recruitment, MLH reported few health and mental health problems, were adherent to medical regimens, did not engage in unprotected sex or drug use acts, and were highly similar to the non-HIV-affected families. MLH were significantly less depressed and anxious, with significant decreases in mental health symptoms over time, compared to the neighborhood controls. Among the MLH, mothers in the intervention condition were significantly more likely to monitor their own health, but were similar on other outcomes compared to control MLH. Intervention children significantly decreased their hard drug use compared to those in the control condition, but were similar on other outcomes. There were significant differences between the intervention and the control condition; yet, there were far fewer challenges for families in 2004 compared to 1994.

HIV has become a chronic disease and the negative impact on families appears reduced in the USA, with families with HIV reporting fewer stressors and fewer problem behaviors than non-HIV-affected families in the same neighborhood. Family interventions in the USA should now be targeted to HIV-affected families who are experiencing problems or are at very high risk of problems.

14.5 Adaptation of HIV Family Interventions in South Africa

14.5.1 Status of HIV in South Africa

South Africa has the highest number of persons living with HIV of any country (UNAIDS 2009). South Africa also has the highest documented rate of Fetal Alcohol Syndrome (FAS) globally (May et al. 2000), and the rate has been increasing over the past 10 years (Viljoen et al. 2005). Simultaneously, hazardous alcohol use is related to child malnutrition; 17% of children have birth weights under 2,500 g, and 24% are stunted and/or malnourished under the age of 5 years, resulting in lifelong negative health outcomes (Le Roux et al. 2010). Although clinics could address alcohol and nutrition problems, there are currently 30% of pregnant women who do not choose to access antenatal care (Rollins et al. 2007; South African Department of Health 2008) and clinics neither screen nor systematically provide care for alcohol use or nutrition. Thus, HIV+ pregnant women in South Africa face intersecting epidemics of alcohol and malnutrition, and continued risk for HIV. We are currently evaluating two projects in South Africa. One is a home-based testing program, and the other is a clinic-based intervention for pregnant HIV+ women that integrates HIV and alcohol prevention with maternal and child health services.

Because perinatal prevention programs are so successful for HIV+ pregnant mothers (Volmink and Marais 2008), the South African government (2008) indicates that 98% of pregnant women are tested for HIV and access to ARV at childbirth is guaranteed. HIV+ mothers have challenges caring for their own compromised health, and the health of their at-risk baby. Specifically, mothers must engage in at least 15 different behaviors to keep their babies safe from HIV: getting HIV tested, getting HIV test results, taking AZT during the last weeks of pregnancy, taking NVP during labor, AZT adherence postnatally, administering AZT to the infant, breastfeeding only, getting the infant tested at 6 weeks, getting the PCR results for the infant, and going to a clinic for one's own health. These behaviors need ongoing support, not easily addressed in a clinic visit.

In addition to concerns about HIV, 30% of pregnant mothers use alcohol at a hazardous level. South Africa has the highest per capita alcohol consumption rate (Warren et al. 2001). Children of mothers with hazardous, dependent, or harmful alcohol use have changes in body and brain morphology; demonstrate deficits in cognitive functioning, verbal fluency, executive functioning, motor development, and school achievement; and have emotional and behavioral problems (Kodituwakku et al. 2001; May et al. 2004; O'Connor and Kasari 2000; Paley et al. 2005; Riley and

McGee 2005. Even low levels of alcohol consumption have been linked to negative developmental sequelae (Sood et al. 2001). Among alcohol users, 75% also smoke cigarettes (May et al. 2005, 2008), which is linked to having underweight babies. In townships, postpartum depression rates exceed 30% (Cooper et al. 1999; Rochat et al. 2006) and are significantly related to alcohol as well. Comorbid alcohol use and depression negatively impact infant outcomes (Kelly et al. 2002), particularly infant malnutrition and stunting in South Africa. Mothers with depressive symptoms demonstrate decreased nurturing behaviors in interactions with their children (Petterson and Albers 2001; O'Connor 1996), similar to that in the USA (Meschke et al. 2003), and are most resistant to alcohol treatment (O'Connor and Whaley 2006).

In South Africa, stunting is 24.5%, wasting rates are 8.9%, and low birth weights are present in 17% of newborns (Zere and McIntyre 2003). Each of these conditions is associated with maternal depression as well as developmental delays, premature death in childhood, and children becoming diabetic and obese adults (45–75% of township adults) (Harvey et al. 2007). About 12% of South African children die before their fifth birthday (Barbarin 2003). Child malnutrition is responsible for 2% of child deaths, 3% of childhood disabilities, and long-term reduction in quality of adjusted life years (Zere and McIntyre 2003). In particular, low birth weights of less than 2,500 g are associated with substantial lifelong impairments in neurocognitive and socio-emotional development (Thompson et al. 1997). In poor households, more than half the children lack sufficient food daily (Myer et al. 2004). Intervening to improve child nutrition is as critical as HIV treatment and alcohol-use prevention.

South Africa has recognized the importance of horizontally integrated services and has developed a funding stream for the management of childhood diseases (i.e., Integrated Management of Childhood Illness [IMCD]). Currently, community health workers are hired in each community, but receive little or no training. The programs we are running in South Africa are *EBI alternatives to the existing IMCD community health workers, one that makes IMCD accountable in new ways.*

14.5.2 Mothers to Mothers HIV Prevention Program

Efficacious HIV prevention programs utilize common components, common processes, and common principles, based on social cognitive theories (Ingram et al. 2008; Rotheram-Borus et al. 2009b). Rather than create a new South African HIV prevention program, this project has adapted existing content, processes, and messages of EBI into a new delivery format: paraprofessional Mentor Mothers in home visits. Paraprofessional counselors are often used by WHO to implement a broad variety of programs (King 1966; Colle 1980), and home visits have been a very effective strategy for HIV testing (Were et al. 2003; Mermin et al. 2004) and are now a strategy for diffusing attitudes toward circumcisions in sub-Saharan Africa, as well as for child adjustment over the life course (Olds et al. 1988, 2002, 2004). Community level interventions that provide access to resources to all families are also important structural interventions (Sumartojo 2000; Jana et al. 2004).

By integrating programs for HIV with alcohol and nutrition, primarily by improving parenting, we are mainstreaming HIV prevention into a framework of "family well-being." Framing the issues of HIV within the context of a non-stigmatizing, community level support program for parenting is aimed at being the next generation of HIV prevention program (Rotheram-Borus and Duan 2003). Our collaborating agency, "Philani," was chosen because it is a nutritional support organization operating in the community for almost 30 years, but not addressing HIV or alcohol. Given their history within the community and focus on nutrition, there is little stigma and neighbors would not know that alcohol use, tuberculosis, or HIV is addressed by the paraprofessional Mentor Mother visits.

In the developing world, home-based support services cannot feasibly be delivered by nurses, as is advocated in the USA by Olds and colleagues (1994, 2002, 2004). To solve this dilemma, we are adopting the model of positive peer deviants, or mothers whose children are thriving as the selection criteria for the home-visiting Mentor Mothers (Aruna et al. 2001; Berggren and Wray 2002; Marsh et al. 2004; Sternin et al. 1998). The theory of positive peer deviants (Berggren and Wray 2002) has guided the selection of Mentor Mothers as a feasible delivery strategy for the services. Mentor Mothers are neighborhood mothers who have been provided training, materials, and skills to address issues of HIV/TB, malnutrition, and alcohol use. Mentor Mothers become sources of social support, making home visits to monitor a baby's progress and provide alcohol and HIV/TB information and skills to mothers to use the clinic-based care and adhere to health care providers' recommendations in daily life on an ongoing basis. Mothers whose children thrive typically have good social skills, an ability to develop caring social relationships, and a sense of pragmatism. Philani has used these criteria since its founding in 1979 to select Mentor Mothers. Mentor Mothers visit the at-risk family or mothers daily when the family is in a crisis and on an ongoing basis. Because the Mentor Mother resides in the community, she may also become a bridge for the mothers to network with her neighbors. Thus, similar to Olds et al. (2002), the Philani Intervention Program is based on the ecology of the African context, building attachment and self-efficacy of mother with her baby.

In addition to providing educational materials, the Mentor Mothers monitor the children's progress over time in all families (e.g., they carry a scale and development charts). The Philani program already has an active training process and assessment protocols that are easy to use by all Mentor Mothers for routinely assessing the mother and infant at each home visit. The written protocol forms show the expected height/weight for each baby, key aspects of the home environment (e.g., mother is dressed, has fed children, home is neat, and children's location is monitored). This chart is updated on each home visit by the Mentor Mother and kept over 18 months by all Mentor Mothers on each family.

14.5.3   Tools Used in Intervention

Several intervention tools were adapted from our US interventions for FAH to the South African context. To increase awareness and skills to regulate emotions, women are taught to use Feeling Cups to calibrate their feelings, which is an adaptation of the commonly used "feeling thermometer" in the USA. A clear glass is filled with different levels of water, depending on their degree of uncomfortable (full) feelings. Tokens are small chips that are not cashed in for any tangible reward; however, they are exchanged during intervention sessions between participants to indicate that the Mentor Mother has a positive feeling toward the mother and her participation. Mothers are provided with an empty jar to store their chips and are able to count the number of times they adhere to their goals. This technique is an adaptation of the self-monitoring diaries used in the USA.

Other activities we identified are related to the intervention messages: (1) showing how an egg poaches in alcohol that is at room temperature to demonstrate the effects of drinking alcohol on the brain of an unborn infant; (2) having a small jar with two different colors of jelly beans in a ratio that reflects the percentage of persons with HIV in the community; (3) showing pictures of women with HIV prior to and following ARV (Lazarus effect); (4) a doll with brown skin that has fetal alcohol syndrome; (5) a normal size baby doll with brown skin (highly realistic); (6) cards that show the HIV test results after their baby is tested; (7) cards to provide to the sister (nurse) at childbirth that says "I am HIV+, please make sure that I get NVP," helping the woman communicate her HIV status without disclosure; (8) pictures taken at each assessment of the mother or the mother and baby that are given immediately to take home; and (9) a workbook that summarizes the mother's experience.

Although AVT is available in South Africa, access and utilization to treatment and prevention services are hindered by high levels of HIV stigma and instrumental barriers around patient-initiated travel from rural or semi-rural areas to centralized treatment clinics for follow-up services. Thus, managing HIV as a chronic disease in South Africa, and similar contexts with limited health care service systems, is not universally or easily achievable. The Mentor Mothers program is an example of an approach to scaling up HIV prevention and treatment services that bridges existing health care services and community health worker capacities to incorporate HIV and comorbid or co-occurring risks. The safety net services and provider training levels are significantly different from those in the USA, yet the core intervention elements are universally applicable and adaptable across context and settings.

14.6 Adaptation of HIV Family Interventions in Thailand

14.6.1 Status of HIV Prevention in Thailand

Thailand once led the way as a model country to combat HIV, with a series of successful campaigns that helped to reduce the national HIV prevalence. In the new millennium, however, there were signs of complacency. Prevention programs received just 8% of the national HIV budget in 2000, and by 2001, the level of domestic funding for HIV prevention was half of what it had been in

1997 (UNDP 2004). By 2006, UNAIDS reported that Thailand government had reduced its HIV prevention budget by two-thirds (UNAIDS 2006).

The declining focus on HIV prevention and treatment had direct impact on putting the public at risk. Recent evidence suggested that condom use had decreased and the transmission rate of sexually transmitted diseases (STDs) had risen (The Nation 2006; Medical News Today 2006). Without new prevention campaigns, there is a risk that safe sex messages would be forgotten and a new generation of young people would grow up complacent of the risks that they may face.

It is estimated that over 610,000 people in Thailand are living with HIV, where a majority of infected are adults older than 15 years of age (41% among women). An astounding 80% of Thailand's HIV infections occur through heterosexual sex (USAID 2005). Since 2000, the government has provided ART to PLH in Thailand through more than 914 public hospitals. An increase in the production of cheap generic drugs within Thailand has allowed the government to obtain medicines at much lower cost, leading to more than an eightfold expansion in treatment provision between 2001 and 2003, with only a 40% increase in budget (Ford et al. 2004).

Thailand has effectively demonstrated, in both prevention and treatment fronts, that it is possible for a developing country to form an effective response to HIV. For all its successes, however, there are still certain regions and groups badly affected by the epidemic. People living with HIV and the needs of their family members need to be addressed, and there is an urgent need for developing interventions that focus on family wellness to assist HIV-affected families in Thailand.

14.6.2   Healthy Families Program

Framing interventions in terms of "Family Wellness" as opposed to HIV prevention helps overcome stigma and marginalization of PLH while supporting the family in addressing common developmental challenges and environmental barriers that drive risks for HIV infection as well as other diseases and life challenges. We describe common elements of EBI for HIV-affected families in Thailand which include the common factors, processes, and tools and activities and how we adapted these common elements.

14.6.2.1   Intervention Target Group

Building on the previous intervention trials in the USA, we aimed to culturally adapt and evaluate the effectiveness of a sustainable family intervention, Family-to-Family (F2F), for families coping with HIV. In Thailand, the intervention target groups consisted of PLH and their family members. The intervention is provided to all adults living in the households of HIV+ parents in which there is a school-age child aged 6–17 years.

14.6.2.2 Adaptation Process

In Thailand, we hypothesized that the social, behavioral, and mental health adjustment of school-age children will be improved when their parents and family caregivers (i.e., HIV+ parents, partners, and family caregivers) participate in a psychoeducational intervention that frames the problem of HIV, provides information about the specific HIV-related stressors (e.g., disclosure, stigma, and transmission acts), builds skills, and provides ongoing social support mechanisms. Drop-in groups in district hospital settings were proposed as the delivery vehicle that will provide routine access to families, as well as an ideal context for delivering ongoing supportive intervention boosters. As children age and present new developmental challenges and parent's HIV disease progresses, the types of stressful situations experienced by families will shift and families will need booster sessions to maintain behavioral gains.

14.6.2.3 Frame the Problem

In Thailand, the F2F program was framed as a support program for persons with chronic illness. We framed the problem (living with HIV) by "normalizing" the types of challenges that all families coping with HIV experience. We designed the intervention to have PLH, partners, and caregivers to be allowed to drop into the same group or different groups to allow families to learn from other families experiencing similar problems.

14.6.2.4 Provide HIV-Specific Information and Encourage Positive Beliefs and Attitudes to Cope with HIV

Interventions need to provide specific information and promote beliefs and attitudes to cope with HIV-related challenges, physical and mental health, and family adjustment. Four domains emerged from focus group discussions regarding the content of family-centered approach to HIV intervention in Thailand: (1) healthy body, (2) healthy mind, (3) healthy families, and (4) healthy community. The format of the intervention session was designed so that each session provided information in an engaging style. The information was tailored to each of the different roles of parents, caregivers, and partners. After reviewing the successes and strengths of the week, the intervention facilitator presents topic information of the day for no more than 15 minutes, accompanied by support materials that can be taken home and reviewed. Given that the issues underlying the content session areas are large and will reemerge in different ways at different stages of illness, the intervention format was designed with highly interactive activities involving family members from different families helping each other.

14.6.2.5   Provide Skills to Cope with the Four Domains

To keep the skills simple, families were asked to rehearse and practice identifying and self-regulating their feelings in HIV-related situations, their thinking patterns in difficult situations, and their social skills. A set of activities, designed so that the participants can learn from each other, was the primary strategy for increasing skills. By asking group attendees to break up into dyads with a participant similar to themselves (HIV+ parents with HIV+ parents, caregivers with caregivers) or complementary dyads (HIV+ parents with caregivers or partners), they were able to increase their skills through practice and role-play.

Children at various levels of development need different things and require different modes of instruction. By allowing only all adults in the families coping with HIV to participate, the power of the intervention was heightened, without the added complication of children of multiple ages attending the same intervention.

14.6.2.6   Address Environmental Barriers to Implementation

The primary environmental barrier for families with HIV was access to ongoing health care. The families were recruited from district hospitals and the Thai government has guaranteed HIV+ persons access to health care. Thus, the intervention consisted of information and skills about when and how to access health care. We also identified other environmental challenges: decreased financial resources associated with parent's illness, access to condoms in order to stop transmission, and transportation costs. In response, we provided access to transportation in the program. Having access to other families experiencing the same challenges also provided instrumental support, in addition to the social support that was included in the program.

14.6.2.7   Provide Support for Maintaining the Behaviors Over Time

Support is being created for all adults in HIV+ families by inviting all adult family members affected by HIV to attend the intervention (if the HIV+ parent provides permission). In addition, the intervention sessions were designed as drop-in sessions so that families can participate in the session on multiple occasions for as long as they desired. District hospitals in Thailand carry out monthly support groups for PLH, which constitutes the standard of care for families living with HIV in Thailand.

14.6.3   Adaptation of Intervention Tools and Activities

Buddhism, which is the religious affiliation claimed by 95% of the Thai population (Jenkins and Kim 2004), played a key role in framing the intervention tools and activities in Thailand. In particular, the pragmatic, empirical aspects of Buddhism proved useful in framing the intervention contents and activities; its emphasis on personal responsibility, its support of personal betterment in the present time, and its attention to impermanence and change all played a key role in framing the intervention (Jenkins and Kim 2004). Key intervention tools and activities, outlined in Table 14.1, were framed in a culturally relevant and acceptable way to ensure intervention acceptability. The tools and activities included relaxation, use of the Feeling Thermometer, Feel-Think-Do (FTD) framework, tokens, role-playing, and pair-sharing. The tools and activities were examined among the workgroups involving the US research team, the Thai research team, and health care providers from Thai provincial and district levels. The workgroup focused on framing the tools and activities to fit the Thai culture.

14.6.3.1   Relaxation

As a country deeply rooted in Buddhism, meditation emerged as a highly relevant and applicable relaxation activity in Thailand (Chuaprapaisilp 1997). Therefore, meditation was employed throughout the pilot sessions as a relaxation activity. In addition, meditation was applied as a stress management tool in several of the intervention sessions. Singing and dancing were incorporated as ice-breaking activities; these were relevant and appropriate in Thai culture, thus promoting group cohesiveness and a supportive environment.

14.6.3.2   Feeling Thermometer

Buddhism advocates self-awareness or being present. Incorporating this element of Buddhism into the intervention, the Feeling Thermometer was framed as an effective tool to help participants understand their current state (feelings). *The application of the Feeling Thermometer made this concept more tangible and concrete.*

14.6.3.3   Feel-Think-Do Model

The FTD model is a concept based on the cognitive behavioral therapy founded on the idea that our feelings, or physiological responses to events, influence our thoughts and behaviors. The benefit of this model is that we can alter the way we think, thus enabling us to feel or act better even if the situation does not change. The FTD model allows us to manage our physiological responses (through awareness and relaxation), facilitating clearer thought and actions in accordance with our intentions. In Thailand, the FTD model was framed within the context of Buddhist belief in self-awareness and the positive cycle of cause and effect. The FTD model is also related and linked to the concept of positive thinking in dealing with HIV-related challenges.

Table 14.1 Common factors and toolkits in family-based interventions for HIV-affected families in Thailand

Common factors	
Establish a framework to understand behavior change	"Normalize" challenges facing HIV-affected families
Convey issue-specific and population-specific information	Address four domains:
	– Maintaining healthy mind
	– Maintaining healthy body
	– Maintaining healthy family relations
	– Improving social and community integration
Build cognitive, affective, and behavioral self-management skills	– Rehearse and practice identifying and self-regulating their feelings in HIV-related situations, their thinking patterns in difficult situations, and their social skills
Address environmental barriers to implementing health behaviors	– Access to ongoing healthcare
	– Access to transportation
Provide tools to develop ongoing social and community support	– Interventions designed as drop-in sessions
	– District hospitals' monthly support groups for HIV-affected families
Common toolkits	
Relaxation and ice-breaking activities	– Meditation
	– Singing
	– Dancing
Feeling thermometer	– Tied to Buddhism advocating self-awareness
	– Effective tool to understand their current state (feelings)
Feel-think-do (FTD) model	– Promoting positive cycle of cause and effect
	– Buddhist philosophy of linking feelings, thoughts, and actions
Tokens	– Yellow color represents loyalty and respect to the King
	– Stars represent culturally accepted symbol for rewards
	– Facilitate expression of kindness and joy
Role-playing	– Effective tool to reduce stress
	– Practice challenging hypothetical scenarios
Pair-sharing	– Effective dyadic exercise to act out situational challenges
	– Rehearse a variety of different problem-solving scenarios with different participants

14.6.3.4 Tokens

We used yellow tokens (small squares of construction paper) with a star, color and symbol accepted by the Thai population, as value-free rewards that are exchanged between group participants and intervention facilitators to acknowledge and encourage participation. Stars in Thailand are culturally accepted symbol for rewards; the color yellow represents loyalty and respect to the king of Thailand (B.B.C. News 2006). For example, in honor of the 60th anniversary of his accession to the throne and continuing until his 80th birthday celebration on 5 December 2007, Thailand has been a veritable sea of yellow as the people of Thailand showed support for their king. Therefore, the yellow token in Thailand carried a much deeper significance and meaning and went beyond a simple token of approval and appreciation. In addition, the use of tokens facilitated the expression of kindness and joy, which are pillars of the Buddhist principles of Phrom Viharn 4 (Phaosavasdi et al. 2006).

14.6.3.5 Role-Playing and Pair-Sharing

Role-playing proved to be an effective and useful tool to reduce stress. It is not common in Thailand to act out certain scenarios. Therefore, role-playing provided participants opportunities to act out certain situations in a safe, comfortable setting and proved to be an effective strategy to practice challenging hypothetical scenarios (e.g., disclosing one's HIV status to a family member). Similar to role-playing activities, pair-sharing activities proved to be an effective dyadic exercise for PLH and family members to act out situational challenges that all HIV-affected families face. By rotating partners in pair-sharing, participants were able to rehearse a variety of different problem-solving scenarios with other PLH or family members. Each role-playing and pair-sharing activity consisted of the application of Feeling Thermometer, FTD models, and the use of tokens.

In summary, mounting an effective family-based intervention in Thailand was accomplished in a systematic, collaborative manner, thus ensuring the intervention's success, cultural relevance, and sustainability. The pragmatic, empirical aspects of Buddhism in Thailand proved useful in framing the intervention contents and activities; its emphasis on personal responsibility, its support of personal betterment in the present time, and its attention to impermanence and change all played a key role in framing the intervention.

14.7 Conclusion

Developing countries cannot broadly mount categorically funded programs, such as HIV prevention. Even with donor funding, the health care budgets are so low as to require horizontally integrated care. Yet, efficacious HIV prevention programs have been designed almost entirely for vertically integrated health care systems only

(Myer et al. 2006). HIV prevention programs typically address a single outcome (reducing HIV transmission) and are categorically funded and vertically integrated (HIV provided at the clinic, hospital, township, provincial, and national levels). The Global Fund, the US HIV funding (PEPFAR), World Bank, and a variety of private donors (Gates, Clinton) fund HIV prevention and care only. In 33 of 41 African countries (70%), the total health care budget is less than 30 USD per person and only two countries spend more than 10% of their annual budgets on health care. In contrast, the USA spends 15.3% of gross domestic product on health care and at 6,714 USD per person annually (http://www.who.int/countries/usa/en/). Although South Africa spends 869 USD per person annually (8.6% of budget), it is insufficient to fund HIV categorically, when there is a 30% infection rate among pregnant women. Additionally, more than 60% of the children who die under the age of 5 years (12% of children) die from malnutrition, dehydration, other infections, or complications related to alcohol use (Statistics South Africa 2008). Prevention must be comprehensive, and families are an ideal social unit to target with comprehensive prevention programs.

The global need for comprehensive family-based HIV interventions exceeds our current capacities to design, deliver, and diffuse programs that are both effective and relevant to local communities. Given increased funding and political will to scale HIV prevention globally, new models of intervention design and adaptation are needed to quicken the adoption and adaptation process in collaboration with service providers, community leaders, and families affected by HIV and related diseases and challenges in local communities. Common factors, processes, and principles operationalize intervention elements in a framework that facilitates adaptation to local priorities while maintaining fidelity to elements that support intervention effectiveness. Family-based interventions provide opportunities to intervene early in the life course, build social support and skills that prevent HIV and promote health broadly throughout life, and overcome stigma that is a significant barrier to HIV-identified service utilization.

Correspondence regarding this chapter should be directed to Mary Jane Rotheram-Borus Ph.D., at 10920 Wilshire Blvd., Suite 350, Los Angeles, CA 90024. Ph: 310.794.8280; Fax: 310.794.8297; E-mail: Rotheram@ucla.edu

References

Abdul-Quader AS, Jarlais DC, Chatterjee A, Hirky AE, Friedman SR. Interventions for injecting drug users. In: Gibney L, DiClemente RJ, Vermund SH, editors. Preventing HIV in developing countries: biomedical and behavioral approaches. New York: Plenum; 2002. p. 283–312.

Aruna M, Vazir S, Vidyasagar P. Child rearing and positive deviance in the development of pre-schoolers: a microanalysis. Indian Pediatr. 2001;38(4):332–9.

B.B.C. News. Thailand marks king's anniversary [on the internet]. Available at: http://news.bbc.co.uk/2/hi/asia-pacific/5062534.stm (2006). Cited 2 Mar 2011.

Bandura A. Social cognitive theory and exercise of control over HIV infection. In: DiClemente RJ, Peterson JL, editors. Preventing AIDS: theories and methods of behavioral interventions. New York: Plenum; 1994. p. 25–59.

Barbarin OA. Social risks and child development in South Africa: a nation's program to protect the human rights of children. Am J Orthopsychiatry. 2003;73(3):248–59.

Benotsch E, Kalichman S. Mental health and quality of life for people with HIV. Focus (San Francisco, California). 2001;16(11):5–6.

Berggren WL, Wray JD. Positive deviant behavior and nutrition education. Food Nutr Bull. 2002;23 Suppl 4:9–10.

Bhana D, Pattman R. Researching South African youth, gender and sexuality within the context of HIV/AIDS. Development. 2009;52(1):68–74.

Chuaprapaisilp A. Thai Buddhist philosophy and the action research process. Educ Action Res. 1997;5(2):331–6.

Colle RD. Paraprofessionals in rural development. Ithaca: Center for International Studies, Cornell University Press; 1980.

Cooper PJ, Tomlinson M, Swartz L, Woolgar M, Murray L, Molteno C. Post-partum depression and the mother-infant relationship in a South African peri-urban settlement. Br J Psychiatry. 1999;175(6):554–8.

Crepaz N, Marks G. Are negative affective states associated with HIV sexual risk behaviors? A meta-analytic review. Health Psychol. 2001;20(4):291–9.

Crepaz N, Marks G. Towards an understanding of sexual risk behavior in people living with HIV: a review of social, psychological, and medical findings. AIDS. 2002;16(2):135–49.

Crepaz N, Horn AK, Rama SM, Griffin T, Deluca JB, Mullins MM, et al. The efficacy of behavioral interventions in reducing HIV risk sex behaviors and incident sexually transmitted disease in black and Hispanic sexually transmitted disease clinic patients in the United States: a meta-analytic review. Sex Transm Dis. 2007;34(6):319–32.

Derogatis LR, Lipman RS, Rickels K, Uhlenhuth EH, Covi L. The Hopkins Symptom Checklist (HSCL): a self report symptom inventory. Behav Sci. 1974;19(1):1–15.

El-Sadr WM, Mayer KH, Hodder SL. AIDS in America – forgotten but not gone. N Engl J Med. 2010;362(11):967–70.

European Collaborative Study. Mother-to-child transmission of HIV infection in the era of highly active antiretroviral therapy. Clin Infect Dis. 2005;40(3):458–65.

Ford N, Wilson D, Bunjumnong O, von Schoen Angerer T. The role of civil society in protecting public health over commercial interests: lessons from Thailand. Lancet. 2004;363(9408):560–3. doi:S0140-6736(04)15545-1 [pii]10.1016/S0140-6736(04)15545-1.

Harvey EA, Friedman-Weieneth JL, Goldstein LH, Sherman AH. Examining subtypes of behavior problems among 3-year-old children, Part I: investigating validity of subtypes and biological risk-factors. J Abnorm Child Psychol. 2007;35(1):97–110.

Ingram B, Flannery D, Elkavich A, Rotheram-Borus M. Common processes in evidence-based adolescent HIV prevention programs. AIDS Behav. 2008;12(3):374–83. doi:10.1007/s10461-008-9369-1.

Jana S, Basu I, Rotheram-Borus M, Newman P. The Sonagachi Project: a sustainable community intervention program. AIDS Educ Prev. 2004;16(5):405–14. doi:10.1521/aeap. 16.5.405.48734.

Jenkins RA, Kim B. Cultural norms and risk: lessons learned from HIV in Thailand. J Prim Prev. 2004;25(1):17–40. doi:10.1023/B:JOPP.0000039937.50357.fc.

Kalichman SC. HIV transmission risk behaviors of men and women living with HIV AIDS: prevalence, predictors, and emerging clinical interventions. Clin Psychol Sci Pract. 2000;7(1):32–47.

Kellerman S, Essajee S. HIV testing for children in resource-limited settings: what are we waiting for? PLoS Med. 2010;7(7):1–5.

Kelly RH, Russo J, Holt VL, Danielsen BH, Zatzick DF, Walker E, et al. Psychiatric and substance use disorders as risk factors for low birth weight and preterm delivery. Obstet Gynecol. 2002;100(2):297–304.

King M, editor. Medical care in developing countries: a symposium from Makerere. London: Oxford University Press; 1966.

Knodel J. Poverty and the impact of AIDS on older persons: evidence from Cambodia and Thailand [proceedings paper]. Econ Dev Cult Change. 2008;56(2):441–75.

Kodituwakku PW, Kalberg W, May PA. The effects of prenatal alcohol exposure on executive functioning. Alcohol Res Health. 2001;25(3):192–9.

le Roux I, le Roux K, Comulada WS, Greco E, Desmond K, Mbewu N, et al. Home visits by neighborhood Mentor Mothers provide timely recovery from childhood malnutrition in South Africa: results from a randomized controlled trial. Nutr J. 2010;9(1):56.

Lester PE, Weiss RE, Rice E, Comulada WS, Lord L, Alber S, et al. The longitudinal impact of HIV+ parents' drug use on their adolescent children. Am J Orthopsychiatry. 2009;79(1):51–9. doi:10.1037/a0015427.

Lightfoot M, Rotheram-Borus MJ. Helping adolescents and parents with AIDS to cope effectively with daily life. In: Pequegnat W, Szapocznik J, editors. Working with families in the era of HIV/AIDS. Thousand Oaks: Sage; 2000. p. 189–200.

Marsh DR, Schroeder DG, Dearden KA, Sternin J, Sternin M. The power of positive deviance. BMJ. 2004;329(7475):1177–9. doi:329/7475/1177 [pii]10.1136/bmj.329.7475.1177.

May PA, Brooke L, Gossage JP, Croxford J, Adnams C, Jones KL, et al. Epidemiology of fetal alcohol syndrome in a South African community in the Western Cape Province. Am J Public Health. 2000;90(12):1905–12.

May PA, Gossage JP, White-Country M, Goodhart K, Decoteau S, Trujillo PM, et al. Alcohol consumption and other maternal risk factors for fetal alcohol syndrome among three distinct samples of women before, during, and after pregnancy: the risk is relative. Am J Med Genet C Semin Med Genet. 2004;127C(1):10–20.

May PA, Gossage JP, Brooke LE, Snell CL, Marais AS, Hendricks LS, et al. Maternal risk factors for fetal alcohol syndrome in the Western Cape Province of South Africa: a population-based study. Am J Public Health. 2005;95(7):1190–9.

May PA, Gossage JP, Marais AS, Hendricks LS, Snell CL, Tabachnick BG, et al. Maternal risk factors for fetal alcohol syndrome and partial fetal alcohol syndrome in South Africa: a third study. Alcohol Clin Exp Res. 2008;32(5):738–53.

Medical News Today. 'Thailand's HIV prevention program absent, endangering country, advocates say'. Available via: http://www.medicalnewstoday.com/articles/44083.php (May 2006). Cited 22 February 2011.

Mermin J, Lule J, Ekwaru JP, Malamba S, Downing R, Ransom R, et al. Effect of co-trimoxazole prophylaxis on morbidity, mortality, CD4-cell count, and viral load in HIV infection in rural Uganda. Lancet. 2004;364(9443):1428–34. doi:S0140673604172255 [pii]10.1016/S0140-6736(04)17225-5.

Meschke LL, Holl JA, Messelt S. Assessing the risk of fetal alcohol syndrome: understanding substance use among pregnant women. Neurotoxicol Teratol. 2003;25(6):667–74.

Mubangizi J, Downing R, Ssebbowa E, Bunnell R, Kalule J, Marum E, et al. (2000). Couples at risk: HIV-concordance and discordance among partners seeking HIV testing in Uganda. Int Conf AIDS. 2000 Jul 9–14;13. Abstract no. TuPeC3465.

Myer L, Ehrlich RI, Susser ES. Social epidemiology in South Africa. Epidemiol Rev. 2004;26(1):112–23. doi:10.1093/epirev/mxh004.

Myer L, Wright TC, Denny L, Kuhn L. Nested case-control study of cervical mucosal lesions, ectopy, and incident HIV infection among women in Cape Town, South Africa. Sex Transm Dis. 2006;33(11):683–7. doi:10.1097/01.olq.0000216026.67352.f9.

O'Connor MJ. The implication of attachment theory for the socioemotional development of children exposed to alcohol prenatally. In: Spohr HL, editor. Alcohol, pregnancy, and the developing child. Cambridge, UK: Press Syndicate of the University of Cambridge; 1996. p. 183–206.

O'Connor MJ, Kasari C. Prenatal alcohol exposure and depressive features in children. Alcohol Clin Exp Res. 2000;24(7):1084–92. doi:10.1111/j.1530-0277.2000.tb04654.x.

O'Connor MJ, Whaley SE. Health care provider advice and risk factors associated with alcohol consumption following pregnancy recognition. J Stud Alcohol. 2006;67(1):22–31.

Olds D, Henderson Jr C, Tatelbaum R, Chamberlin R. Improving the life-course development of socially disadvantaged mothers: a randomized trial of nurse home visitation. Am J Public Health. 1988;78(11):1436–45.

Olds DL, Henderson CR, Tatelbaum R. Prevention of intellectual impairment in children of women who smoke cigarettes during pregnancy. Pediatrics. 1994;93(2):228–33.

Olds DL, Robinson J, O'Brien R, Luckey DW, Pettitt LM, Henderson CR, et al. Home visiting by paraprofessionals and by nurses: a randomized, controlled trial. Pediatrics. 2002;110(3):486–96. doi:10.1542/peds.110.3.486.

Olds DL, Robinson J, Pettitt L, Luckey DW, Holmberg J, Ng RK, et al. Effects of home visits by paraprofessionals and by nurses: age 4 follow-up results of a randomized trial. Pediatrics. 2004;114(6):1560–8. doi:114/6/1560 [pii] 10.1542/peds.2004-0961.

Paley B, O Connor MJ, Kogan N, Findlay R. Prenatal alcohol exposure, child externalizing behavior, and maternal stress. Parenting. 2005;5(1):29–56.

Pearson CR, Micek M, Simoni JM, Matediana E, Martin DP, Gloyd S. Modified directly observed therapy to facilitate highly active antiretroviral therapy adherence in Beira, Mozambique: development and implementation. J Acquir Immune Defic Syndr. 2006;43:S134–41.

Petterson SM, Albers AB. Effects of poverty and maternal depression on early child development. Child Dev. 2001;72(6):1794–813.

Phaosavasdi S, Taneepanichsicul S, Tannirandorn Y, Pupong V, Pruksapong C, Kanjanapitak A. Muted ethics. J Med Assoc Thai. 2006;89(6):904.

Ravishankar N, Gubbins P, Cooley RJ, Leach-Kemon K, Michaud CM, Jamison DT, et al. Financing of global health: tracking development assistance for health from 1990 to 2007. Lancet. 2009;373(9681):2113–24.

Remien RH, Rabkin JG. Topics in review: psychological aspects of living with HIV disease: a primary care perspective. West J Med. 2001;175(5):332–5.

Rice E, Lester P, Flook L, Green S, Valladares ES, Rotheram-Borus MJ. Lessons learned from "integrating" intensive family-based interventions into medical care settings for mothers living with HIV/AIDS and their adolescent children. AIDS Behav. 2009;13(5):1005–11.

Riley E, McGee C. Fetal alcohol spectrum disorders: an overview 18. with emphasis on changes in brain and behavior. Exp Biol Med (Maywood). 2005;230(6):357–65.

Rochat TJ, Richter LM, Doll HA, Buthelezi NP, Tomkins A, Stein A. Depression among pregnant rural South African women undergoing HIV testing. JAMA. 2006;295(12):1376–8.

Rollins NC, Coovadia HM, Bland RM, Coutsoudis A, Bennish ML, Patel D, et al. Pregnancy outcomes in HIV-infected and uninfected women in rural and urban South Africa. J Acquir Immune Defic Syndr. 2007;44(3):321–8.

Rotheram-Borus MJ, Duan N. Next generation of preventive interventions. J Am Acad Child Adolesc Psychiatry. 2003;42(5):518–26. doi:S0890-8567(09)60936-9 [pii] 10.1097/01.CHI.0000046836.90931.E9.

Rotheram-Borus M, Miller S. Secondary prevention for youths living with HIV. AIDS Care. 1998;10(1):17–34.

Rotheram-Borus MJ, Murphy DA, Miller S, Draimin BH. An intervention for adolescents whose parents are living with AIDS. Clin Child Psychol Psychiatry. 1997;2(2):201–19. doi:10.1177/1359104597022003.

Rotheram-Borus MJ, Lee M, Zhou S, O'Hara P, Birnbaum JM, Wright W, et al. Variation in health and risk behavior among youth living with HIV. AIDS Educ Prev. 2001;13(1):42–54.

Rotheram-Borus MJ, Lee M, Leonard N, Lin YY, Franzke L, Turner E, et al. Four-year behavioral outcomes of an intervention for parents living with HIV and their adolescent children. AIDS. 2003;17(8):1217–25.

Rotheram-Borus MJ, Flannery D, Lester P, Rice E. Prevention for HIV-positive families. J Acquir Immune Defic Syndr. 2004;37:S133–4.

Rotheram-Borus MJ, Lester P, Song J, Lin YY, Leonard NR, Beckwith L, et al. Intergenerational benefits of family-based HIV interventions. J Consult Clin Psychol. 2006;74(3):622–7. doi:2006-08433-021 [pii]10.1037/0022-006X.74.3.622.

Rotheram-Borus MJ, Ingram BL, Swendeman D, Flannery D. Common principles embedded in effective adolescent HIV prevention programs. AIDS Behav. 2009a;13(3):387–98. doi:10.1007/s10461-009-9531-4.

Rotheram-Borus MJ, Swendeman D, Flannery D, Rice E, Adamson DM, Ingram B. Common factors in effective HIV prevention programs. AIDS Behav. 2009b;13(3):399–408.

Rotheram-Borus MJ, Richter L, Van Rooyen H, van Heerden A, Tomlinson M, Stein A, et al. Project Masihambisane: a cluster randomised controlled trial with peer mentors to improve outcomes for pregnant mothers living with HIV. Trials. 2011;12(1):2.

Sood B, Delaney-Black V, Covington C, Nordstrom-Klee B, Ager J, Templin T, et al. Prenatal alcohol exposure and childhood behavior at age 6 to 7 years: I. dose-response effect. Pediatrics. 2001;108(2):e34.

South African Department of Health. South African PMTCT policy (revised, 2008). Available via: http://www.doh.gov.za/docs/policy/pmtct.pdf (2008). Cited 4 March 2011.

Statistics South Africa. Mortality and causes of death in South Africa, 2006: findings from death notification. Available via: http://www.statssa.gov.za/publications/P03093/P030932003,2004. pdf (2008). Cited 4 Mar 2011.

Sternin M, Sternin J, Marsh D. Designing a community-based nutrition program using the hearth model and the positive deviance approach: a field guide. Westport, CT: Save the Children Federation/US; 1998.

Sumartojo E. Structural factors in HIV prevention: concepts, examples, and implications for research. AIDS. 2000;14:S3.

Swendeman D, Ingram BL, Rotheram-Borus MJ. Common elements in self-management of HIV and other chronic illnesses: an integrative framework. AIDS Care. 2009;21(10):1321–34.

The Nation. HIV prevention forgotten, now verging on crisis. Available via http://nationmultimedia. com/2006/05/24/national/national_30004762.php (May 2006). Cited 23 Feb 2011.

Thompson RJ, Gustafson KE, Oehler JM, Catlett AT. Developmental outcome of very low birth weight infants at four years of age as a function of biological risk and psychosocial risk. J Dev Behav Pediatr. 1997;18(2):783–92.

UNAIDS. Report on the global AIDS epidemic. Geneva, Switzerland: UNAIDS; 2006.

UNAIDS. AIDS epidemic update – December 2009. Geneva, Switzerland: UNAIDS; 2009.

UNDP. Thailand's response to HIV/AIDS. Bangkok, Thailand: UN Development Programme; 2004.

USAID. HIV program in Thailand. Available via: http://www.usaid.gov/our_work/global_health/ aids/Countries/asia/thailand_profile.pdf (2005). Cited 6 Mar 2011.

Viljoen DL, Gossage JP, Brooke L, Adnams CM, Jones KL, Robinson LK, et al. Fetal alcohol syndrome epidemiology in a South African community: a second study of a very high prevalence area. J Stud Alcohol. 2005;66(5):593–604.

Volmink J, Marais B. HIV and AIDS. Lancet. 2008;372(9635):300–13.

Warren KR, Calhoun FJ, May PA, Viljoen DL, Li TK, Tanaka H, et al. Fetal alcohol syndrome: an international perspective. Alcohol Clin Exp Res. 2001;25:202S–6.

Were W, Mermin J, Bunnell R, Ekwaru J, Kaharuza F. Home-based model for HIV voluntary counselling and testing. Lancet. 2003;361(9368):1569. doi:S0140-6736(03)13212-6 [pii]10.1016/S0140-6736(03)13212-6.

Wolitski RJ, Valdiserri RO, Stall R. Unequal opportunity: health disparities affecting gay and bisexual men in the United States. New York: Oxford University Press; 2008.

Zere E, McIntyre D. Inequities in under-five child malnutrition in South Africa. Int J Equity Health. 2003;2(1):7.

Chapter 15
Promoting Family-Focused Evidenced-Based Practice in Frontline HIV/AIDS Care

Bruce Rapkin and Claude Mellins

Abstract This chapter addresses challenges involved in disseminating evidence-based interventions to frontline HIV/AIDS care settings, to encourage more high-quality services for families affected by HIV/AIDS. In order to inform this discussion, this chapter examines the many ways in which HIV affects families, the rationale for reaching families through HIV-related service settings, and the many barriers that must be overcome. Next, we provide an overview of the Special Needs Clinic, which offers an exemplary model of a continuum of services organized to support families coping with HIV/AIDS alongside co-morbid medical and mental health problems, poverty, and substance use. Lessons learned at the Special Needs Clinic highlight some inherent difficulties in dissemination of behavioral and psychosocial interventions for families affected by HIV/AIDS, even under the best of circumstances. Next, we turn to results of the Family ACCESS to Care Study, based on interviews with 68 providers, 622 persons living with HIV/AIDS (PLHA), and 195 of their family members from 22 different community service agencies in New York City. Findings of this study demonstrate those PLHAs and their family members express high levels of unmet need for marital and family therapy and other family-focused services. Despite relevant training and experience, agency staff members perceive a mismatch between family-focused interventions and agencies' mission. Staff and family members also differ in the priorities they ascribe to different evidence-based interventions. Dissemination research focused on local experimentation and problem solving is needed to overcome challenges, bridge differences in perspectives, and build a strong foundation of support and care for families affected by HIV/AIDS.

15.1 Introduction

HIV/AIDS is understood to be an illness that affects families, with families affected by HIV/AIDS requiring access to a wide range of prevention and support services (Havens and Mellins 2008). There is considerable interest on the part of

W. Pequegnat and C.C. Bell (eds.), *Family and HIV/AIDS: Cultural and Contextual Issues in Prevention and Treatment*, DOI 10.1007/978-1-4614-0439-2_15, © Springer Science+Business Media, LLC 2012

NIMH and academic researchers to understand how successful programs like those presented in this book can be adopted by HIV/AIDS service providers. To be sure, providers working with families today do use practices and treatments that are grounded in literature and theory. However, the connections between research and practice are sporadic and loose. Systematic attempts to scale up evidence-based mental health and support services for families affected by HIV/AIDS are rare.

HIV/AIDS-related medical and social services are typically organized around individuals. There are few institutional or financial incentives to involve families in care or to offer them supportive services. In fact, there are potential disincentives, including demanding caseload pressures, limited funding streams for services for family members of people living with HIV/AIDS (PLHA), limited clinic space, difficulty engaging families in care, and reticence to address needs that are not AIDS-specific. Yet, research summarized in this volume and elsewhere has demonstrated the significant benefits associated with incorporating families into HIV/AIDS prevention and treatment efforts. This chapter examines factors influencing the provision of family-based services in frontline HIV/AIDS care. In particular, we are interested in understanding what would be involved in disseminating evidence-based interventions to agencies on the frontline, to support their work with PLHA and their families. This means using dissemination methods to encourage more services for families affected by HIV/AIDS, and getting the science out in ways that are most useful to both new and experienced programs. Getting a handle on the "who, what, when, where and how" of dissemination is critical if we ever hope to realize the benefits promised by family-focused intervention research.

In order to inform our discussion of dissemination research, we first review the ways that HIV affects families, the evidence supporting the rationale for reaching families through HIV-related service settings, and the many barriers that must be overcome. Next, we provide an overview of the Special Needs Clinic, an exemplary family-based model of mental health service delivery for HIV-affected families. Examination of the Special Needs Clinic provides lessons about how a continuum of services can be organized to support families coping with HIV/AIDS, alongside co-morbid medical and mental health problems, poverty, and substance use. At the same time, this example highlights many of the challenges that must be considered in bringing evidence-based interventions into frontline care.

Based on experiences of the Special Needs Clinic and elsewhere, we turn to the notion of dissemination research as a strategy to promote evidence-based programs for families in community settings. We summarize results of interviews conducted with 68 providers, 622 PLHAs, and 195 family members receiving services at 22 community service agencies in New York City (NYC). This work identified factors that would contribute to successful dissemination of evidence-based, family-focused programs to frontline service settings and their clients.

We close this chapter with a discussion of the dissemination research necessary to create and sustain the evidence-supported continuum of family-based services. Through a directed program of "comprehensive dynamic trials" (Rapkin and Trickett 2005), we believe that academic centers can forge collaborative partnerships with community providers and stakeholders to effectively address the psychosocial needs of families coping with HIV/AIDS.

15.2   The Family Dimension of HIV/AIDS

Problems related to HIV/AIDS do not occur in isolation, and are often compounded by other personal and family issues (Rapkin et al. 2000). Throughout this chapter, we use the definition of family as a "network of mutual commitment" as adopted by the NIMH Consortium on Families and HIV/AIDS (Pequegnat and Bray 1997; Pequegnat and Szapocznik 2000). This definition is intended to encompass the wide diversity in family composition (Mellins et al. 1996). The particular mix of problems that families face will depend on their environment and living situation, family structure, developmental stages of individual members, and the families' unique narrative and history (Boyd-Franklin and Boland 1995). As with any illness, many factors can impede a family's attempts to cope with HIV/AIDS as outlined herein.

15.2.1   Family Dynamics

- Lack of knowledge of HIV and the PLWHA's health care needs: Family members may be uncertain about how to help (Levine et al. 2010).
- Competing demands: Family member's time, energy, and resources must often be shared among multiple problems (Stoller and Pugliesi 1989; Boyd-Franklin and Boland 1995).
- History of interactions: Family members are coping with a new situation against the backdrop of their relationship history and previous attempts to cope with a host of stressors (Atwood and Weinstein 2010).
- Caregiver support: Family members may assume caregiving roles for individuals with advanced illness, often with minimal support which leads to high levels of stress and ultimately fatigue (Litwak and Sudit 1992; Smith and Rapkin 1996).
- Custody planning: Families may have difficulty making custody plans for children that are legally viable and acceptable to the family (Bauman et al. 2007; Havens and Mellins 2008).

15.2.2   Prevention Issues

- Maintaining safe sexual practices: Serodiscordant couples face the challenge of maintaining sexual precautions on an ongoing basis, which can interfere with intimacy and disrupt relationships (Remien and Mellins 2007).
- Addressing alcohol/substance use: Problems with substance abuse may compound family functioning, including disrupted relationships, and make it difficult to engage families in prevention, treatment, and care (Shulman et al. 2000; Calsyn et al. 2004).
- Parenting aging perinatally infected children: Managing adolescent risk behavior is compounded when the child is living with HIV (Donenberg and Pao 2005).

15.2.3   Testing, Disclosure, and Stigma

- HIV disclosure: The disclosure process is stressful for children and adults. Learning about illness can disrupt family roles and relationships (Simoni et al. 1995; Weiner et al. 2007; Adedimeji 2010).
- Spouse/partner HIV notification: Even though it is now mandatory in some states for providers to notify the spouse or partner of someone diagnosed with an STD, it can have adverse consequences in a family (Rothenberg and Paskey 1995; El-Bassel et al. 2010).
- Positive prenatal/newborn HIV screening results: Learning of one's HIV at the time of delivery presents a mother with the double stress of dealing with her HIV+ diagnosis as well as with the possibility that her baby may be HIV+ (Havens and Mellins 2008).
- HIV-related Stigma: Stigma can affect not only the seropositive person but the entire family, leading to isolation and rejection in some communities (Fullilove and Fullilove 1989; Bor et al. 1993; Remien and Mellins 2007).

15.2.4   Health Status and Treatment Issues

- HIV medication management/adherence: A complex treatment regimen may require family support, while patient nonadherence can become a source of family conflict (Rapkin et al. 2000; Mellins et al. 2004; Havens and Mellins 2008).
- Longer-term survival: Treatment advances have improved the functional health of people living with HIV and have led to families renegotiating household roles, work responsibilities, and future plans (Remien and Mellins 2007).
- Coping with changing function: However, disease progress can lead to cognitive or psychiatric changes that have a negative impact on family members and their roles (Havens and Mellins 2008; Donenberg and Pao 2005).

- Advancing illness: As the seropositive individual becomes more ill, family members may withdraw due to burden or over-identification with the patient (Namir et al. 1989; Rosen et al. 1997; Lyon et al. 2009).
- Palliative care: AIDS patients and families often have little access to palliative care, and may fear that requesting it will lead to withdrawal of treatment (Breitbart et al. 1996; Krug et al. 2010).
- Death/bereavement: Despite the availability of effective treatments, families affected by AIDS may still deal with untimely death and bereavement (Havens and Mellins 2008).

Many of the problems listed above can be addressed by comprehensive, evidence-based models of family-focused care such as those described in this book. Frontline AIDS service providers are the best candidates for dissemination of evidence-based family interventions in the context of ongoing services, as they have a structure to deliver the specialized assistance that these problems require (Rothenberg and Paskey 1995; Domek 2006; Marks et al. 2004). However, reaching families affected by HIV/AIDS with evidence-based interventions represents a double challenge. First, there are significant barriers involved in identifying or creating appropriate venues for delivering services to families. Second, even in venues designed to serve families affected by HIV/AIDS, there are major impediments to introducing evidence-based interventions. We shall examine each of these challenges in turn.

15.3 Barriers to Incorporating Serving for Family in Frontline HIV/AIDS Care

Brach and colleagues (1995) identified categories of barriers that interfered with linkage of mental health services to primary care. Their categories pertain to families affected by HIV/AIDS.

15.3.1 Provider Resistance and Lack of Professional Expertise

Providers may view working with families as a distraction from their primary goal of helping the person with HIV/AIDS (Allen and Petr 1998). This may be especially true when additional effort is needed to engage and retain families in care, as is often the case with families affected by AIDS, who are often from disenfranchised impoverished communities that have experienced discrimination and racism. Moreover, providers are often only trained to deliver individual services (Allen and Petr 1998). Providers may not feel they have the skills to address multiple, simultaneous problems, particularly across medical and psychosocial domains. In pediatric care, McKee and colleagues (2011) found that providers felt tension between providing confidential care to their adolescent patients and fostering effective communication with parents.

15.3.2   Lack of Cultural Competence

Providers may have the cultural competence to work with diverse patients, yet lack the training to address the potential diversity in many family systems. For example, agency staff accustomed to advocating for women may find it difficult to accommodate their partners or their parents. Adult-oriented providers may have difficulty working with children and adolescents. Gay and lesbian patients may also face insensitivity, homophobia, and discrimination in health care.

15.3.3   Client Resistance

Family members may be uncomfortable seeking services at places identified with AIDS or mental illness due to stigma. Others may dislike clinical settings. Alternatively, some people living with HIV may be reluctant to include their family in clinical care.

15.3.4   Logistical Problems

Space allocated for provision of services to individuals may be inadequate or inappropriate for working with families, who may introduce new kinds of clients that require different kinds of space (e.g., children in adult care facilities; male partners at women's health centers). Introduction of children also raises issues around scheduling of appointments after school or concerns about children sharing spaces with adults. For example, it may be necessary to keep immune-compromised adults away from children exposed to infections in school or daycare. Conversely, parents may be uncomfortable bringing children to settings that serve people who are visibly ill or affected by substance abuse or mental illness. Reimbursement for clinical services may not support services for family members, although this varies across states and service types.

15.3.5   Interagency Coordination

Efforts to integrate family-oriented services may increase the need for coordinated care across agencies, clinics, or departments. For example, nursing and social work may need to work together to help clients bridge systems of care (Andersen et al.

1999; Francouer et al. 1999). Establishing these networks takes time and effort, and they do not always run smoothly.

15.4 Models of Service Integration That Have Overcome Barriers to Serving Families

From the earliest days of the AIDS epidemic in the United States, innovative models of integrated service delivery have been developed to overcome barriers to serving families. For example, Feingold and Slammon (1993) describe the NOAH program (No One Alone with HIV), a hospital-based program that supplemented mental health services offered by HIV primary care providers with more intensive interventions offered by "family health facilitators." In 1994, the Title IV of the Ryan White Care Act was initiated to improve coordination of medical care and supportive services for women, children, and families (Health Resources and Services Administration 2011). Brach and colleagues (1995) discuss the multi-site Integrated Primary Care and Substance Abuse Treatment Program sponsored by HRSA and NIDA, to link health services with substance use treatment, including HIV care. Although oriented primarily to individuals, family and collateral counseling were part of the services provided by sites. The Langone Inpatient Cooperative Care Unit was established at New York University prior to HAART to deliver a system of acute inpatient hospital care characterized by a live-in family member or friend acting as a "care partner" (Grieco 1988; Smith and Rapkin 1996).

After the advent of HAART, efforts to support families expanded into outpatient and social service settings. Ryan White Title IV programs were charged with providing the full range of comprehensive medical, mental health, developmental and logistical support for PLHAs and their families, going beyond primary medical and specialty care to include substance abuse and mental health services, case management, transportation, child care, and housing assistance (Abramowitz and Greene 2005). Ryan White also supports specialized training of providers necessary to deliver and manage these integrated services.

In New York State, the Department of Health has developed an integrated model of care management and financing for Medicaid recipients living with HIV/AIDS, known as Special Needs Plans (Feldman et al. 2002; The Lewin Group 2009; Rapkin et al. 2008). Special Needs Plans were developed as an adjunct to hospital-based care provided at the State's Designated AIDS Centers. Special Needs Plans make provisions for a full range of medical, mental health, and social services for adults living with HIV/AIDS and their dependents. Moreover, the state requires that linkages with family-centered clinical and social support services must be incorporated into each Special Need Plan's network (Feldman et al. 2002).

15.5   The Special Needs Clinic Model of Family Services in AIDS Mental Health Care

It is noteworthy that services for families affected by HIV/AIDS developed over the same time period as the research supported by the NIMH, as reflected in this volume and its predecessor. Throughout this history there have been relatively few points of contact between the research to develop evidence-based interventions for families and public policy initiatives to reach families with mental health and supportive care. In other words, although these integrated models meet the challenge of serving families, they do not necessarily address the challenge of incorporating evidence-based practices. Examining the Special Needs Clinic (Havens et al. in press), a long-standing model of integrated services for families affected by HIV/AIDS, helps shed light on the complexities of service integration and associated difficulties in integrating research-based interventions into routine care.

15.5.1   Overview and Rationale for the Special Needs Clinic Model

The Special Needs Clinic (SNC), a sub-specialty service in the Division of Child and Adolescent Psychiatry at Columbia University Medical Center, was founded in 1992 to serve the complex mental health need of the growing numbers of HIV-affected women and children in New York City (Havens et al. 1997, Havens et al. in press). Over the past 19 years, the SNC has developed a model of care specifically designed to overcome fragmentation of care that impedes effective treatment of HIV-affected families (Havens et al. in press). Outpatient mental health care has not generally been coordinated with medical care. This limits the identification, engagement, and retention of PLHA in need of mental health services. While there have been some efforts to use the primary care setting as an opportunity to screen patients for mental health problems, the mental health needs of other family members, which may be a source of significant stress to the identified patient, are generally not considered. Further fragmentation results from the separation of mental health and substance abuse services. Substance abusers may be excluded from mental health care until they are abstinent, or receive their substance abuse treatment in a setting which may be distant from their ongoing mental health care. Finally, in traditional care, child and adult services are kept separate, with distinct administration, clinical staff and sites. Adult mental health providers typically lack expertise in the assessment and treatment of children. Child mental health providers often treat adult family members only as collaterals to the child client. Although pervasive, a fragmented system of services is not in the best interests of families affected by HIV/AIDS. Rather, multi-modal, multi-generational and long-term mental health services may be necessary to address the often entrenched psychosocial and psychiatric problems of families as they confront the stresses of HIV illness.

The SNC utilizes a multi-disciplinary team (e.g., psychiatrists, psychologists, clinical social workers, case managers, and educators) to provide multi-generational, family-based, long-term mental health treatment for children and adult family members that is coordinated with support services and medical care. The SNC recognizes that problems prevalent in the target population – including active substance use, psychiatric impairment, or psychological difficulties – are barriers to adults' accessing and adhering to the complicated regimens for themselves and their children (Mellins et al. 2003, 2004; Uldall et al. 1994). Close communication among the client, mental health provider, and HIV health care staff is essential for addressing multiple families' problems. This level of coordination ensures that families are actively connected to the full range of necessary services. Commonly, several family members representing two or three generations are engaged in ongoing individual mental health treatment with several different SNC clinicians, along side a range of other services, including family and group therapy, after school programs, case management, tutoring, psychopharmacology, etc. Co-location of the SNC with adult and child medical care allows the SNC patients to be engaged on site in the medical clinic by SNC clinicians. Treatment of uninfected family members at the SNC, particularly children, is a critical piece as recent studies have indicated high rates of mental health problems in uninfected siblings or children of HIV+ mothers (Bauman et al. 2007; Malee et al. 2011; Mellins et al. 2009).

15.5.2   *Impediments to Intervention Research and Dissemination at the Special Needs Clinic*

The SNC presents a very special case, with a specific mission to address the needs of families affected by HIV/AIDS. The SNC staff has worked hard to develop a model of family-based care that overcomes many of the barriers described earlier, including systems for monitoring and tracking family needs and making referrals as needed to medical sub-specialty and substance use treatment, as well as community-based programs. Many SNC services draw upon therapeutic approaches and principles that have been widely studied, such as cognitive behavioral therapy, family ecology and developmental/life course perspectives. Yet despite considerable attention to meeting the needs of families in a comprehensive matter, the SNC has not typically participated in research-based trials or dissemination research of short-term manualized interventions such as those described in this book. There are multiple reasons for this lack of participation.

First, many research-based programs with focused targets were developed as stand-alone programs. The procedures for incorporating such interventions into ongoing treatment, including funding requirements, have rarely been considered and tested. Few SNC patients have only one behavioral problem or diagnosis, typically required in many intervention trials and even in many evidence-based approaches.

Second, stressors in families' lives and their multigenerational needs often preclude use of only one treatment. Families may have competing needs, including crises that need immediate attention or that involve different treatments simultaneously or sequentially. This requires a shift in focus that can derail a specific short-term intervention focused on one problem (e.g., sexual risk reduction). Studies of short-term, stand-alone evidence-based interventions typically emphasize fidelity over accommodation of real-world circumstances. There is no guidance about how to modify intervention protocols in response to all too common disruptions that occur in work with families.

Using traditional research models to develop interventions in the context of the SNC also presents challenges. Providers may be reluctant to participate in clinical trials of new approaches because of concerns about untested programs, randomization, and insufficient numbers of eligible patients/families with the target diagnoses. Most intervention trials do not address integration of short-term evidence-based practices into ongoing therapy. Providers may not believe it is clinically advisable to interrupt ongoing work. There is also concern about the rigid time frames required for many manualized interventions when applied to patients in ongoing treatment. Logistic problems are compounded when multiple family members are involved.

Finally, the adaptation of many of the interventions described in this book into the SNC would require some level of operational research to assess the feasibility of a particular strategy in a new or different context with a potentially different population or culture. The SNC has not typically had the resources to undertake this sort of preparatory work. Burden on staff time to carry out activities in research-based projects that do not result in billable encounters (e.g., nonbillable services, research-based paper work, supervision and training on research activities) is another impediment to participation in research-based trials.

In other words, there are both clinical barriers to the incorporation of stand-alone family-focused evidence-based interventions that were developed elsewhere for specific problems, and structural barriers to conducting research in the context of real work clinics, that do not have dedicated research funds to protect staff time. Despite these considerations, the SNC represents a "best case" for testing and disseminating family-focused interventions because of the ongoing relationships between families and patients, already established trust, user-friendly services, and a large number of engaged patients. Understanding how to overcome barriers to implementation and research participation in clinics like the SNC is critical to dissemination of evidence-based family programs.

15.6 The Challenge of Transferring Evidence-Based Programs for Families to Frontline Clinics

Although clinicians and other staff in the SNC and similar settings might significantly benefit from the arsenal of tools described in this book, how to accomplish this has been difficult to conceptualize and implement due to the mismatch between the scientifically driven demands of multi-session evidenced-based HIV interventions and the real world demands of clinical practice. The barriers that interfere with implementing services to families in AIDS service organizations are compounded when transferring an evidence-based program from randomized controlled trials (RCT). The success of such efforts hinges on the answers to a number of key questions: Are there community partners interested in providing support for families? Do they have the expertise and resources necessary to undertake programs developed in randomized clinical trials? What are the barriers to adoption of evidence-based programs? What services would be most helpful to families affected by HIV? What steps must be taken to engage and retain families in prevention, treatment, and care?

Rapkin and colleagues (Lounsbury et al 2007; Reich et al. 2010; Floyd et al. 2010; Zaid-Muhammad 2010) initiated the Family ACCESS to Care Study (FACS) to explore questions that bear on the dual challenges of integrating services for families and implementing evidence-based family interventions in settings that provide frontline services to individuals living with HIV/AIDS. Participating agencies included 22 private nonprofits, selected and recruited at random from a list over 160 HIV/AIDS agencies in New York City in 2003 and providing continuous service to PLHA for at least 3 years. Working with these agencies, FACS gathered data from HIV+ clients, their families, providers, and agency administrators in order to better understand whether and how research could be used to stimulate and enhance services to families as a standard of care.

15.6.1   Administrative and Clinical Staff

15.6.1.1   Staff Characteristics

Rapkin and colleagues were concerned about community providers' readiness and capacity to undertake family programs. They were also interested in community providers' willingness to partner with academic researchers to develop new family interventions (for a detailed discussion of FACS community partnerships see Lounsbury et al. 2007). They interviewed a total of 68 administrative and clinical staff affiliated with agencies providing direct service to PLHAs (see Table 15.1 describing Staff Characteristics).

15.6.1.2   Staff Interest in Family-Based Research

Given the interest in the feasibility of disseminating evidence-based programs for PLHA and their families, we examined staff members' relevant training and experience. We asked staff about their desire to get more involved in research in their current jobs. Interest was quite high, but differed by category of involvement, with 77% expressing at least some interest in working directly with participants in

Table 15.1 Staff characteristics (*N*=68)

Staff roles	
Social worker	16%
Clinician (nurse or physician)	18%
Case manager	21%
Administrator	45%
Staff demographic characteristics	
Female	58%
African American	33%
White	30%
Latino	15%
Asian	12%
Mixed/other	10%
Areas of training	
Family case management	68%
Family therapy	53%
Family medicine	12%
Experience working with	
Children	63%
Adolescents	68%
Adults	94%
Elders	71%
Service provided to	
Family members of PLHAs	77%
Families as a unit	62%
Research training and experience	
Formal coursework	56%
On the job research training	38%
Attended workshops/seminars	29%
Member of a research team	41%
Supervision of research	22%

research projects, 59% interested in developing research protocols and proposals, 56% wanting to publish and present research at meetings, 57% wanting to take a role in participant recruitment, and 44% interested in training and supervising research staff.

We also asked staff to provide their perspective on the readiness and capacity of organizational leadership, staff, and clients to participate in research to expand services for families affected by HIV/AIDS. Overall, respondents believed that leadership would be favorable to undertaking research (69% positive, 15% mixed, 4% negative). However, respondents anticipated that clinical staff would be much less favorable (38% positive, 44% mixed, 8% negative) and that clients would be even more wary (29% positive, 54% mixed, 8% negative).

When we introduced the idea of conducting dissemination research through collaborations with outside academic institutions, respondents believed that this would not only be favorable to leadership (67% positive, 17% mixed, 2% negative) but also considerably more acceptable to both agency staff (54% positive, 25% mixed, 6% negative) and clients (40% positive, 38% mixed, 8% negative) than doing research without an academic partner. Respondents also raised concerns about practical and tangible barriers to providing programs for families in the agency (e.g., child care, space, insurance). The greatest barrier involved staff concerns with the fit of family-oriented programs with their agencies' missions which they viewed as individual-focused service.

15.6.2 PLHAs and Their Families

15.6.2.1 Family Characteristics

We also conducted interviews with up to 30 PLHAs receiving services at a given agency for a total of 622 individuals and we attempted to recruit one member of each PLHA's family, as a proxy for families' availability and willingness to participate in HIV-related programs at a given agency. Over half of PLHAs (53%) were not willing or able to provide contact information for potential family participants. Out of those families we were given permission to contact, 33% refused participation. Thus, we were able to recruit a total of 195 adult family members, including 43% who were themselves HIV+ (see Table 15.2 for family characteristics). Interviews for PLHAs and family members included measures that are reported elsewhere in greater detail, including psychosocial well-being and unmet needs (Zaid-Muhammad 2010), social support networks (Reich et al. 2010), and attitudes toward participation in research (Floyd et al. 2010).

PLHA and family members in this study reported significant needs for assistance, particularly related to their families. We asked respondents to identify concerns and problems that they had faced over the past 4 weeks (see Table 15.3). Financial problems, emotional distress, and housing problems were prevalent for both PLHAs and family members. PLHAs were significantly more likely to report problems with health care providers, while family members experienced more problems with employment and benefits. On average, PLHAs and their adult family members mentioned dealing with just under two significant life events over the past month.

15.6.2.2 Mental Health Service Use and Unmet Needs

PLHAs were heavy users of available mental health and supportive services. Figure 15.1 summarizes PLHA's use of different services into three categories: (1) those who are currently receiving satisfactory services, (2) those receiving unsatisfactory services, and (3) those who are interested in receiving services. For example, 24% reported satisfaction with the individual psychotherapy that they received, about 1% of respondents were dissatisfied, and 30% would like to receive individual

Table 15.2 Family member characteristics

	Index PLHAs			Family members	
	Participated without family member	Could not recruit family member	Would not invite a family member	Seropositive	Seronegative
N	195 (31.4%)	97 (15.6%)	330 (53.1%)	84 (43.1%)	111 (56.9%)
Mean age (SD)	45.63 (7.97)	45.87 (7.35)	45.23 (10.01)	46.23 (9.40)	41.17 (11.22)
Female	90 (46.2%)	26 (26.8%)	125 (38.0%)	36 (42.9%)	67 (60.4%)
African American[a]	140 (33.5%)	66 (15.8%)	212 (50.7%)	61 (44.9%)	75 (55.1%)
Latino/a[a]	54 (29.0%)	30 (16.1%)	102 (54.8%)	23 (42.6%)	31 (57.4%)
White[a]	25 (25.3%)	15 (15.2%)	59 (59.6%)	11 (44.0%)	14 (56.0%)
Born in USA	185 (94.9%)	88 (90.7%)	298 (90.3%)	79 (94.0%)	103 (92.8%)
GED/HS diploma	85 (44.2%)	44 (45.3%)	156 (48.1%)	37 (44.0%)	67 (60.3%)
Employed	17 (8.7%)	12 (12.4%)	31 (9.4%)	14 (16.7%)	39 (35.1%)
Children in family	126 (64.6%)	51 (52.6%)	190 (57.6%)	52 (66.7%)	87 (78.4%)
Past research experience	107 (54.9%)	51 (52.6%)	198 (60.0%)	35 (41.7%)	22 (19.8%)

[a]Proportions within racial/ethnic group

Table 15.3 Recent life events identified by families

Life events	Index PLHA%	Family members	χ2	Sig.
	622	189		
% had any new medical problems or injuries?	18.17%	19.05%		
% hospitalized?	8.20%	7.41%		
% problems without how you were treated by a provider?	9.81%	3.70%	8.26	$p<0.004$
% experienced prejudice or discrimination?	9.66%	8.47%		
% had any housing problems?	25.88%	22.75%		
% problems without benefits, entitlements, or insurance?	15.11%	24.87%	8.94	$p<0.003$
% employment or work-related problems?	4.02%	10.05%	9.14	$p<0.002$
% major financial problems?	31.35%	37.04%		
% important people in your life died?	15.59%	13.23%		
% experienced a serious emotional crisis?	28.78%	31.75%		
% victim of domestic violence?	8.68%	6.35%		
% victim of a crime?	4.34%	1.60%		
% arrested, charged with a crime, or put in jail?	2.09%	2.65%		
Mean number of life events (SD)	1.82 (1.80)	1.89 (1.85)		

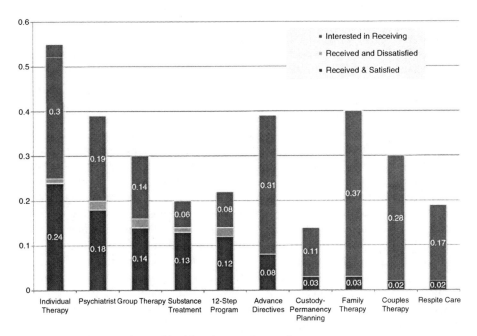

Fig. 15.1 PLHAs use of mental health and supportive services

therapy. Several important trends are evident in this figure. First, across the board, proportions of respondents dissatisfied with mental health and supportive services were quite low (0–2%). Further, individual and group mental health services were the most widely used. In contrast, family-oriented services including family and marital therapy, custody-planning, and respite care were used by only about 2–3% of respondents. These family-oriented services were in very high demand, with 37% desiring family therapy, 28% wanting couples therapy and 31% of respondents wanted help with advanced directives. Interest in custody planning and respite care were somewhat lower, perhaps due to their associations with advanced illness.

15.6.3   Priorities for Dissemination of Evidence-Based Programs

We asked index PLHAs, family members, and agency staff members to rank 25 different evidence-based programs in terms of their importance to families affected by HIV/AIDS. These findings are presented in Table 15.4. As this table demonstrates, PLHAs placed the greatest importance on programs related to living with HIV for the long term, drawing on faith and spirituality, and support for people affected by HIV. Coping with psychological issues, making treatment decisions and communication skills were also rated highly. PLHAs ranked most programs explicitly involving partners and families in the middle, including disclosure, household management skills, advanced directives, family problem solving, and addressing abuse. Programs for youth and teens tended to receive the lowest priority among adult PLHAs, with several noteworthy exceptions: stopping teens' risky sexual behavior and alcohol/substance use. In fact, concern about teens' risk was given much greater priority than personal risk reduction (e.g., prevention for positives). Overall, priorities of PLHAs' family members were similar to PLHAs. Rank-order correlation between PLHA and family members' priorities was 0.80.

However, agency staff members' rankings differed substantially from those of index PLHAs and their families, with rank-order correlations of 0.26 and 0.19, respectively. Staff placed greatest emphasis on managing HIV medications, sexual risk behavior, and HIV treatment decisions. Other highly ranked programs included those for reducing alcohol/substance use, addressing abuse in the family, and helping people cope with the consequences of abuse. Mental health, family problem solving, household management and life skills, and skills for living long term with HIV/AIDS were also ranked highly. Given that we sampled agencies that primarily serve adults, providers placed most programs for children in the middle ranks, with the exception of youth smoking which was ranked near the bottom. Staff placed low priority on programs related to end-of-life issues (advanced directives, permanency planning, and bereavement) as well as spirituality and faith-based programs. Staff were also less interested in interventions to address stigma and discrimination and to promote tobacco cessation for adults.

Table 15.4 Dissemination of evidence-based programs for families affected by HIV/AIDS: PLHA, family, and agency staff priorities

Evidence-based programs	Index PLHAs	Family members	Providers	PLHA vs. family	PLHA vs. provider	Family vs. provider	Provider: fit with agency mission? (%)
	Rank of importance for families			Discrepancies in rank			
Skills for living with HIV over the long-term	1.0	1.5	10.0	-0.5	-9.0	-8.5	73.6
Drawing on faith and spirituality	2.0	4.0	24.0	-2.0	-22.0	-20.0	58.9
Support for people infected or affected by HIV	3.0	1.5	7.0	1.5	-4.0	-5.5	71.7
Coping with depression/anxiety in adults	4.0	3.0	9.0	1.0	-5.0	-6.0	67.3
HIV treatment decisions	5.0	9.5	3.0	-4.5	2.0	6.5	71.7
Communication	6.0	9.5	15.0	-3.5	-9.0	-5.5	63.0
Risky sexual behaviors in children or teens	7.0	7.0	8.0	0.0	-1.0	-1.0	42.9
Disclosure	8.0	20.0	13.0	-12.0	-5.0	7.0	67.9
Managing HIV medications	9.0	8.0	1.0	1.0	8.0	7.0	69.8
Household management and life skills	10.0	5.0	11.5	5.0	-1.5	-6.5	53.6
Reducing or quitting alcohol/drugs	11.0	16.0	5.0	-5.0	6.0	11.0	66.0
Advanced directives/living will	12.5	18.0	24.0	-5.5	-11.5	-6.0	63.0
Alcohol or drug use in children or teens	12.5	11.0	17.0	1.5	-4.5	-6.0	36.4
Reducing or quitting tobacco	14.0	6.0	24.0	8.0	-10.0	-18.0	53.7
Family problem solving	15.0	12.5	11.5	2.5	3.5	1.0	53.7
Grieving/bereavement	16.0	17.0	19.0	-1.0	-3.0	-2.0	66.0
Stopping abuse within the family	17.0	19.0	4.0	-2.0	13.0	15.0	58.2
Reducing risky or unsafe sexual behavior	18.0	14.5	2.0	3.5	16.0	12.5	59.3

(continued)

Table 15.4 (continued)

Evidence-based programs	Index PLHAs	Family members	Providers	PLHA vs. family	PLHA vs. provider	Family vs. provider	Provider: fit with agency mission? (%)
	Rank of importance for families			Discrepancies in rank			
Overcoming discrimination	19.0	24.0	21.0	-5.0	-2.0	3.0	61.1
Programs for children's learning problems	20.0	12.5	19.0	7.5	1.0	-6.5	32.1
Programs for children's emotional problems	21.0	22.0	14.0	-1.0	7.0	8.0	33.9
Coping with abuse and victimization	22.0	22.0	6.0	0.0	16.0	16.0	56.6
Programs for children's behavioral problems	23.0	22.0	16.0	1.0	7.0	6.0	32.1
Custody planning (permanency planning)	24.0	14.5	19.0	9.5	5.0	-4.5	56.4
Tobacco use in children or teens	25.0	25.0	22.0	0.0	3.0	3.0	39.3
Spearman rank-order correlations between columns				0.80	0.26	0.19	

Large discrepancies in priority between agency staff and PLHAs were evident in respect to managing medications (rank of 1 for staff versus 8 for PLHAs), coping with abuse (rank of 6 versus 22) and stopping abuse within the family (rank of 4 versus 17), reducing HIV risk behavior among adults (rank of 2 versus 18), and dealing with children's problems with emotions (rank of 14 versus 21) and learning (rank of 16 versus 23). Conversely, staff placed less priority than their clients on programs drawing on faith and spirituality (rank of 24 versus 2), establishing advanced directives (rank of 24 versus 12.5), tobacco cessation for adults (rank of 24 versus 14), and communication skills training (rank of 15 versus 6). Discrepancies in priorities between agency staff and family members were similar to those between staff and PLHAs, with several key exceptions. Staff members were more interested in programs around treatment decision making (rank of 3 for staff versus 9.5 for family members) and HIV disclosure (rank of 13 versus 20). Compared to family members, agency respondents placed lower priority on tobacco cessation (rank of 24 versus 6), household management and life skills (rank of 11.5 versus 5), and children's learning problems (rank of 19 versus 12.5). In general, staff priorities emphasized HIV risk and medical management concerns compared to PLHAs and their family members focus on spirituality, communication, and strategies for living long term with the virus.

15.6.4 The Fit of Family-Oriented Services and Research to Agency Mission

Perhaps the greatest potential barrier involved staff concerns about the fit of family-oriented intervention with agencies' missions. We asked staff to rate whether each of the 25 types of interventions fit with their agencies' mission statement. As Table 15.4 indicates, staff respondents' perception of the appropriateness of different interventions for their settings varied greatly and depended upon the category of service. About 70% of agency respondents rated individual-focused services for adults as fitting their agencies' missions, including managing medication, assisting with treatment decisions, teaching skills for living with HIV as a chronic disease, and providing support. Most respondents also agreed that programs for mental health, substance use, bereavement, and HIV disclosure were appropriate. Family-specific programs for adults were seen as somewhat less appropriate, including family problem solving, household management, abusive behavior, and custody planning. Most striking programs for children and teens were rated as outside the agencies' scope by more than half of all respondents. Of course, it is very important to acknowledge that the agencies included in FACS largely served individual adults. Staff at programs like the SNC which explicitly focus on families affected by HIV, with child and adult family members, would likely rank these priorities differently. Nonetheless, these findings highlight the fragmentation that still exists between medical and mental health care, and even more importantly between child/family and adult services.

15.7 Dissemination Research to Foster Service Integration and Evidence-Based Practice

Evidence-based interventions have been developed to address many of the problems and challenges experienced by PLHA and their families. Despite the availability of these interventions, families do not have routine access to the necessary continuum of services and supports. The fragmented organization of services continues to make it difficult to serve adults and children in one setting, to care for seropositive and seronegative adult family members together, and to integrate medical, mental health, and substance use treatment. Although many providers have interest and expertise in working with families, serving families is not central to the missions of many organizations delivering services to PLHA. Moreover, as our FACS findings show, service providers' priorities revolve around medication adherence and sexual risk reduction, compared to families' emphasis on living with HIV, spirituality, and support. Although agency leaders, staff and family members are generally favorable about partnering with researchers to develop services for families, the gap between research and practice is considerable. Even at a setting like the Special Needs Clinic that is explicitly designed to meet the needs of HIV-affected families, it is not clear how to incorporate manualized programs into ongoing therapy with families whose needs are complex and rapidly changing.

Recent work in dissemination and implementation research has the potential to foster service integration and overcome the gaps between research and practice in order to foster more effective and comprehensive programs for families affected by HIV/AIDS (Fixsen et al. 2005; Glasgow et al. 2004; Wandersman et al. 2008). Often, dissemination has been viewed as simply getting the word out or encouraging practice settings to make use of evidence-based interventions (Mrazek and Haggerty 1994). However, this approach to dissemination has very limited utility with respect to complex psychosocial, behavioral, or mental health interventions. There is considerable variation in settings where PLHA receive care and no established methods to introduce innovations for families into practice. Community service settings may serve a very diverse group of PLHAs, including individuals who would not have been eligible for original trials to test evidence-based practices due to substance use, psychiatric problems, or medical co-morbidities (Green 2001; Green and Glasgow 2006). Due to the wide differences in capacities of settings and the heterogeneity of families, evidence-based family-focused HIV programs may need to be reinvented, combined, or woven together with ongoing clinical strategies. These necessary modifications in procedures and inclusion criteria represent violations of "fidelity" in the traditional sense (Bauman et al. 1991). In short, the notion of taking a program directly from research to widespread practice will generally not work when it comes to development of services for families affected by HIV/AIDS (McKleroy et al. 2006).

Rather than direct transfer of programs, dissemination of evidence-based programs to support HIV-affected families may be viewed as a process of collaborative research involving service organizations, community stakeholders, and academic researchers (Rapkin and Trickett 2005; Miller and Shinn 2005). The goal of such research is to figure out how to best apply available intervention technology to address families' needs in a given setting. Collaborative dissemination research of this sort is necessary because available data provide very little information on how to implement, optimize, and sustain evidence-based family-focused interventions in new settings. It is useful to consider the kinds of research questions that must be addressed to get interventions for HIV-affected families into widespread practices.

First, it is necessary to address organizational readiness to undertake programs for families affected by HIV/AIDS (Goodman and Steckler 1990; Chinman et al. 2005; Livet et al. 2008). Leadership and staff may be encouraged to consider family interventions by research showing how family factors impinge on outcomes for their agency's clients. Data showing families' unmet needs and interest in services may also be persuasive. Organizations will also want to know about how new programs for families would fit into the local service ecology. For example, are there competing programs? Would new programs attract referrals? What funding sources are available to cover costs of these programs? Academic collaborators can play an important role in helping service organizations conduct preparatory research at this level, especially if organizations do not have in-house capacity for this level of assessment (Glasgow and Emmons 2007).

Second, academic collaborators have a critical role to play in helping organizations identify and adapt family-focused evidence-based interventions to meet local needs. As highlighted in our discussion of the Special Needs Clinic, families' needs are often complex and rarely map onto a single evidence-based program. Rather than be hamstrung by existing off-the-shelf protocols, agencies and academics need as many degrees of freedom as possible to devise the package of strategies, services and referrals that is most workable in a particular setting (Kreuter and Wray 2003; Collins et al. 2004). This is a problem solving approach to dissemination, because the evidence base is used to help generate alternative solutions to meet local needs. For example, an agency might decide to adopt structural ecosystems therapy (Szapocznik et al. 2004) as a general model for engaging and maintaining contact with families, and then orchestrate in other evidence-based practices for issues like HIV disclosure, sexual risk or permanency planning when and if they are needed. Alternatively, an agency may determine that it wants to provide a more focal program for families, such as a caregiver support group. They may also decide to use validated assessment measures to ensure that potential members are appropriate for the group. In any event, agencies and researchers must use the available evidence base combined with local expertise to determine the right treatment algorithm for their setting.

Third, incorporation of new programs and practices may pose considerable practical and logistical challenges to community service delivery settings. Intervention identification and adaptation must be informed by operations and systems research to determine how to implement the intervention in a given service environment (Hawe et al. 2009; Yoshikawa et al. 2003). In addition, the assessment of staff members' ability to carry out programs is critical. Results of the Family Access to Care study suggest that staff members in many agencies already have training and experience working with families, but it may be necessary to modify agency roles or to re-organize services to make it possible to offer services for families. Schein (1999) discusses the use of ongoing process consultation to help agencies incorporate new innovations. Process consultation is intended to engage key organizational personnel in identification of challenges to the adoption of innovations such as family-focused interventions, in order to carry out necessary training, leadership development, and organizational capacity building (Lambrechts et al. 2009).

Fourth, academic researchers, agencies and community stakeholders must collaborate closely to ensure that interventions adopted and adapted for new service settings and new populations are performing as intended (Grimshaw et al. 2006; Epstein et al. 2010). Whether interventions are directly replicated or completely reinvented, it is necessary to track how they are working in new settings (Green 2001). Rapkin and Trickett (2005) proposed the use of "comprehensive dynamic trial" designs to study the implementation of interventions in community settings. In a "comprehensive dynamic trial," data on intervention reach, efficacy and costs are gathered and tracked on an ongoing basis, along with information on fidelity and process. Community stakeholders and agency representatives continually monitor and query data to identify potential ways in which intervention performance might be improved. With assistance from academic collaborators, stakeholders' suggested changes to the intervention are implemented as "embedded experiments" to determine whether changes are warranted. Incorporating methods for continuous improvement into the dissemination process makes it possible to evolve interventions as much or as little as necessary to meet the needs of particular settings. This process can be continued until a suitable level of performance is achieved. Along with process consultation to foster necessary organizational capacities, using comprehensive dynamic trial methods to optimize intervention performance is intended to maximize the likelihood that family-focused interventions can and will be sustained.

15.8   Conclusion

The evidence is clear that the family has a direct and immediate role in helping to mitigate the burden of HIV/AIDS, and that HIV/AIDS has implications for the health and well-being of the family as a whole. The program of dissemination research envisioned here is intended to maximize the uptake, effectiveness, and sustainability of services for families affected by HIV/AIDS. This research agenda is highly consistent with the recent emphasis on the study of comparative effectiveness. The only way to determine what interventions are most appropriate for different families in different service delivery contexts is to gather lessons learned from experimentation in local settings. Our focus on dissemination of evidence-based interventions must be inextricably combined with intervention adaptation, quality improvement, and community capacity building efforts. At this writing, major changes are being discussed in terms of the national HIV/AIDS strategy, multifaceted strategies to improve health quality, and of course improved access to care for underserved populations. This alignment of health quality, health financing, and research priorities suggests that resources can and should be made available to support dissemination research to provide effective services for families affected by HIV/AIDS.

References

Abramowitz S, Greene D. Ryan White CARE Act Title IV programs: a preliminary characterization of benefits and costs. AIDS Public Policy J. 2005;20(3–4):108–25.

Adedimeji A. To tell or not to tell: managing HIV/AIDS disclosure in a low-prevalence context. SAHARA J. 2010;7(1):16–23.

Allen R, Petr C. Rethinking family-centered practice. Am J Orthopsychiatry. 1998;68(1):4–15.

Andersen MD, Smereck GA, Hockman EM, Ross DJ, Ground KJ. Nurses decrease barriers to health care by "hyperlinking" multiple-diagnosed women living with HIV/AIDS into care. J Assoc Nurses AIDS Care. 1999;10(2):55–65.

Atwood JD, Weinstein E. Chronic illness and the family meaning system. In: Atwood JD, Gallo C, editors. Family therapy and chronic illness. New Brunswick, NJ: Aldine Transaction Publishers; 2010. p. 27–56.

Bauman LJ, Stein REK, Ires T. Reinventing fidelity: the transfer of social technology among settings. Am J Community Psychol. 1991;19(4):619–39.

Bauman LJ, Silver EJ, Draimin BH, Hudis J. Children of mothers with HIV/AIDS: unmet needs for mental health services. Pediatrics. 2007;120(5):e1141–7.

Bor R, Miller R, Goldman E. HIV/AIDS and the family: a review of research in the first decade. J Fam Ther. 1993;15:187–204.

Boyd-Franklin N, Boland M. A multisystems approach to service delivery for HIV/AIDS families. In: Boyd-Franklin N, Steiner G, Boland M, editors. Children, families, and HIV/AIDS: psychosocial and therapeutic issues. New York: Guilford Press; 1995. p. 199–215.

Brach C, Falik M, Law C, Robinson G, Trent-Adams S, Ulmer C, et al. Mental health services: critical component of integrated primary care and substance abuse treatment. J Health Care Poor Underserved. 1995;6(3):322–41.

Breitbart W, Rosenfeld BD, Passik SD. Interest in physician-assisted suicide among ambulatory HIV-infected patients. Am J Psychiatry. 1996;153(2):238–42.

Calsyn RJ, Klinkenberg WD, Morse J, Miller J, Cruthis R. Recruitment, engagement, and retention of people living with HIV and co-occurring mental health and substance use disorders. AIDS Care. 2004;16 Suppl 1:S56–70.

Carillo J, Green A, Betancourt J. Cross cultural primary care: a patient-based approach. Ann Intern Med. 1999;130:829–34.

Chinman M, Hannah G, Wandersman A, Ebener P, Hunter S, Imm P, et al. Developing a community science research agenda for building community capacity for effective preventive interventions. Am J Community Psychol. 2005;35:143–58.

Collins LM, Murphy SA, Bierman KL. A conceptual framework for adaptive preventive interventions. Prev Sci. 2004;5:185–96.

Domek GJ. The social consequences of antiretroviral therapy: preparing for the unexpected futures of HIV-positive children. Lancet. 2006;367:1367–9.

Donenberg GR, Pao M. Youths and HIV/AIDS: psychiatry' role in a changing epidemic. J Am Acad Child Adolesc Psychiatry. 2005;44(8):728–47.

El-Bassel N, Gilbert L, Witte S, Wu E, Vinocur D. Countering the surge of HIV/STIs and co-occurring problems of intimate partner violence and drug abuse among African American women: implications for HIV/STI prevention. African Americans and HIV/AIDS. 2010;Part 2:113–30. doi:10.1007/978-0-387-78321-5_7.

Epstein JN, Langberg JM, Lichtenstein PK, Kolb RC, Stark LJ. Sustained improvement in pediatricians' ADHD practice behaviors in the context of a community-based quality improvement initiative. Child Health Care. 2010;39(4):296–311.

Feingold A, Slammon WR. A model integrating mental health and primary care services for families with HIV. Gen Hosp Psychiatry. 1993;15(5):290–300.

Feldman IS, Cruz H, DeLorenzo JP, Sharp MJ. HIV special needs plans: New York State's unique Medicaid managed care model. Paper presented at International Conference on AIDS, 14, abstract no. F12318; 2002, July.

Fixsen DL, Naoom SF, Blase KA, Friedman RM, Wallace F. Implementation research: a synthesis of the literature. Tampa, FL: University of South Florida, Louis de la Parte Mental Health Institute, The National Implementation Research Network. (FMHI Publication #231); 2005.

Floyd T, Patel S, Weiss E, Zaid-Muhammad S, Lounsbury D, Rapkin B. Beliefs about participating in research among a sample of minority persons living with HIV/AIDS in New York City. AIDS Patient Care STDs. 2010;24(6):373–80.

Francouer R, Copley C, Miller P. The challenge to meet the mental health and biopsychosocial needs of the poor: expanded roles for hospital social workers in a changing healthcare environment. Soc Work Health Care. 1999;26(2):1–13.

Fullilove MT, Fullilove RE. Stigma as an obstacle to AIDS action: the case of the African American community. Am Behav Sci. 1989;42(7):1117–29.

Glasgow RE, Emmons KM. How can we increase translation of research into practice? Types of evidence needed. Annu Rev Public Health. 2007;28:413–33.

Glasgow RE, Goldstein MG, Ockene J, Pronk NP. Translating what we have learned into practice: principles and hypotheses for addressing multiple behaviors in primary care. Am J Prev Med. 2004;27:88–101.

Good M, Good B, Schaffer C, Lind S. American oncology and the discourse on hope. Cult Med Psychiatry. 1990;12:59–79.

Goodman RM, Steckler A. A model for the institutionalization of health promotion programs. Fam Community Health. 1989;11(4):63–78.

Goodman RM, Steckler A. Moblizing organizations for health enhancement: theories of organizational change. In: Glanz K, Lewis FM, Rimer BK, editors. Health behavior and health education: theory, research and practice. San Francisco: Jossey-Bass; 1990. p. 314–41.

Green LW. From research to "best practices" in other settings and populations. Am J Health Behav. 2001;25:165–78.

Green LW, Glasgow RE. Evaluating the relevance, generalization, and applicability of research: Issues in external validity and translation methodology. Eval Health Prof. 2006;29:126–53.

Grieco AJ. Home care/hospital care/cooperative care: options for the practice of medicine. Bull N Y Acad Med. 1988;64(4):318–26.

Grimshaw J, Eccles M, Thomas R, MacLennan G, Ramsay C, Fraser C, et al. Toward evidence-based quality improvement: evidence (and its limitations) of the effectiveness of guideline dissemination and implementation strategies 1966–1998. J Gen Intern Med. 2006;21:S14–20.

Havens JF, Mellins CA. Psychiatric aspects of HIV/AIDS in childhood and adolescence. In: Rutter M, Taylor E, editors. Child and adolescent psychiatry. 5th ed. Oxford, UK: Blackwell; 2008.

Havens JF, Mellins CA, Ryan S. The mental health treatment of children and families affected by HIV/AIDS. In: Wicks L, editor. Psychotherapy and AIDS. Washington, DC: Taylor and Francis; 1997.

Havens J, Ryan S, Mellins C, Ng W. A model of mental health Service delivery for children and families and families affected by HIV/AIDS. HIV Soc Serv. In press.

Hawe P, Shiell A, Riley T, Gold L. Methods for exploring implementation variation and local context within a cluster randomised community intervention trial. J Epidemiol Community Health. 2009;58:788–93.

Health Resources and Services Administration. U.S. Department of Health and Human Services. The Ryan White HIV/AIDS Program: Biennial Progress Reports. Available via: http://hab.hrsa.gov/publications/progressreports.htm (2011). Cited 5 Mar 2011.

Kreuter MW, Wray RJ. Tailored and targeted health communication: strategies for enhancing information relevance. Am J Health Behav. 2003;27:S227–32.

Krug R, Karus D, Selwyn PA, Raveis VH. Late-stage HIV/AIDS patients' and their familial caregivers' agreement on the Palliative Care Outcome Scale. J Pain Symptom Manage. 2010;39(1):23–32.

Lambrechts F, Grieten S, Bouwen R, Corthouts F. Process consultation revisited: taking a relational practice perspective. J Appl Behav Sci. 2009;45(1):39–58.

Levine C, Halper D, Peist A, Gould DA. Bridging troubled waters: family caregivers, transitions, and long-term care. Health Aff (Millwood). 2010;29:116–24.

Litwak E, Sudit M. Task-specific theoretical framework for the design of optimal caregiving structures for minority women with AIDS. Paper presented at the Annual Meeting of the American Sociological Association, Pittsburgh, PA; 1992.

Livet M, Courser M, Wandersman A. The prevention delivery system: organizational context and use of comprehensive programming frameworks. Am J Community Psychol. 2008;41:361–78.

Lounsbury DW, Murphy P, Robinson J, Rapkin BD. Managing multi-site collaborative research with community-based agencies. In: Loue S, Pike E, editors. Case studies in ethics and HIV research. New York: Springer; 2007. p. 184–204.

Lyon ME, Garvie PA, McCarter R, Briggs L, He J, D'Angelo LJ. Who will speak for me? Improving end-of-life decision-making for adolescents with HIV and their families. Pediatrics. 2009;123:e199–206.

Malee KM, Tassiopoulos K, Huo Y, Siberry G, Williams PL, Hazra R, Smith RA, Allison SM, Garvie PA, Kammerer B, Kapetanovic S, Nichols S, Van Dyke R, Seage III GR, and Mellins CA for the Pediatric HIV/AIDS Cohort Study Team. Mental health functioning among children and adolescents with perinatal HIV infection and perinatal HIV exposure. AIDS Care, Jun 27, 2011. [Epub ahead of print].

Marks G, Mason HR, Medley A, Garcia-Moreno C, McGill S, Maman S. Rates, barriers and outcomes of HIV serostatus disclosure among women in developing countries: implications for prevention of mother-to-child transmission programmes. Bull World Health Organ. 2004;82(7):552.

McKee MD, Rubin SE, Campos G, O'Sullivan L. Challenges of providing confidential care to adolescents in urban primary care: clinician perspectives. Ann Fam Med. 2011;9:37–43.

McKleroy VS, Galbraith JS, Cummings B, Jones P, Harshbarger C, Collins C, et al. Adapting evidence-based behavioral interventions for new settings and target populations. AIDS Behav/AIDS Educ Prev. 2006;18(Suppl A):59–73.

Mellins C, Ehrhardt A, Newman L, Conard M, editors. Selective kin: defining the caregivers and families with HIV disease. New York: Plenum; 1996.

Mellins CA, Kang E, Leu CS, Havens JF, Chesney MA. Longitudinal study of mental health and psychosocial predictors of medical treatment adherence in mothers living with HIV disease. AIDS Patient Care STDs. 2003;17(8):407–16.

Mellins CA, Brackis-Cott E, Dolezal C, Abrams EJ. The role of psychosocial and family factors in adherence to antiretroviral treatment in human immunodeficiency virus infected children. Pediatr Infect Dis J. 2004;23:1035–41.

Mellins CA, Brackis-Cott E, Leu CS, Elkington KS, Dolezal C, Wiznia A, et al. Rates and types of psychiatric disorders in perinatally human immunodeficiency virus-infected youth and serorevertors. J Child Psychol Psychiatry. 2009;50:1131–8.

Miller RL, Shinn M. Learning from communities: overcoming difficulties in dissemination of prevention and promotion effort. Am J Community Psychol. 2005;35(3–4):169–83.

Mrazek PJ, Haggerty RJ. Reducing risks for mental disorders: frontiers for preventive intervention research. Washington, DC: National Academy Press; 1994.

Namir S, Alumbaugh M, Fawzy F, Wolcott D. The relationship of social support to physical and psychological aspects of AIDS. Psychol Health. 1989;3:87–92.

Pequegnat W, Bray J. Families and HIV/AIDS: introduction to the special section. J Fam Psychol. 1997;11(1):3–10.

Pequegnat W, Szapocznik J. Working with families in the era of HIV/AIDS. Thousand Oaks. CA: Sage; 2000.

Rapkin BD, Trickett EJ. Comprehensive dynamic trial designs for behavioral prevention research with communities: Overcoming inadequacies of the randomized controlled trial paradigm. In:

Trickett E, Pequenaut W, editors. Increasing the community impact of HIV prevention interventions. New York: Oxford University Press; 2005. p. 249–77.

Rapkin BD, Murphy P, Bennett JA, Munoz M. The family health project: strengthening problem
solving in families affected by AIDS to mobilize systems of support and care. In: Pequegnat W,
Szapocznik J, editors. Working with families in the era of HIV/AIDS. Thousand Oaks, CA:
Sage; 2000. p. 213–42.

Rapkin B, Weiss E, Chhabra R, Ryniker L, Patel S, Carness J, Adsuar R, Kahalas W, DeLeMarter C,
Feldman I, DeLorenzo J, Tanner E. Beyond satisfaction: Using the Dynamics of Care assess-
ment to better understand patients' experiences in care. Health & Quality of Life Outcomes,
March 2008.

Reich WA, Lounsbury DW, Zaid-Muhammad S, Rapkin B. Forms of social support and their relationships to mental health in HIV-positive persons. Psychol Health Med. 2010;15(2):135–45.

Remien RH, Mellins CA. Long-term psychosocial challenges for people living with HIV: let's not
forget the individual in our global response to the pandemic. AIDS. 2007;21 Suppl 5:S55–63.

Richardson JL. Women's self-disclosure of HIV infection: rates, reasons, and reactions. J Consult
Clin Psychol. 1995;63(3):474–8.

Rosen L, Mellins CA, Ryan S, Havens J. Family therapy with HIV/AIDS affected families.
In: Wicks L, editor. Psychotherapy and AIDS. Washington, DC: Taylor and Francis; 1997.

Rothenberg KH, Paskey SJ. The risk of domestic violence and women with HIV infection: implications
for partner notification, public policy, and the law. Am J Public Health. 1995;85(11):1569–76.

Ruiz MS, Ryan S, Havens J, Mellins CA. Psychotherapy with HIV-affected adolescents. In: Wicks
L, editor. Psychotherapy and AIDS. Washington, DC: Taylor and Francis; 1997.

Schein EH. Process consultation revisited, building the helping relationship. Reading, MA:
Addison-Wesley; 1999.

Shulman LH, Shapira SR, Hirshfield S. Outreach developmental services to children of patients in
treatment for substance abuse. Am J Public Health. 2000;90(12):1930–3.

Simoni JM, Mason HRC, Marks G, Ruiz MS, Reed D, Richardson JL. Women's self-disclosure of
HIV infection: Rates, reasons, and reactions. Journal of Consulting and Clinical Psychology,
Vol 63(3), Jun 1995, 474–78.

Smith M, Rapkin B. Social support and barriers to family involvement in caregiving for persons
with AIDS: implications for patient education. Patient Educ Couns. 1996;27(1): 85–94.

Stoller E, Pugliesi K. Other roles of caregivers: competing responsibilities or supportive resources?
J Gerontol. 1989;44:31–8.

Szapocznik J, Feaster DJ, Mitrani VB, Prado G, Smith L, Robinson-Batista C, et al. Structural
ecosystems therapy for HIV-seropositive African American women: effects on psychological
distress, family hassles, and family support. J Consult Clin Psychol. 2004;72(2):288–303.

The Lewin Group. Evaluation of New York's HIV special needs plan program: cost and usage
impacts. Available via: http://www.health.state.ny.us/diseases/aids/resources/snps/docs/hiv_
snp_research_paper.pdf 2009. Cited 3 Mar 2011.

Uldall KK, Koutsky LA, Bradshaw DH, Hopkins SG, Katon W, Lafferty WE. Psychiatric comorbidity and length of stay in hospitalized AIDS patients. Am J Psychiatry. 1994;151:1475–8.

Wandersman A, Duffy J, Flaspohler P, Noonan R, Lubell K, Stillman L, et al. Bridging the gap
between prevention research and practice: the interactive systems framework for dissemination
and implementation. Am J Community Psychol. 2008;41:171–81.

Weiner L, Mellins CA, Marhefka S, Battles HB. Disclosure of an HIV diagnosis to children: history, current research, and future directions. J Dev Behav Pediatr. 2007;28:155–66.

Yoshikawa H, Wilson PA, Hsueh J, Rosman EA, Chin J, Kim JH. What front-line CBO staff can
tell us about culturally anchored theories of behavior change in HIV prevention for Asian/
Pacific Islanders. Am J Community Psychol. 2003;32:143–58.

Zaid-Muhammad SA. Transactional ecosystems framework of HIV positive fathers' perceptions
of their children's psychosocial and health needs: implications for family and school-focused
therapeutic interventions for children affected by HIV. Pace University, ETD Collection for
Pace University. Paper AAI3436598. Available via: http://digitalcommons.pace.edu/dissertations/
AAI3436598 (2010 Jan). Cited 7 Mar 2011.

Part V
Challenges for the Future

Chapter 16
Future Directions for Family-Based Prevention and Treatment Research: Challenges and Emerging Issues

Carl C. Bell and Willo Pequegnat

Abstract This chapter reviews the emerging issues in family-based prevention programs and future research directions. Despite the fact that there are many universal family attributes, there are some important cultural and contextual issues that require "tailor made" approach for some issues. However, the culturally tailored intervention must be grounded in core behavior change principles or they will not have the intended benefit for families. This chapter reviews the challenges of family-based combination and multilevel intervention which combine biomedical and behavioral approaches that optimize the HIV prevention benefits for families. There are some challenges in research strategies that must be addressed. For example, the current studies have a short follow-up period and if we are going to learn how the family impacts the long-term protective factors, we must have cohorts that are followed while children age into more risky periods of social development. Strategies need to be identified that ensure sustainability of effective family-based programs. If family based programs are going to be adopted by public health agencies, it is important to generate cost effectiveness data. There are also challenges in new settings that need to be explored; for example, foster care and juvenile systems, African American and Hispanic churches, and workplaces. There are also some populations that would benefit from family-based prevention program such as mentally ill children, young men who have sex with men (YMSM), rural families, and children in blended families. Researchers are challenged by the promising new directions of the third decade of the HIV epidemic.

16.1 Introduction

The chapters in this book review state-of the-art family-based HIV prevention and treatment research conducted over the last 18 years. There have been major accomplishments since the publication of *Working with Families in the Era of AIDS*

W. Pequegnat and C.C. Bell (eds.), *Family and HIV/AIDS: Cultural and Contextual Issues in Prevention and Treatment*, DOI 10.1007/978-1-4614-0439-2_16, © Springer Science+Business Media, LLC 2012

(Pequegnat and Szapocznik 2000) which describes interventions being tested in the field at the time. Families are essential to the healthy development of children because of their slow brain development. Protective families ensure optimal survival and develop cognitive, social, emotional, and behavioral competencies in children. (See Chap. 2 for a fuller discussion of these issues.) Families develop the capacity for learning, socialization, connectedness, and self-esteem. Parents provide mastery experiences across developmental stages: infancy, childhood, adolescence, and young adulthood. Parents inculcate healthy behaviors and stave off illness-generating behaviors with their children (Pequegnat and Stover 2000).

In this chapter we would like to discuss some of the contextual issues for future research and practice and end with challenges and emerging issues for family-based research.

16.2   Challenges of Adapting Existing Prevention Programs Versus Developing New Programs

Since 1993, the NIMH Consortium on Families and HIV/AIDS and other researchers have been developing family-based prevention strategies to prevent HIV infections in adolescents and young adults and to help families adapt to HIV infection in its members. There are frequent discussions in academic and practice communities about whether evidence-based family prevention programs can be adapted for the cultural and contextual issues in diverse families or whether new studies need to be conducted. These conversations focus on whether there are common elements in prevention programs that can be used to adapt an evidence-based intervention. In our experience it is more helpful to have "both/and" conversations than "either/or" conversations because both approaches have merit.

There are some universal protective factors and strengths within families that can benefit from adaptations of evidence-based prevention programs conducted with one group of families. These protective family factors are nested within communities and environments. Family members teach one another social and emotional skills; reinforce individual self esteem by providing a sense of power, uniqueness, and models; monitor and protect one another; and provide a network to help when needed.

Despite the universality of these healthy family attributes, there are important cultural and contextual attributes of families that require a "tailor made" approach for some issues. For example, while the need to eat is universal, what individuals choose to eat is determined by cultural backgrounds and contextual experiences. While a good relationship between the health care provider and client/patient transcends culture as a necessary component to optimize health outcomes, health care services need to be delivered in a language and approach that is tailored to the client or the client may not adhere to the recommended treatment regimen. If the provider speaks Spanish and does not communicate the benefits of the treatment to the English-speaking client, it will not have the intended effect. Thus, despite the universality of the benefits, the lack of cultural specificity can undercut the delivery of the prevention program. On the other hand, if a culturally tailored intervention is not grounded in core behavior change principles, it will not have the intended benefit either.

The core principles of evidence-based prevention programs for families need to be adapted to the cultural and contextual circumstances of the targeted families. (For a fuller discussion of this approach, see Chap. 14.) CHAMP was originally developed on the Southside of Chicago but when it was implemented in Durban, South Africa, the research team took great pains to ensure the intervention was embedded in Zulu culture. The team ensured that the packaging of the intervention was familiar, the individuals in program material were dressed appropriately, and the exercises were approved by the Zulu Community Advisory Board (Paruk et al. 2005).

16.3 Challenges of Family-Based Combination and Multilevel Interventions

16.3.1 Family-Based Combination Biomedical and Behavioral Interventions to Optimize HIV Prevention

As new biomedical prevention opportunities become available (e.g., microbicides, PEP, PrEP, male circumcision), it is important that we do not abandon existing prevention strategies that have had an important impact on the epidemic. Most biomedical interventions raise issues of congruence with age, gender, culture; maintaining mental health; having attitudinal arguments; accessing accurate information; ensuring good decision making, having the proper behavioral skill set, and implementing long-term adherence – all of which are part of a good family-based behavioral intervention. Family-based combination behavioral and biomedical approaches can optimize HIV/STD prevention outcomes.

In situations without effective combination prevention approaches, there has been poor uptake. For example, Parent to Child Transmission (PTCT) studies have found that simply offering a drug during a brief counseling program is not sufficient because the woman and her husband often do not show up at the clinic until they are ready to deliver the baby. Even if the drug is officered at pre-natal visits, this may not also be sufficient because the prospective parents may be suspicious of the drugs. To address these issues, Rotheram and colleagues have initiated an outreach program called Mentor Mothers program to work with pregnant women in their community to ensure better uptake of programs to prevent Parent to Child Transmission PTCT.

There is evidence that there has been poor uptake of Gardasil (e.g., a vaccine for preventing HPV which is a sexually transmitted disease causing cancer) among adolescents who could benefit the most. When asked about it, adolescents said that if their mother had encouraged them, they would have been vaccinated (Chao et al. 2009).

There are growing numbers of adults and children living with HIV worldwide who must adhere to complex antiretroviral therapy which requires combination approaches. In the case of pediatric HIV infection, family factors include caregiver psychosocial and material resources, knowledge and beliefs about the medications, and self-efficacy to support the child's adherence. By contrast, research on ART adherence among adults considers the individual living with HIV in isolation apart from their family and partners. Research on barriers and facilitators of adherence largely ignores the potential impact of family structure and processes and significant others. (For a fuller discussion of the issue of adherence, see Chap. 10.)

16.3.2   Family-Based Multilevel Interventions

The Triadic Theory of Influence informs us that behavior is multi-determined (Bell et al. 2007; Flay et al. 2009). Thus, to achieve larger effect-sizes we need more multilevel impact of family-based programs using social ecology models/social fabric models along with family- and individual-based influences. Developing a quality research project evaluating a multilevel family-based prevention program is difficult because the theoretical underpinning, design, methodology, statistical analysis, and operationalization of the research plan (e.g., sample attrition, contamination, ethics, etc.) are complex.

When HIV/AIDS family-based interventions were first rolled out, there were many researchers who doubted whether there would be any indication of efficacy. However, the research highlighted in the book has proved them wrong. Then, CHAMP which is a multilevel intervention was able to demonstrate changes in individual, family, and community dynamics (Bell et al. 2002; Flay et al. 2009; National Research Council and Institute of Medicine 2009). Multilevel family-based intervention also cultivates changes in communities and services that can support parenting and reduction of youth risks.

16.4   Challenges of Research Strategies

16.4.1   Long-Term Follow-Up of Current Family-Based Cohorts

Currently, many of the outcomes of family-based HIV/AIDS prevention programs have focused on the proximal outcomes of increased communication, increased closeness, parental monitoring, and social and emotional skills among parents and their children and increased social fabric surrounding at-risk families. Unfortunately, although important, these proximal outcomes do not provide the distal outcomes that would decrease HIV/STDs over the 5–10 years that adolescents may be sexually active prior to a committed relationship or marriage. Accordingly, long-term follow-up of current family-based HIV/AIDS experimental cohorts must be undertaken.

16.4.2   Sustainable Family-Based Interventions

Future family-based HIV prevention research needs to identify strategies that diminish intervention decay. One way to sustain positive outcomes may be to teach family members to reinforce one another's changes, rather than focusing on a single family member. Moving beyond individual-level changes within families (knowledge, attitudes, beliefs) and toward modifying familial systems may produce more protracted change. (For a fuller discussion of structural ecological interventions, see Chap. 11.) Family-based interventions need to be integrated into community settings (e.g., physician's offices, workplaces, schools) and into public health agencies but technology transfer is a challenge. (For a fuller discussion of this issue, see Chap. 15.) More research on how to implement family-based prevention programs into these settings is needed. Another research direction is to incorporate family-based programs (such as Project STYLE discussed in Chap. 13) into empirically supported individually focused interventions (e.g., broadening the scope of individual interventions to target families).

16.4.3   Cost Effectiveness of Family-Based Prevention Programs

An important component of implementing evidence-based prevention programs in public health settings is demonstrating cost-effectiveness of the approach. It is critical that more cost effectiveness studies be integrated into family-based prevention programs so this evidence is available when Directors of public agencies are making a decision whether to implement these evidence-based programs.

16.5   Challenges of New Settings for Family-Based Prevention

16.5.1   Foster Care and Juvenile Systems

Dr. David Satcher's *Report of the Surgeon General's Conference on Children's Mental Health: A National Action Agenda* (U.S. Public Health Service 2000) suggested that we focus our public health attention on the most vulnerable children in our society who are in protective services, correctional facilities, and mental health settings. Research on HIV/AIDS prevention in children in foster care, juvenile detention centers, and in children in special education is limited. These are risky settings because the children's family-systems are disrupted and strained by their removal from their family systems (Redd et al. 2005).

16.5.2 African American and Hispanic Churches

After three decades of HIV/AIDS in the U.S., the epidemic is continuing to spread rapidly in African American and Hispanic subpopulations. Often churches provide the focal point for spiritual, social, political, and health-related matters in these communities. Churches may be a vehicle for reaching these subpopulations with effective HIV/STD prevention programs in an appropriate cultural approach and in overcoming HIV stigma. Religious leaders have great influence in providing information and guidance to their parishioners. While African American churches have begun to incorporate HIV/STD prevention programs into their ministry activities but Hispanic churches are lagging behind. Research to demonstrate effective strategies to develop, test, and integrate prevention programs for African American and Hispanic families would make a major impact in controlling the spread of the HIV epidemic.

16.5.3 Workplace

The economic impact of AIDS shifts to the workplace as companies are faced with employees who are being treated for HIV through their health insurance and are less available for working. The recent court cases and anti-discrimination legislation, such as Americans with Disabilities Act of 1990, expose firms to liabilities for discrimination against employees with HIV. It therefore is in their best interest to prevent HIV infection among their employees and families. While there has been some focus on family-based prevention programs in the workplace, this is an area that could benefit from additional programs. AIDS education and information programs can reduce the probability of HIV infection and reduce the likelihood of infection and to minimize employee fears and disruptions in the workplace. A strategy to increase in these programs is to offer HIV prevention for parents teaching them how to talk to their children about sex and STD prevention.

16.6 Challenges for New Populations and Their Families

16.6.1 HIV Family-Based Prevention Programs for Mentally Ill Children

Another challenge is addressing HIV prevention in children who are at risk for or are experiencing mental issues that impair their judgment and result in their engaging in HIV-related risky behaviors. Children who grow up in contexts where they experience adverse childhood experiences (Felitti et al. 1998) and trauma develop poor affect regulation. We have learned that childhood adversities stemming from "maladaptive family functioning clusters" (including parental mental illness, substance abuse disorder, and criminality; family violence; physical and sexual abuse; and neglect) may be associated with subsequent psychological distress and poor school performance. These experiences can also put children at risk of triggering mental disorders if they are vulnerable (e.g., Borderline Personality Disorder, Conduct Disorder, etc.) (Green et al. 2010; McLaughlin et al. 2010).

16.6.2 Family-Based HIV Prevention Programs for Young Men Who Have Sex with Men

In 2008, young men who have sex with men (YMSM) represented 68% of infections among all adolescents and young adults (male and female) and were one of the only HIV risk groups showing an increasing rate of infection (Centers for Disease Control and Prevention (CDC) 2010). Despite this fact, there is no CDC-endorsed intervention for this population (Centers for Disease Control and Prevention (CDC) 2010). Family-based approaches have great potential because they address both HIV/AIDS risk for the youth and provide skills to families that may be struggling with supporting their sexual minority children. (See Chap. 12 for a discussion of these issues.) Family-based approaches are also needed to enhance family acceptance, parenting skills, and working together to prevent adverse outcomes (e.g., depression, suicide) in families with gay and bisexual sons (Ryan et al. 2010).

16.6.3 Rural Families

New prevention strategies are needed for working with families in rural areas. The epidemic was first identified in urban areas, but the spread of the epidemic to rural areas is becoming a new challenge. (See Chap. 11 for a discussion of Section 11.4.1.1) HIV/AIDS tends to be diagnosed in later stages of the disease in infected persons in rural areas because they do not have access to health care providers that recognize the HIV-related symptoms. There is also the challenge of stigma and disclosure because these families live in small towns where rumors can spread rapidly which results in not seeking HIV prevention or treatment services. In some cases, people who were infected in urban areas, return to their hometown as they become more sick. Rural families are less likely to have public or private health insurance. There are also issues around conducting research because these families are not as familiar with the research process and do not understand the concept of confidentiality and are reluctant to share family information with interviewers. All of these issues present new challenges for HIV prevention researchers.

16.6.4   Children in Blended Families

With the increasing divorce and remarriage rate, there are increasing numbers of blended families which can be a challenge. It requires not only mixing different cultures, rules, and expectations, it may also mix together unrelated older children who act as role models for younger children. If the older children are becoming sexually active, this can be a challenge for good parental monitoring of HIV risk behaviors as younger children may try to emulate their new older siblings. In blended families there is often conflictual family communication around integrating children into one family that can lead to early sexual debut and HIV risk behavior. Some parent–child HIV prevention programs need to be tailored for the special challenges for these blended families.

16.7   Conclusion

As demonstrated in this book, AIDS has presented families with new challenges, and researchers, service providers, and families have developed new family-based strategies that have implications for other families handling the chronic disease. This book presents families and service providers with new options for working with families around prevention and treatment issues. Family-oriented programs can enhance the quality of life of families infected and affected by HIV. They also offer public health clinics with new options for services and they may ultimately prove to be cost effective if they keep new persons from becoming HIV. As outlined in this chapter, it also provides researchers in the third decade of this epidemic promising new directions in which to pursue research.

References

Bell CC, Bhana A, McKay MM, Petersen I. A commentary on the triadic theory of influence as a guide for adapting HIV prevention programs for new contexts and populations: the CHAMP-South Africa story. Soc Work Mental Health. 2007;5(3/4):243–67.

Bell CC, Flay B, Paikoff R. Strategies for health behavioral change. In: Chunn J, editor. The health behavioral change imperative: theory, education, and practice in diverse populations. New York: Kluwer Academic/Plenum Publishers; 2002. p. 17–40.

Centers for Disease Control and Prevention (CDC). HIV surveillance in adolescents and young adults (2010). Atlanta, GA: US DHHS. Available via: http://www.cdc.gov/hiv/topics/surveillance/resources/slides/adolescents/index.htm. Cited 2 Dec 2010.

Chao C, Slezak JM, Coleman KH, Jacobsen SJ. Papanicolaou screening behavior in mothers and human papillomavirus vaccine update in adolescent girls. Am J Public Health. 2009;99(6):1137–42.

Felitti VJ, Anda RF, Nordenberg D, Williamson DF, Spitz AM, Edwards V, et al. Relationship of child abuse and household dysfunction to many of the leading causes of death in adults – The Adverse Childhood Experiences (ACE) Study. Am J Prev Med. 1998;14(4):245–58.

Flay BR, Snyder F, Petraitis J. The theory of triadic influence. In: DiClemente RJ, Kegler MC, Crosby RA, editors. Emerging theories in health promotion practice and research. 2nd ed. New York: Jossey-Bass; 2009. p. 451–510.

Green JG, McLaughlin KA, Berglund PA, et al. Childhood adversities and adult psychiatric disorders in the national comorbidity survey replication I. Arch Gen Psychiatry. 2010;67:113–23.

McLaughlin KA, Green JG, Gruber MJ, Sampson NA, Zaslavsky AM, Kessler RC. Childhood adversities and adult psychiatric disorders in the national comorbidity survey replication II. Arch Gen Psychiatry. 2010;67:124–32.

National Research Council and Institute of Medicine. Preventing mental, emotional, and behavioral disorders among young people: progress and possibilities. In: O'Connell ME, Boat T, Warner KE, editors. Washington, DC: The National Academies Press; 2009.

Paruk Z, Petersen I, Bhana A, Bell C, McKay M. Containment and contagion: how to strengthen families to support youth HIV prevention in South Africa African. J AIDS Res. 2005;4(1):57–63.

Pequegnat W, Stover E. Behavioral prevention is today's AIDS vaccine! AIDS. 2000;14 Suppl 2:S1–7.

Pequegnat W, Szapocznik J. Working with families in the era of HIV/AIDS. Thousand Oaks, CA: Sage Publications; 2000.

Redd J, Suggs H, Gibbons RD, Muhammad L, McDonald J, Bell CC. A plan to strengthen systems and reduce the number of African-American children in child welfare. Illinois Child Welfare. 2005;2(1 and 2):1–13.

Ryan C, Russell ST, Huebner D, Diaz R, Sanchez J. Family acceptance in adolescent and the health of LGBT young adults. J Child Adolesc Psychiatr Nurs. 2010;23(4):205–13.

U.S. Public Health Service. Report of the surgeon general's conference on children's mental health: a national action agenda. Rockville, MD: US Department of Health and Human Services; 2000.

About the Contributors

Susannah Allison, Ph.D., is a program officer at the National Institute of Mental Health within the Infants, Children and Adolescents Research Program in the Center for Mental Health Research on AIDS. The program supports neurobehavioral and psychosocial studies involving infants, children, and adolescents who are infected with HIV, affected by HIV (such as born to an HIV+ mother or living in an household with an HIV+ person), or at-risk for HIV. Prior to working at NIMH, Dr. Allison worked with children and families infected and affected by HIV/AIDS for a number of years in Baltimore, Miami, and Washington, DC. She completed her doctorate at the George Washington University where she received her Ph.D. in Clinical Child Psychology with an emphasis in child health psychology.

Bita Amani, Ph.D., is currently a postdoctoral scholar in the National Institutes of Mental Health AIDS Research Training Program at University of California, Los Angeles. She received her doctorate from UCLA School of Public Health in the Department of Epidemiology and her MHS from the Johns Hopkins Bloomberg *School of Public Health*. Her research interests include HIV and methodological biases in biomedical research. Additionally, she is interested in how scientific literature (and biases) shape understandings of disease.

Cady Berkel's, Ph.D., research interests relate to the impact of discrimination on adolescent health and social disparities, and the protective influence of cultural factors. She is also interested in improving interventions that may reduce disparities via research on program implementation, with specific attention to cultural adaptations.

Clair Blake is currently a doctoral student at Florida International University. She has previously served as a research assistant at the Mount Sinai School of Medicine.

Larry K. Brown, M.D., is a professor in the Department of Psychiatry and Human Behavior at Brown University and director of research in the Division of Child and Adolescent Psychiatry at Rhode Island Hospital. Dr. Brown has expertise in HIV prevention for at-risk youth and psychological issues of infected or affected youth and families with more than 100 publications in this area. He is the PI of on-going or recent NIMH projects that investigate programs for youth in the criminal justice setting, those in alternative/therapeutic schools, and families in mental health treatment. He is also a member of the NIH Adolescent Trials Network (ATN) Behavioral Leadership Group, program director of a NIMH T32 program in child and adolescent biobehavioral HIV research training, and co-director of the Prevention Core of the Lifespan/Tufts/Brown Center for AIDS Research.

Scott C. Brown, Ph.D., is a research assistant professor of Epidemiology and Public Health at the University of Miami, Miller School of Medicine in Miami. Brown is interested in the neighborhood built (physical) and social environment as a pervasive contextual factor in relation to a variety of health outcomes, including mental health, physical functioning, obesity, drug abuse, and HIV risk. He has been co-PI or investigator on multiple studies of the built environment in relation to health in Hispanic children, adults, and elders.

Nicole Cano, B.S., a graduate student in public health at the University of Miami, Miller School of Medicine, serves as a clinical research coordinator in the prevention division. She has published in the areas of medical neglect and child maltreatment and specializes in maternal and child health. Cano has worked with preventive programs focusing on child development, in addition to interventions with Hispanic adolescents to prevent alcohol use, drug use, and risky sexual behavior. Her primary interests are in family-based interventions for the prevention of childhood obesity and child development.

Barbara L. Dancy, R.N., Ph.D., F.A.A.N., is a professor at the University of Illinois at Chicago College of Nursing in the Department of Health Systems Science. Barbara Dancy has substantial experience in working with minority communities, in developing and conducting qualitative and quantitative research studies, and in tailoring prevention programs. Her program of research focuses on developing and testing culturally sensitive intervention for vulnerable underserved populations in the area of HIV prevention, mammography screening, and health promotion. She has conducted research both nationally and internationally and has published extensively in the area of HIV risk reduction for low-income African American woman and for African American mother–daughter pairs.

Ralph DiClemente, Ph.D., is a Charles Howard Candler professor of Public Health and Associate Director, Emory Center for AIDS Research. He holds concurrent appointments as professor in the School of Medicine, Department of Pediatrics, in the Division of Infectious Diseases, Epidemiology, and Immunology, and the Department of Medicine, in the Division of Infectious Diseases, and the Department of Psychiatry. He was most recently selected as Chair, Department of Behavioral Sciences and Health Education at the Rollins School of Public Health, Emory University. He is currently the President of the Georgia Chapter, Society for Adolescent Medicine, and an executive board member of the American Sexually Transmitted Disease Association. He is also on the Board of Scientific Counselors to the CDC Center for Infectious Diseases and the National Advisory Council for the National Institute of Mental Health. He has published extensively in the area of

HIV/STD prevention, particularly among African American adolescents and young adults. He is the author, along with Gina Wingood, on six CDC-defined evidence-based HIV interventions that are currently being disseminated nationally. He is the author of more than 350 publications and has edited or written 16 books.

Coleen DiIorio, Ph.D., R.N., F.A.A.N., is a professor in the Department of Behavioral Sciences and Health Education at the Rollins School of Public Health. She has an extensive experience in the study of health behaviors including the psychosocial aspects of health and health behaviors. Her primary area of study is self-management. Her work has included the study of psychosocial factors associated with medication adherence and self-management practices and factors associated with quality of life among those with chronic illnesses including HIV. Her work has included the study of self-efficacy, coping, and spirituality. She has received funding for her work from the National Institutes of Health, Centers for Disease Control and Prevention, and the Epilepsy Foundation of America.

Geri R. Donenberg, Ph.D., is a professor and director of the Healthy Youth Program in the Department of Psychiatry and director of the Community Outreach Intervention Projects in the Division of Epidemiology and Biostatistics in the School of Public Health at the University of Illinois at Chicago. Dr. Donenberg is the PI or co-investigator of recent or ongoing NIH-funded studies of HIV/AIDS risk and prevention with families and youth in mental health services, juvenile offenders, men who have sex with men, injection drug users, and youth in South Africa and Indonesia. Dr. Donenberg is also a recent Fulbright scholar and fellow in the Executive Leadership in Academic Medicine program.

Nabila El-Bassel, Ph.D., is a professor at the Columbia University School of Social Work and director of the Social Intervention Group (SIG), a multidisciplinary research center focusing on developing and testing HIV prevention intervention approaches and disseminating them to local, national, and international communities. Dr. El-Bassel is also the director of the Columbia University Global Health Research Center of Central Asia (GHRCCA), focusing on health and social issues in Central Asia through research, education, training, and policy and dissemination. She has designed and tested HIV intervention and prevention models for women, men, and couples, which have been disseminated nationally and internationally.

Jay Fagan, D.S.W., is a professor in the School of Social Work at Temple University. His research has focused on at-risk fathers (nonresident, head start, adolescent fathers), parent education and co-parenting interventions for fathers, fathers and early childhood programs, fathering in the context of family processes, and the relationship between childcare and work–family balance among low-income women. He has published more than 50 peer-reviewed research papers.

Kathryn Flavin, B.A., received her B.A. from Duke University where she studied English and Music. Following that, she came to the University of Miami where she assisted the Department of Epidemiology and Public Health with various studies involving the built environment, metabolic syndrome, HIV risk, and cigarette use in adolescents and adults in the Hispanic community. She is currently pursuing her M.D. degree at the University of Miami Miller School of Medicine.

Wendy Hadley, Ph.D., is an assistant professor in the Department of Psychiatry and Human Behavior at Brown University and a staff psychologist in the Division of Child and Adolescent Psychiatry at Rhode Island Hospital. Dr. Hadley has expertise in HIV prevention interventions with at-risk youth and with parents with psychiatric disorders.

Ikkei Hirama, M.P.H., received his master's degree in public health, with a concentration in epidemiology from Florida International University. Hirama is currently a medical student at the West Virginia School of Osteopathic Medicine. His research interests include impacts of neighborhood built (physical) and social environments on residents' health and well-being. Hirama has been part of the built environment and health team at the University of Miami Miller School of Medicine which is conducting research on neighborhoods and Hispanics' health.

Joyce Hunter, D.S.W., has been a human rights activist, researcher, and clinician for over 30 years, specializing in issues relating to youth, women, HIV/AIDS, and LGBT communities. A research scientist, HIV Center for Clinical and Behavioral Studies/New York State Psychiatric Institute/Columbia University, she is also a Principal Investigator, "Working It Out," HIV prevention for LGB adolescents. Dr. Hunter is also an assistant clinical professor, Department of Psychiatry, College of Physicians and Surgeons and assistant clinical professor of Public Health, Sociomedical Sciences, at Columbia University.

Larry Icard, Ph.D., is a professor in the College of Health Profession and Social Work at Temple University where he also serves as a director of the Center for Intervention and Practice Research. He received his doctorate from the School of Social Work at Columbia University. His research and publications focus on developing and testing interventions to reduce health problems experienced by at-risk population including low-income urban African American families, pre-release incarcerated men, African American men on the down low, South African men who have sex with men, and HIV-positive African American men and women.

Chisina Kapungu, Ph.D., is an assistant professor in the Department of Obstetrics and Gynecology at the University of Illinois at Chicago. She has an extensive experience in the development, implementation, and evaluation of culturally sensitive HIV prevention interventions in community-based settings. Her research is focused on the multisystemic factors associated with sexual risk behaviors among African American girls and women.

Sheila Kaupert, M.P.H., is a senior research manager in the Department of Epidemiology and Public Health at the University of Miami Miller School of Medicine in Miami. Ms. Kaupert is interested in social epidemiology and structural interventions that may affect a broad range of health outcomes in marginalized communities within the USA and in developing countries. She has been working with the National Hispanic Science Network on Drug Abuse since 2005.

Beatrice J. Krauss, Ph.D., is a professor of Public Health at the City University of New York School of Public Health at Hunter College and executive director of the Center for Community and Urban Health. Dr. Krauss co-chairs the nongovernmental organization committee on HIV/AIDS and serves as the special project associate for the American Psychological Association on HIV-related issues at the United Nations. She was PI of the Parent/Preadolescent Training for HIV Prevention (PATH, NIMH R01 53834). PATH has informed interventions in the USA, Mexico, India, and Africa in community, school, clinic, and hospital settings.

Sung-Jae Lee, Ph.D., is an associate professor in-residence in the Department of Psychiatry and Biobehavioral Sciences, Semel Institute for Neuroscience and Human Behavior, University of California at Los Angeles. Dr. Lee's research focuses on developing family-based interventions for HIV-affected families in Thailand. He is currently a principal investigator on a Mentored Research Scientist Development Award funded by NIMH. The goal of his study is to develop and pilot culturally tailored family-focused HIV disclosure intervention for people living with HIV in Thailand.

Celia Lescano, Ph.D., is a research associate professor in the Department of Mental Health Law and Policy, received her B.S., M.S., and Ph.D. (Clinical and Health Psychology – concentration in Clinical Child/Pediatric area) from the University of Florida, and completed an APA-approved internship in clinical psychology at the University of Miami. Following internship, she completed a NIMH T32 postdoctoral fellowship in pediatric psychology at the Brown University School of Medicine and subsequently received an appointment at Brown University as assistant professor in the Department of Psychiatry and Human Behavior, where she served as a faculty member from 2000 to 2010. Dr. Lescano has published widely, has been actively involved in professional psychology activities at the national level, and has successfully developed a program of funded research, focused primarily on HIV prevention work with at-risk adolescents and families.

Gabriel M. Lopez is a Government and Sociology double major at Dartmouth College, from which he is graduating in the spring of 2011. Lopez is interested in the role of culture in HIV/STD family-based preventive interventions for Hispanic adolescents. He will be pursuing graduate school in the fall of 2012.

Dominica F. McBride, Ph.D., is a co-founder/co-president and evaluation specialist of the HELP Institute, Inc. Dr. McBride also heads the research division of the Community Mental Health Council, Inc. She has conducted domestic and international program development and evaluation projects with underserved communities, including rural communities in Tanzania, East Africa, African American communities, Hispanic communities, urban native American communities, and women.

Mary McKay, Ph.D., is a professor of Psychiatry and Preventive Medicine at the Mount Sinai School of Medicine in New York and internationally recognized for her research on interventions that meet the needs of inner-city youth and families. The Collaborative HIV Prevention and Adolescent Mental Health Project (CHAMP), one of her most successful efforts, is a university and community collaborative research study that focused on the collaborative design, delivery, and testing of a family-based HIV prevention program.

Claude Mellins, Ph.D., is a clinical psychologist with research and clinical expertise in psychosocial aspects of HIV disease in children and families living in impoverished urban environments. She is a research scientist at the HIV Center for Clinical and Behavioral Studies at the New York State Psychiatric Institute and Columbia University and professor of Clinical Psychology in the Departments of Psychiatry and Sociomedical Sciences at Columbia University. Over the past 20 years, she has completed projects examining individual and family psychosocial factors mediating medical adherence in HIV-infected women and children; sexual and drug use risk behavior in uninfected youth with HIV-infected mothers; and psychiatric and psychological functioning in HIV-infected mothers and children. She has also become involved in intervention efforts to address the mental health and risk behavior needs of HIV-infected and -affected children in the USA and Africa. In addition to her research, Dr. Mellins is the co-founder and co-director of the Special Needs Clinic (SNC) at New York Presbyterian Hospital (NYPH), one of the first and currently one of the largest mental health clinics for HIV-infected women, children, and families. The SNC has provided care to over 1,600 patients since 1992 and has served as a model for the Ryan White Care Act mental health programs.

Kim S. Miller, Ph.D., is the senior advisor for Youth Prevention at the Centers for Disease Control and Prevention, Center for Global Health, Division of Global HIV/ AIDS Prevention. She is well known for her work with *Parents Matter* and *Families Matter*, evidence-based programs that were developed to engage parents in HIV prevention efforts by enhancing their ability to speak to their children about sexual health. She is also a co-developer of *Project AIM*, a youth development sexual risk prevention intervention. She is currently implementing these evidence-based programs in the USA and in eight African countries.

Velma McBride Murry, Ph.D., has an extensive expertise on adversity that includes race, ethnicity, and poverty; with a background in the role that parenting plays in addressing the needs of rural African American youth. She has completed an efficacy trial, the Strong African American Families (SAAF) program that targets the prevention of early sexual onset and substance use among rural youth. She has created a second generation version SAAF, Pathways for African American Success (PAAS), designed to test the feasibility and efficacy of delivering a family-based computer-based interactive technology to increase assessibility and diffusion of HIV risk reduction programs for rural African American families.

Brian Mustanski, Ph.D., is a faculty at Northwestern University, where he directs the IMPACT LGBT Health and Development Program. He received his doctorate in Clinical Psychology from Indiana University, where he trained extensively at the Kinsey Institute. He has been the principal investigator for multiple National Institutes of Health, National Science Foundation, and other foundation research and training awards, including being named a William T. Grant Foundation Scholar.

The majority of his research focuses on the health and development of gay, lesbian, bisexual, and transgender (LGBT) youth.

Hadiza Osuji is a senior research coordinator at the Mount Sinai School of Medicine and holds a master degree in Public Administration from Columbia University. She is actively involved in the development, delivery, and testing of research intervention programs for youth and families and coordinates the Champions Program which is currently testing the delivery of three evidence-based HIV prevention and early pregnancy prevention interventions for urban youth and families by community HIV educators.

Hilda Pantin, Ph.D., a clinical associate professor at the University of Miami Miller School of Medicine, serves as the executive chair of the Department of Epidemiology and Public Health, the associate director of the Center for Family Studies (CFS), and the director of the Prevention Division at the CFS. As director of the CFS Prevention Division, she launched a systematic program of research for the prevention of problem behaviors in Hispanic adolescents. She has over 45 scholarly publications and has served as principal or co-principal investigator on several grants from the National Institutes of Health. Her primary interests are in designing and evaluating family-based preventive interventions to prevent drug use, sexual risk behaviors, and related problem behaviors in Hispanic adolescents.

Maura Porricolo, R.N., Dr. N.P.(c), is a certified pediatric nurse practitioner, providing both HIV specialty care and primary care to children with HIV for 20 years. In addition to being a clinician, Ms. Porricolo has been a co-investigator on multiple federally funded research programs involving pharmacological interventions, medication adherence, and more recently disclosure in HIV. She also taught, at New York University, a postgraduate certificate program for NPs learning the art and science of caring for children with special needs.

Guillermo ("Willy") Prado, Ph.D., is an associate professor of Epidemiology and Public Health, acting chief of the Division of Epidemiology, and director of the Doctoral Epidemiology Program, all at the University of Miami Miller School of Medicine in Miami. His research focuses on the prevention and reduction of substance use and HIV risk behaviors among Hispanic youth. His research has been recognized by the Society for Prevention Research, the National Hispanic Science Network on Drug Abuse, and the Miami Herald, which selected him as one of the Top 20 Leaders and Innovators in South Florida under the age of 40.

Bruce Rapkin, Ph.D., is a professor of Epidemiology and Population Health in the Division of Community Collaboration and Implementation Science at the Albert Einstein College of Medicine. He is a community psychologist, focused on improving access to care, quality of care, and quality of life with diverse, medically underserved patients and families through community–academic partnerships. This collaborative research has contributed to the development of new research designs and assessment methods needed to disseminate and adapt evidenced-based interventions.

Robert H. Remien, Ph.D., is a professor of Clinical Psychology (in Psychiatry) at Columbia University. He is the director of the HIV Center's Global Community

Core, faculty mentor for HIV Center Postdoctoral Fellows, and clinical supervisor to psychiatric residents in training. His research is focused on mental health, sexual risk behavior, and adherence to treatment and care among individuals and couples, and he has developed and tested several behavioral interventions in these domains in both domestic and international settings.

Mary Jane Rotheram-Borus, Ph.D., is the director of the Global Center for Children and Families and Bat-Yaacov professor in Child Psychiatry and Biobehavioral Sciences at UCLA. Over the past 30 years, Dr. Rotheram-Borus has directed and implemented several landmark intervention studies that have demonstrated the benefits of providing behavior change programs and support to families in risky situations, specifically families affected by HIV. Several of these programs have received national and international recognition, including designation as model programs by the American Psychological Association, the American Medical Association, and the Centers for Disease Control and Prevention.

Jane M. Simoni, Ph.D., is a clinical psychologist and professor in the Department of Psychology at the University of Washington in Seattle. For the past decade, her NIH-funded research program has addressed ART adherence, focusing on practical and sustainable ways to promote lifelong adherence. She has developed and evaluated peer support, pager, and counseling interventions in New York City, Seattle, and Miami, as well as China and the USA–Mexico border

Dallas Swendeman, Ph.D., is an assistant professor in-residence in the Department of Psychiatry and Biobehavioral Sciences at the David Geffen School of Medicine at UCLA. His research has focused on interventions for adolescents and young adults living with HIV in the USA and sex workers in India. More recently, he has worked on teams developing mobile phone applications for self-monitoring and self-management of health behaviors and mental health factors related to obesity and HIV. Dr. Swendeman recently received a William T. Grant Scholars award to develop and validate new mobile phone tools for ecological momentary assessment and intervention for children's and families' daily routines, relationship processes, and well-being.

Maria I. Tapia, M.S.W., L.C.S.W., is a senior research associate in the Department of Epidemiology and Public Health at the University of Miami Miller School of Medicine in Miami, FL. Mrs. Tapia is a family therapist with many years of experience as a supervisor and clinical trainer in the prevention and treatment of adolescent substance use, behavioral problems, and HIV prevention.

Mari Umpierre, Ph.D., is the coordinator of the Center for Collaborative Inner City Child Mental Health Services Research at the Mount Sinai School of Medicine. Dr. Umpierre trained at the University of Puerto Rico Medical School's Behavioral Sciences Research Institute and holds a Ph.D. in Clinical Social Work from New York University. Her clinical work and research interests include cross cultural issues in mental health and access to care for minorities.

Joyce P. Yang, M.A., is a graduate student of Clinical Psychology in the Department of Psychology at the University of Washington in Seattle. Her research interests span multicultural psychology, the development of culturally relevant interventions, and global mental health. She is pursuing work using participatory action research methods with broad social justice advocacy goals.

About the Editors

Carl C. Bell, M.D., is a clinical professor of Psychiatry and Public Health and the director of the Institute for Juvenile Research (IJR), University of Illinois at Chicago (UIC). IJR is a century-old, multimillion dollar academic institute providing child and family research, training, and service, employing 257 academic faculty and support staff. Dr. Bell is the president and CEO of Community Mental Health Council (CMHC) and Foundation, Inc., in Chicago. CMHC is a large multimillion comprehensive community mental health center employing 390 social service geniuses. During 40 years, he has published more than 450 articles, chapters, and books on mental health and authored *The Sanity of Survival*. He has been interviewed by *Ebony; Jet; Essence; Emerge; New York Times; Chicago Tribune Magazine; People Magazine; Chicago Reporter; Nightline*; *ABC News*; *NPR*; *CBS Sunday Morning*; *The News Hour with Jim Lehrer; the Tom Joyner Morning Show*; *Chicago Tonight*; and the *Today* show. A 1967 graduate of UIC, he earned his M.D. from Meharry College in Nashville, Tennessee, in 1971. He completed his psychiatric residency in 1974 at the Illinois State Psychiatric Institute/Institute for Juvenile Research in Chicago.

Willo Pequegnat, Ph.D., is an associate director of the International AIDS Prevention Research in the NIMH Division of AIDS Research at the National Institutes of Health (NIH). Dr. Pequegnat has a range of experience with both national and international HIV/STD prevention research and has expertise in primary and secondary behavioral preventive interventions, stress and coping, psychological, neuropsychological, and physical functioning, and quality of life. Her research involves multilevel social organization and complex relationships: couples, families, communities, societal (media, policy), technological (internet, web, smart phones, etc.). She is working on the issue of social instability, such as consequences of war, terrorism, migration, female, and drug trafficking on HIV/STD transmission. She took the initiative to develop a research program on the role of families in preventing and adapting to HIV/AIDS and chairs the only annual international research conference on families and HIV/AIDS. She co-edited the book on this program of research entitled, *Working with Families in the Era of AIDS*. Dr. Pequegnat initiated and is a co-editor of *How to Write a Successful Research Grant Application: A Guide for Social and Behavioral Scientists, 2nd edition, Community Interventions and AIDS, and From Child Sexual Abuse to Adult Sexual Risk: Trauma, Revictimization, and Intervention*. She has developed three special issues of *AIDS* and one of *JAIDS*. She plans and implements national and international workshops, conferences, and symposia on HIV/STD and represents NIMH on science policy-making committees and workgroups in the Public Health System on a broad range of HIV/STD issues.

Index

A

ABLE. *See* Attention, Behavior, Language, and Emotions (ABLE) tool
Abuse. *See* Substance abuse
Access to care. *See* Family ACCESS to Care Study (FACS)
Adaptation of interventions
  in New York City and Los Angeles, 286–288
  PATH, 110
  in South Africa
    HIV status, 288–289
    Mothers to Mothers HIV Prevention Program, 289–290
    tools used in intervention, 290–291
  in Thailand
    healthy families program, 292–294
    status of HIV, 291–292
    tools and activities, 294–297
Adherence
  ART, in couple, 159–160
  cultural values incorporation, 220–221
  family issues, 221–222
  family role, 210–211
  among HIV-affected adults
    clinical setting aspects, 216
    disease characteristics, 215
    familial context, 216–217
    patient-provider relationship, 215
    patient variables, 215
    treatment regimen variables, 215
  among HIV-affected children
    caregiver-related factors, 213
    child-related factors, 212–213
    familial context, 213–214
    medication regimen-related factors, 212
  interventions to promote adherence, 217–220
  pyramid, 210–211
Administrative and clinical staff
  characteristics, 313, 314
  family-based research, interest in, 313–315
Adolescence
  economic empowerment program, 185
  girls, 180
  HIV prevalence rates, 174
  HIV-risk reduction interventions
    CHAMP program, 129
    ImPACT program, 128–129
    MDRR program, 126–127
    a mother–adolescent HIV prevention program, 126
    PARE program, 129–130
    Saving Sex for Later program, 127–128
  most affected group, 174
  orphans, 180, 184–185
  phase in, human development, 48
  with psychiatric disorders
    affective characteristics of families, 264
    instrumental characteristics of families, 264–265
    mental health and HIV/AIDS, 261–262
    parent-teen communication, 265–266
    peer and partner relationships, 266–267
    personal attributes, 263–264
    Project STYLE, 267–271
  risk behaviors, HIV, 180
  school and substance abuse, 75–76

CPSIA information can be obtained at www.ICGtesting.com
Printed in the USA
LVOW100232070612

285043LV00004B/58/P